Critical Participatory Inquiry

Sara Miller McCune founded Sage Publishing in 1965 to support the dissemination of usable knowledge and educate a global community. Sage publishes more than 1000 journals and over 600 new books each year, spanning a wide range of subject areas. Our growing selection of library products includes archives, data, case studies and video. Sage remains majority owned by our founder and after her lifetime will become owned by a charitable trust that secures the company's continued independence.

Los Angeles | London | New Delhi | Singapore | Washington DC | Melbourne.

Critical Participatory Inquiry

An Interdisciplinary Guide

Meagan Call-Cummings

Johns Hopkins University

Giovanni P. Dazzo

University of Georgia

Melissa Hauber-Özer

University of Missouri-Columbia

Sage

Sage

FOR INFORMATION:

2455 Teller Road
Thousand Oaks, California 91320
E-mail: order@sagepub.com

1 Oliver's Yard
55 City Road
London, EC1Y 1SP
United Kingdom

Unit No. 323-333, Third Floor, F-Block
International Trade Tower
Nehru Place, New Delhi – 110 019
India

18 Cross Street #10-10/11/12
China Square Central
Singapore 048423

Printed in the United States of America

ISBN: 978-1-0718-2586-0

This book is printed on acid-free paper.

Acquisitions Editor: Leah Fargotstein

Content Development Editor: Cassie Carey

Production Editor: Vijayakumar

Copy Editor: Diane DiMura

Typesetter: TNQ Technologies

Indexer: TNQ Technologies

Cover Designer: Scott Van Atta

Marketing Manager: Victoria Velasquez

23 24 25 26 27 10 9 8 7 6 5 4 3 2 1

BRIEF CONTENTS

DETAILED CONTENTS

PREFACE

Each of us came to critical participatory inquiry (CPI) in different ways, through different life experiences, and as different people, yet we share a common idealism in the potential for inquiry to provoke social transformation.

MEAGAN

I grew up in a White, middle-class, suburban, Christian bubble. My dad has a PhD and, when I was young, had a job that supported our family just fine. My mom had gotten married before she finished her bachelor's degree and so attended college in each location where we lived as I grew up. I'm sure she had hundreds of credits by the time she graduated—the same year I graduated from high school. I remember my parents taking seriously the Christian values of helping others, not judging others' circumstances, and giving even if it made oneself uncomfortable or if it was inconvenient. I remember my dad bringing people who were experiencing homelessness to our home to sleep. My mom volunteered as an English language tutor for newcomers. My older brothers (I have three) were always joining in on some service project to raise money for a family or an organization. This idea of giving was instilled in me at an early age. I had a vague knowledge that I could give, that I should help.

Since then, various life experiences led to an interest in anti-oppressive education. As I began my doctoral program at a college of education, I began to take research methodology courses and started to consider ways in which research can be (and has been) violent, particularly how research has been wielded as a weapon in and against communities of Color and among indigenous people. How numbers and statistics have been treated as neutral, how data analysis (both quantitative and qualitative) is seen as detached and therefore objective and "true," how we are so often told inquiry has to look a particular way—measure up to standards set by White men—in order to be counted as valid or valuable. I began to question whose knowledge counts in everything I did. I started looking at participatory action research as a possibility in my desire to deconstruct, reconstruct, and repair in and through inquiry—to really turn academia on its head, to rethink whose knowledge counts, to demand that we pay attention to and honor those whose knowledges have been so often violently stolen, repackaged, commodified, and resold to people in power—in an effort to remain in power over those from whom it was stolen. It has been through my research with youth and practitioners that I have come to see a necessity for research to be participatory.

GIOVANNI

Growing up in a household with immigrant parents and grandparents, from Sicily, and in a rural town with a majority Hispanic population provided me with an early outlook on racial, ethnic, and socioeconomic equities. Like many immigrant families, my parents stressed the importance of education; they believed it was the greatest way to obtain the social and economic mobility that had motivated them to leave their homes. While education was important, my family stressed the necessity to look back on where we came from—an economically under-resourced area in Sicily, with little access to formal education, but with a linguistic, social, cultural, and culinary history that we could take pride in.

When I am asked about my experience growing up in this area, I often recall two experiences. The first was with my paternal grandfather, who was always interested in reminding me that we did not have a history of wealth. At the age of 5, I asked my grandfather for money to purchase a toy. He agreed and told me that we were going to the bank. After driving through town and passing every bank, we arrived at a cherry orchard. He calmly announced that we had arrived at the bank. He then handed me a 5-gallon bucket, instructing me that it needed to be completely full before being taken to the weighing station. That day, I worked alongside migrant laborers, moving up and down ladders to fill the plastic pail. After weighing my bucket and receiving the little money I did, my grandfather asked if I still wanted to purchase that toy. I simply said that I wanted to keep my money and go home. The second experience includes the many Sicilian card games I would play with my maternal grandmother, who lived with us and was my best friend until the day she passed. Of all my grandparents, my maternal grandmother was the most highly educated, having advanced to the third grade before having to drop out due to illness and the obligations of helping her family. During these card games, I was constantly humbled (and sometimes humiliated) by a witty and wonderfully sarcastic woman who taught me small life lessons and the necessity to push forward, even when it was likely I would not win. In reflecting on these experiences, although I became a fairly competitive person, it also taught me to never underestimate anyone—to respect and honor the words and experiences of everyone, no matter their upbringing, level of formal education, economic standing, and many of the other categories that society tells us are important ways to measure success and expertise.

The conversations I had at home, these instances of life and labor, and the opportunity to learn from so many people of diverse backgrounds from such an early age affected how I viewed the world. There are also a number of experiences that defined me by my deficits and led me to doubt myself: being categorized as low income or at risk; being told I would never get a PhD because it was for smart people; being told that I was not fully White—sometimes said as a compliment (by minoritized people), sometimes as an insult (by those considering themselves fully White)—because of my Sicilian parents and the fact we did not solely speak English at home. I see all of these incidents as the motivating factors behind the value I place on the knowledge held by all people, especially those who hold knowledge from their practical and lived experiences. I also see the privileges I have held, continue to hold, and those I was able to take advantage of living in a society that deems itself postcolonial but continues the entrenchments of racialized capitalism.

When speaking about my own research, especially when it comes to the PAR projects I have facilitated, I began this work outside of academia. My first PAR project in Burma/Myanmar, conducted alongside former political prisoners, was successful in some respects (e.g., changing financial assistance policies for this population), but failed in having a bigger impact, such as using evidence to advocate for fundamental rights and freedoms. In an effort to improve my work, I felt the need to start a doctoral program and question the transformative and restorative potential for inquiry. I was blessed here to meet Meagan and Melissa. Through our countless conversations and their guidance, I learned that I was enough, even without a PhD. Although I came late to this lesson, as a methodologist, I continue to stress it to the communities I work alongside: We are all enough; the everyday methods we use to learn and create knowledge are enough; there is a necessity to revolutionize and democratize how we conduct inquiry and what we see as evidence. I hope these lessons are evident in this book.

MELISSA

Like Meagan, I grew up in a White, suburban, Christian bubble, albeit in an aspiring middle-class family descended just a few generations from European immigrants. My dad, a vocational high school graduate trained as a mechanic, and my mom, a registered nurse trained in a hospital (not college) program were determined to provide my older sister and me with the educational opportunities they hadn't had and to steep us in the conservative Evangelical values they had embraced as young adults. We were homeschooled until transitioning to private Christian middle and high school, when my parents felt they'd reached the limits of their knowledge and had scrimped, saved, and secured enough financial aid to make it feasible. My formative elementary years, however, were filled with independent, self-directed and group learning experiences with other homeschool families. I read thousands of books, acted out historical events with my Barbies (complete with hand-sewn period costumes!), went on dozens of field trips, experimented with pulleys and levers under my dad's instruction, watched my mom and Dr. Snyder dissect a cow's heart, painted with Mrs. Leaman, and studied music theory with Mrs. Hawthorn. This type of schooling was doubtless pivotal in fostering my respect for different types of expertise and my inclination toward hands-on, student-centered learning. We were also actively involved in our church, where I listened with rapt attention to missionaries' accounts of far-off countries and volunteered to "serve" low-income communities in nearby Philadelphia. I *loved* learning, a fact that was only slightly tempered by formal schooling, had an insatiable curiosity about other cultures and languages, and felt a strong obligation to make a difference in the world, rooted in the values of our faith.

When I was in high school, my parents decided to expand our family by adopting a young child from Romania in need of a loving home. Over the next 6 years, my new brother was joined by two of his biological siblings and then a pair of sisters from Russia, giving us a crash course in second language acquisition, learning disabilities, and the effects of childhood trauma, all of which we were naively unprepared to handle as a family. Along with these experiences, my interests and commitment to doing good led me to study languages in college and then teach in several nonformal, community-based adult literacy and English as a second language (ESL) programs in Philadelphia after graduating. Breaking out of my White, Christian bubble for the first time, my eyes were opened to intersectional barriers I would never face through my interactions with these adult learners who were experiencing severe poverty, deeply entrenched structural racism, interactions with the criminal justice system, struggles with addiction, undiagnosed learning disabilities, a lack of legal documentation, or the challenges of forced migration and resettlement in a foreign country.

Feeling a need for formal teacher education, I completed a master's degree and then, keeping one foot in the nonformal world by launching an adult ESL program at my community development association, started teaching university-based ESL courses. There, I learned about the set of challenges my international students—most of them Muslim—faced in a post–9/11 world rife with Islamophobia and racialized controversy over immigration. A desire to understand and address culturally and linguistically diverse learners' challenges with them—not for them—drew me to participatory research and to my doctoral program, where I met and began working with Meagan. My learning journey through and now beyond the PhD have cemented my conviction that research should do good through honoring diverse forms of knowledge, calling out injustice, and working for meaningful change.

WHY CRITICAL PARTICIPATORY INQUIRY?

Since 2017, we have worked together to craft research methodology courses that could help students and practitioners feel a sense of confidence in their own knowledge and ways of knowing. We did not want to offer courses that sought to teach the vocabulary of methods or the techniques of so-called validity. We wanted to develop a course that would help students see their own identities and commitments as intrinsically linked and entangled with the methods they use. In 2019, we published a paper together in *The Qualitative Report* that concluded participatory inquiry requires a kind of becoming that is often uncomfortable since almost all of us have been socialized to consider expertise as something achieved through the acquisition of formal accolades rather than through everyday experience. We learned that novice researchers experience a kind of "mental oscillation" (p. 2193) as they seek to stay true to their own epistemological commitments to equitable and participatory inquiry while navigating rigid neoliberal "institutional and social structures that can make them feel as if wholehearted adoption of and engagement with these methodologies is impossible" (p. 2193). We then wrote this book to help students, practitioners, and research collectives see their knowledge as valid and valuable and to uncover new possibilities of inquiry that do not bow to status quo pressures but that deconstruct them, exposing the capitalist and colonial agendas that undergird them. Ultimately, our goal is to reconstruct a new inquiry that is simultaneously critical and humble, caring and daring, dialogic and disruptive.

AUDIENCE(S)

We wrote this book as a guide for people who feel committed to inquiry that is equitable at its core but who may feel unsure how to enact those commitments. We have drawn on literature and used examples from public health, social work, psychology, education, criminal justice, conflict resolution, and more, so that instructors of graduate research methods courses in a variety of disciplines could use it as a core text. Graduate students—in both practice-based and research-oriented programs—could use this text as a step-by-step manual as they dive into CPI projects. Indeed, we have included "Recommended Practices" in each chapter that will guide readers through their own CPI projects, as well as "Step-by-Step" instructions on how to facilitate several methods (e.g., community consultations, storyboards). Practitioners may use this book as they form community advisory boards for specific projects or longer term social change agendas. Our goal was to create a guidebook that can bridge the academia–practice divide, speaking to the typical differences in purpose and procedures but also recognizing similarities.

CHAPTER 1: WHOSE KNOWLEDGE COUNTS?

In this chapter, we lay the groundwork of the book by clarifying the ontological and epistemological roots of CPI. We discuss CPI as part of a larger movement of knowledge democratization, which seeks to break the colonial, capitalist monopoly of knowledge valued by those historically in positions of power. We then move to describe the many strands of CPI and discuss how it has been both adopted and adapted in and by academic disciplines. We conclude this chapter with a brief discussion of how CPI have been and continue to be coopted and appropriated in ways that are not in keeping with its critical, emancipatory roots.

CHAPTER 2: WHAT IS CRITICAL PARTICIPATORY INQUIRY?

After laying the ontological and epistemological groundwork in Chapter 1, Chapter 2 establishes CPI as an epistemological commitment, not just one of many research methods. This chapter really delves into the ways in which a CPI approach can play a role in advancing the people's knowledge for liberation and transformation. We explore the messiness, fluidity, and flexibility of the CPI process and conclude the chapter with some of the major critiques of CPI.

CHAPTER 3: ETHICS AND VALIDITY IN PARTICIPATORY INQUIRY

This chapter takes a deep dive into how ethics and validity are intertwined in research in general, and how this can be seen clearly in CPI. We review core concepts like praxis, objectivity, subjectivity, bias, and access and how they are reconceptualized in and through CPI. We survey the major theories and philosophies that anchor CPI, including indigenous theories of knowledge, critical race theory, feminist theories, and more.

CHAPTER 4: BUILDING (ON) RELATIONSHIPS

While the first three chapters of the book go through some heavy theoretical and philosophical concepts, Chapter 4 starts a more practically oriented section of the book, aimed at providing useful tools for engaging CPI while at the same time integrating theory throughout. In Chapter 4, we offer opportunities to reflexively analyze your insider–outsider status within the communities you seek to conduct CPI. We discuss the various types of relationships that can give rise to CPI. As in each chapter, we review key ethical considerations as you seek to build relationships in and through CPI. Finally, we discuss concrete ways to build equitable inquiry relationships.

CHAPTER 5: GETTING STARTED

As part of the second section of the book, Chapter 5 offers strategies for reflexively starting a CPI project. We first offer opportunities to reflect on the ways in which power dynamics may have implications for your CPI work. We discuss the role critical consciousness and dialogue play in the CPI process. We offer several concrete tools and approaches to beginning a CPI project, including co-creating consent forms and an inquiry plan.

CHAPTER 6: GATHERING DATA AND MAKING MEANING: MAKING TRADITIONAL APPROACHES MORE PARTICIPATORY

Chapters 6, 7, and 8 all provide tools for gathering data (data collection) and making meaning (data analysis). While these two aspects of the research process are often treated as separate and distinct, we know from experience that they most often occur simultaneously. Thus, we present ways in which this blurred data collection and analysis process can happen productively in CPI.

The main thrust of Chapter 6 is to provide several tools for making surveys, interviews, and focus groups more participatory and in keeping with the ontological and epistemological commitments CPI practitioners make to knowledge democracy. Of course, before getting into the concrete tools, we review key theoretical concepts like intersubjectivity and intersubjective understanding, and we again point out how and in what ways ethics and validity are linked as we gather data and make meaning in CPI.

CHAPTER 7: GATHERING DATA AND MAKING MEANING: ARTS-BASED APPROACHES

Chapter 7 continues discussions started in Chapter 6 but through the lens of arts-based inquiry techniques for gathering data and making meaning. We again start by teasing apart key concepts like impact before turning to the ethical and validity considerations in arts-based approaches. We cover visual arts inquiry like murals, street art, and storyboards. We then turn to the ways in which we may use poetry; memoir, and narrative as well as theatre and other arts-based techniques to gather data and make meaning. As we review each approach, we offer examples and discuss how negative impacts may be foreseen and mitigated.

CHAPTER 8: GATHERING DATA AND MAKING MEANING: DIGITAL AND MULTIMEDIA APPROACHES

As in previous chapters, we begin Chapter 8 by reviewing key concepts connected to digital and multimedia approaches to gathering data and making meaning. We cover how to use virtual and online ethnography as participatory tools for inquiry. We also review how social media, websites, and blogs can be great opportunities to gather data and make meaning in efficient ways, broadening the idea of what a CPI collective might look like. We also discuss radio, podcasting, digital storytelling, and photographic methods like photovoice.

CHAPTER 9: TAKING ACTION

In Chapter 9, we switch gears to discuss what it means to take action with co-researchers and others as a vital part of the CPI process. We identify several opportunities for CPI collectives to take action within and outside of academia. Finally, we discuss the implications of taking action for social and organizational change.

CHAPTER 10: STAYING COMMITTED AND IN SOLIDARITY

In this final chapter, we address the importance of as well as the complexity of staying committed to and with co-researchers and others. We discuss opportunities to stay committed and in solidarity with co-researchers in ways that they and the community in which you conduct CPI value. Finally, we consider the many implications of staying committed or potentially agreeing to move on.

APPENDICES

Our Appendices offer several resources including a glossary, sample syllabi, and samples of tools introduced within the book's chapters. In addition, we also offer three case studies that are mentioned in the chapters. By including the full stories of each of these cases, we hope that readers will be able to reference these as they read the chapters. Here we offer brief descriptions of each case:

Case Study 1: *Amigas de la Comunidad*, a community-based participatory research project that began in October 2014 focused on early childhood education and early literacy among and in immigrant families, is a partnership between Central American immigrant mothers of young children, many of whom are undocumented and all of whom are low income ("Amigas"), local community agencies, nonprofit organizations, and schools ("community partners"), and faculty and students at George Mason University.

Case Study 2: *Women's Empowerment Project*, is an empowerment-oriented CPI project focused on the enhancement of wellness among adult women in the Bahamas who have experienced and survived trauma. An emphasis is placed on supporting and informing survivors through a holistic approach that not solely focuses on the women's experiences of violence and abuse, but also their experiences and readiness for recovery and healing as part of the process of empowerment.

Case Study 3: *Everyday Friends Research Group*, a critical participatory inquiry project to study college programs labeled "inclusive" with higher education students with intellectual and developmental disabilities (IDD). The study focused on the following questions: (1) What are experiences of inclusion held by individuals with IDD at college? (2) What are the recommendations and expectations of inclusive college experiences held by young adults with IDD? and (3) How do we navigate and reconcile imbalances of power and equity and the dilemma of creating a research community that did not ask to be created?

In addition to these three case studies that are referenced throughout the book, we often reference each of our most recent CPI projects. Because we refer to them so extensively in many of the chapters, we will provide brief introductions to them here to give readers some context.

COURAGEOUS CONVERSATIONS IN THE UNITED STATES

Meagan has been involved with the *Courageous Conversations* youth participatory action research (YPAR) group since 2017, when she approached her local high school principal with a vague idea of forming a group of student and teacher co-researchers to work together on a project oriented toward social justice. The principal gave several possible ideas for the focus of such a group. After consulting with several teachers and students in after school meetings, a collective of two teachers, 10 students, Meagan, and two of Meagan's doctoral students identified an area of concern that they wanted to conduct research around: a sense of belonging among students of color. The school is a large, public high school in the suburbs of Washington D.C. and is quite diverse along many lines, including race, ethnicity, immigration status, and socioeconomic status. It is also a magnet school; that is, its specialty programs in biotechnology allow students from outside its geographical zone to enroll in the school. Because students often travel up to an hour to attend school, they are typically not able to stay after school to attend sports games or club meetings. According to the principal and several teachers, this has led to a difficulty creating a sense of cohesion and community at the school. According to students, however, there is a racial aspect to this lack of community that was not being addressed.

So, in Fall 2017, our research collective came together to gather and analyze data with the goal of offering actionable recommendations to the school's administrators to address the situation. We created a questionnaire (see Chapter 6 this volume) that went out to the entire student body and garnered over 500 responses, and student co-researchers conducted interviews and focus groups. Our collaborative data analysis brought out several possibilities for celebrating the diversity of the student body and starting "courageous conversations" about equity and inclusion. And yet, after we presented our ideas and recommendations to the principal, we felt, as one co-researcher said, that we were "asking the wrong questions." We all agreed that our research needed to be deepened to better understand and grapple with the nuances of the experiences of students of color at the school.

Since that first year, we have used arts-based methods like Theatre of the Oppressed (see Chapter 7), spoken-word poetry (see Chapter 7), creative writing, and photovoice (see Chapter 8) to encourage students to express themselves in ways that feel natural and less hygienic than what we had done previously. Most significantly, we founded an annual all-day workshop that has brought students from area schools to create and perform or display artwork that represents their school experiences, inviting teachers, parents, peers, and policymakers to view the art created as a form of social change advocacy.

CPI IN GUATEMALA

Giovanni's CPI project spans national boundaries, with co-researchers based across the United States and Guatemala. It is situated on Kaqchikel Maya land in San Juan Comalapa, Guatemala; near the site of Iximche', the capital of the former Kaqchikel Maya kingdom. The objectives of the project are threefold: understanding the Kaqchikel community's priorities for a memorial site—the San Juan Comalapa Memorial for Victims of Enforced Disappearance—that commemorates the lives of those who disappeared during the country's 36-year armed conflict (1960–1996); documenting Indigenous views of justice and ways of knowing; and exploring the transformative and restorative potential for inquiry (i.e., the concept of restorative validity).

To begin, it is necessary to acknowledge and recognize the time and knowledge shared by the Kaqchikel Maya community members involved in this work. In addition to Giovanni, the CPI collective is comprised of an intergenerational group of 43 Kaqchikel community members, many of whom are members of the *Coordinadora Nacional de Viudas de Guatemala* (National Coordination of Widows of Guatemala, CONAVIGUA); and approximately a dozen nonprofit staff members from the *Fundación de Antropología Forense de Guatemala* (Forensic Anthropology Foundation of Guatemala, FAFG), which includes community investigators, forensic anthropologists, and geneticists.

Prior to the development of the memorial, it should be noted that this land was already a sacred site for the Kaqchikel. However, due to the armed conflict, it comes with a painful history. This sacred land where the memorial now sits was commandeered by paramilitary forces during the armed conflict, becoming a military detachment where community members were forcibly executed and buried. This history, however, has led to a longstanding relationship between FAFG, CONAVIGUA, and the Kaqchikel community. For over three decades, FAFG has worked alongside Indigenous communities to investigate and document disappearances that occurred during the armed conflict. FAFG collaborates with communities to learn the stories of the forcibly disappeared, identify mass grave sites where they may have been buried, exhume remains, and match the DNA from remains with samples from living family members. After identifying and confirming the identity of a missing person, FAFG then returns the remains to the family so they can hold a traditional ceremony.

This painful history, however, is met with the continued strength of those from the Kaqchikel community, who along with FAFG and CONAVIGUA, have turned this site into a living site, a memorial that community members visit, and a meeting place to hold traditional ceremonies to commune with ancestors. On this land, the community has built a lodge (*nimajay* in Kaqchikel), on which they have painted murals depicting symbols from Mayan cosmology and scenes representing violence during the armed conflict—a visual contact zone that shows how a relatively peaceful present continues to grapple with a painful past. Many of our participatory data collection and analysis activities—for example, community consultations, storytelling sessions, Ripples of Change, ranked choice voting (see Chapter 6)—have taken place in and around the nimajay. Through these sessions, we have come to understand our priorities as a collective and the ways in which we can work together to motivate change.

ADVOCACY ETHNOGRAPHY IN TURKEY

Melissa's dissertation research with Syrian refugees studying in Turkish universities was motivated by her prior experiences teaching English to refugee learners in the United States and facilitated by her ties to a university near her home in southern Turkey. Based on her concerns about conducting critical research with participants living under precarious legal status and rising hostility among the host population, she designed the study to employ participatory ethnographic and narrative inquiry methods. Her goal was, as a less vulnerable advocate, to facilitate the production of counternarratives about refugee experiences that challenged dominant discourses about refugees globally and Syrians in Turkey.

With the help of a Syrian friend, Samar (pseudonym), Melissa planned to recruit a collective of student co-researchers at the local university in the early spring of 2020; however, COVID-19 lockdowns forced her to shift to a virtual approach in which Samar took a central role as co-researcher (and was paid as a research assistant). The process entailed a questionnaire, in-depth, semistructured interviews, and photovoice workshops, all conducted virtually and in participants' preference of Turkish, English, or Arabic. Samar provided an insider perspective on data collection topics, instruments, and methods; recruited participants from her networks; translated documents and interpreted when participants chose to use Arabic (which Melissa does not speak well); collaboratively analyzed data; and copresented findings at practitioner conferences.

In Melissa's dissertation, each participant's narrative portrait is presented using a common story arc to preserve their individual voices while highlighting similar experiences in coming to Turkey, learning Turkish and gaining access to university, overcoming academic and social barriers, and finding a way to participate on their own terms. Their powerful photovoice images and accompanying texts are woven into the stories, bringing their challenges, dreams, and successes to life. She continues to seek out opportunities to share these stories formally and informally with friends, relatives, faculty members, and fellow scholars in order to change minds, inform pedagogies, and, hopefully, influence policies.

ACKNOWLEDGMENTS

This book would not have been written and published without the support of family, friends, colleagues, students, and so many, many others. We would all like to thank our colleagues and friends who pushed our thinking and offered such clear and bold examples and experiences that figure in the book: Sharrell Hassell-Goodman, Khaseem Davis, Jen Rainey, Maria Rybicki-Newman, Betsy Scotto-Lavino, Sascha Reed, Elisabeth Chan, Becca Brusseau, Rob Graham, Jeff Keller, Terrie Galanti, Christie Byers, and so many more. We thank Leah Fargotstein and Audra Bacon at SAGE and the many reviewers who were so helpful in their suggestions to improve each chapter, including the following:

Shannon Alpert, Northeastern University
Heidi R. Bacon, Southern Illinois University Carbondale
Johanna P. Bishop, Wilmington University
Shannon Calderone, Washington State University
Samuel Collins, Towson University
Elizabeth Currin, University of South Carolina
Steven D. Drouin, Stanislaus State University
Ryan Flessner, Butler University
Kirk A. Foster, University of South Carolina
Anne M. Hornak, Central Michigan University
Louise Jezierski, Michigan State University
Maryam Kia-Keating, University of California, Santa Barbara
S. Jay Kuder, Rowan University
Margaret Lombe, Boston College
John Lupinacci, Washington State University
Joseph McNabb, Northeastern University
Kelly Melekis, Skidmore College
Sarah Mountz, University at Albany
Linnea L. Rademaker, Abilene Christian University
Julie Steinkopf, New Mexico State University
Felicia J. Tuggle, Auburn University
Leticia Villareal Sosa, Dominican University
Nancy A. Watkins, California State University Fullerton
Jessica Wendorf Muhamad, Florida State University
Joseph Zompetti, Illinois State University

Meagan: I thank my parents, for never doubting my ability to do anything and everything. Thank you to my partner and kids for their endless patience, love, and encouragement as I locked myself in my bedroom–office for hours on end writing and revising the book, as dinner was sometimes late or the TV was on for way too long. Robert, thank you for supplying me with Diet Dr. Pepper, for getting the kids out of my hair when I was losing my mind, and for giving me time and space. Dye Dye, thank you for all the free babysitting and movies late at night. Derek, thank you for always hugging me right when I needed it. Macey, thank you for all the artwork that surrounds my office. Tabby, thank you for being willing to introduce yourself to my Zoom friends. Corey, you have been such a sweet addition. I thank kind friends for watching and entertaining my children on the days I couldn't. I thank my co-authors, who have become such close friends and whom I admire. I thank my Indiana University people: Barbara Dennis, Karen Ross, Peiwei Li, Pengfei Zhao, for all the quick responses, encouraging Zoom calls and text messages, and co-authorships on other projects that helped form a foundation for this work. And for the "no" necklace, Karen. Finally, thank you to "Mrs. Beardsley" and the many brilliant students of the Courageous Conversations project who became friends through social justice inquiry. I have learned so much from and with you.

Giovanni: Thank you to my spouse, Smita, for providing me with the time to co-author a textbook while I was still a doctoral student, held a full-time job, and raised a toddler with her. I am amazed at your patience each time I take on a new project. I am ever grateful to my parents, grandparents, and ancestors, who sacrificed so I could succeed. To Ravi Luca and Rishi Giona, for bringing light into our lives and showing me why I continue to do this work, so we can better ourselves and do better for the next generation. Last, none of my research would be possible without the many community co-researchers who have allowed me to learn from and with them. Thank you to the former political prisoners in Burma/Myanmar, who taught me about the realities and limitations of participatory inquiry; the Kaqchikel Maya community members who have shared their traditional forms of knowing and have welcomed me into their community; and, the many high school students across the Washington, D.C. metropolitan area who have shown me that our collective future is bright.

Melissa: Thank you to my parents and grandparents for igniting a love of learning and instilling a commitment to the greater good, the combination of which led me to CPI. To Mehmet Onur, who unfailingly believes in me, encourages me to pursue my goals, and picks up the slack at home when I'm tied to my laptop. To Meagan, who took on an idealistic doctoral student and made a methodologist out of her, and to Becky and Kathy for understanding and supporting my dissertation vision. To my students and research participants, past and present, who educate me about the world and how to make it a better place.

ABOUT THE AUTHORS

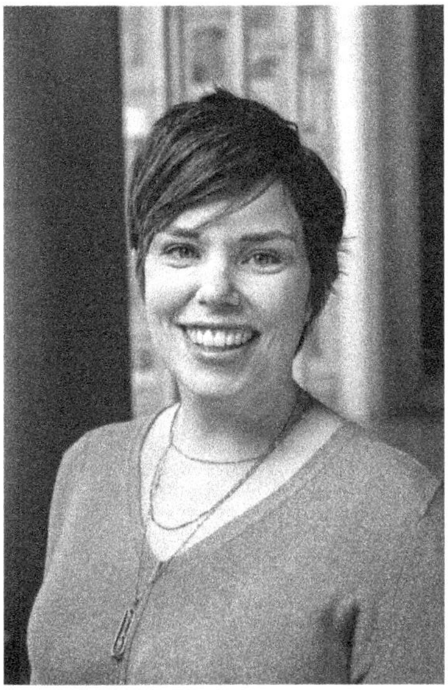

Meagan Call-Cummings is an associate professor in the School of Education at Johns Hopkins University. She specializes in critical, participatory, and feminist methodologies and teaches doctoral-level courses in critical qualitative inquiry. Her research engages participatory, narrative, ethnographic, and visual methods to explore issues of equity, justice, and peace with groups that are often silenced or harmed by traditional research practices. She has published articles in journals including *Qualitative Inquiry, Qualitative Research*, the *International Journal of Research and Method in Education, The Qualitative Report, Educational Action Research, High School Journal, Action Research*, and the *International Journal of Qualitative Studies in Education*.

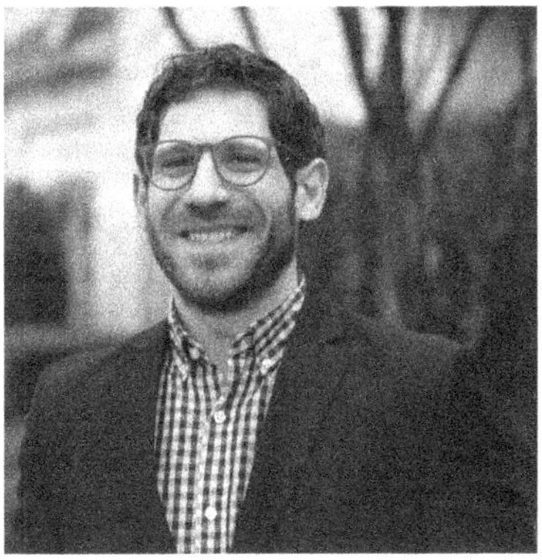

Giovanni P. Dazzo is an assistant professor of qualitative research and evaluation methodologies in the Mary Frances Early College of Education at the University of Georgia. He employs critical forms of participatory action research, ethnography, narrative and visual inquiries, and program evaluation, and teaches doctoral-level courses in qualitative methods, mixed methods, program evaluation, and critical participatory inquiry. As a methodologist, he focuses on restorative forms of inquiry (i.e., research that heals), epistemic justice, and critical and standpoint theories. He has published in journals including *The Qualitative Report, Educational Action Research, Conflict Resolution Quarterly*, and *New Directions for Evaluation*. His work on the concept of (re)imagining inquiry as restorative practice is currently funded by the Robert Wood Johnson Foundation.

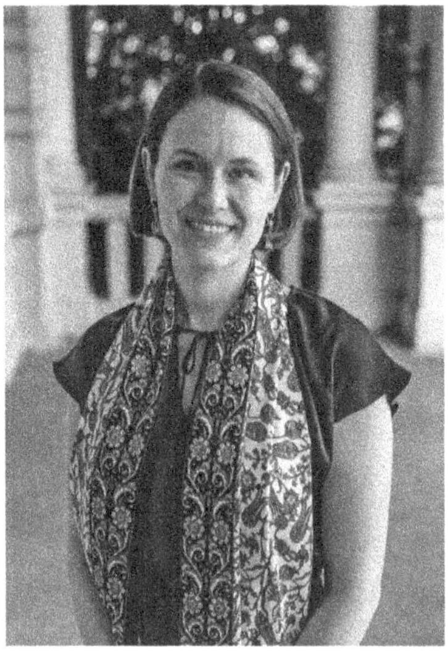

Melissa Hauber-Özer is an assistant professor of qualitative inquiry in the Department of Learning, Teaching, and Curriculum at the University of Missouri-Columbia. She teaches graduate courses in qualitative research methods, critical participatory inquiry, and educational philosophy. Her research employs critical participatory, ethnographic, and narrative methodologies to examine issues of educational access and equity for linguistically and culturally diverse learners. She has published in several edited volumes and journals, including the *International Journal of Qualitative Studies in Education*, the *Journal of Adolescent & Adult Literacy, Action Research*, and the *International Journal of Research and Method in Education.* Melissa's current work addresses community-identified needs in partnership with a local nonprofit organization supporting refugees and immigrants in mid-Missouri.

1 WHOSE KNOWLEDGE COUNTS?

LEARNING OBJECTIVES

By the end of this chapter, you will be able to

- Articulate the ontological and epistemological roots of critical participatory inquiry (CPI).
- Explain CPI's goal of knowledge democratization.
- Describe the various strands of CPI and how it is adopted and adapted by and in academic disciplines.
- Recognize how CPI has been and continues to be coopted and appropriated.

FOCUS ACTIVITY 1.1: WHO AM I?

Conduct a researcher positionality inventory. Some questions you may ask yourself are listed below, but do not limit yourself to these. Refer to the Appendix for a sample researcher positionality inventory.

1. What are all the identities I hold?
2. How are these identities salient to who I am as a researcher?
3. How might some of these identities help my CPI?
4. How might some of these identities hinder my CPI?
5. What can I start doing now to become aware of how my identities play a role in my inquiry and research?

Have you ever sat in a classroom, conference room, religious space, family gathering, or other social situation and thought, "It doesn't really matter if I say anything," or "They know way more than I do about this"? We all have. Meagan has told a story to some of her students about a time a few years ago when she was sitting around a large dining table with her family at an annual family reunion. The group had begun what they typically referred to as a "family meeting," which they would have toward the end of each of their reunions to reflect on what went well that year as well as what could be improved in years to come, and then to start planning for the next reunion. Her parents could not make it that year because they were traveling elsewhere, so they had asked that her oldest brother lead the meeting. As she sat there, she felt herself becoming quieter and quieter. She describes it as an almost out-of-body experience. She realized in that moment that she, as the only daughter and youngest of the four siblings, would have never been asked to lead such a discussion. It was seen as "normal" to ask one of the brothers to lead. Even though it was completely unspoken, it was taken for granted that a man would lead the family in their process of knowledge creation.

We begin with this short vignette because it highlights how we often make assumptions about **knowledge creation** even in our everyday lives. Often these assumptions are ingrained into our daily practices, and they can make their way into our research practices without us knowing. The overarching goal of this book is to help you develop a keen understanding of the principles of critical participatory inquiry so that you are positioned to create knowledge with communities effectively and ethically. We will question the definition of knowledge, whose knowledge has traditionally been seen as valuable, and who determines this, introducing the guiding concept of **knowledge democratization**. We will define central concepts of **positionality**, **ontology**, and **epistemology** and situate CPI within its historical, cultural, and conceptual contexts. In the second part of the chapter, we will introduce the lineage of the CPI ecosystem—from its roots in Indigenous, Global South, and activist knowledge systems around the world—through the development of what is often referred to as action research and carefully consider how the action research approach has been coopted for various goals.

Before getting started, though, we want to offer a brief note about these first few chapters that may appear somewhat daunting or perhaps peripheral to a reader's interest in getting to the "nuts and bolts" of CPI. We want to clearly state that we are not trying to intimidate you with what may appear to be highly theoretical concepts, but rather to engage theory in a way that is meaningful and that illustrates how CPI is radically different from most forms of research. We understand the tendency for methodologists to become obsessed with theory at the risk of alienating practitioners and those who really need "tools in their toolbox." While we do offer tools, it is imperative to understand and grapple with the underlying roots of CPI because it is not a one-size-fits-all method, nor is it a set of methods from which to choose depending on what you are doing or who you are working with. To "do" CPI is to make a commitment to unlearning and relearning what we think knowledge is, what is "normal" in the knowledge creation process, and which knowledge(s) is or are valuable and useful for meaningful social change.

WHAT IS KNOWLEDGE AND WHOSE KNOWLEDGE COUNTS?

We began this chapter with Meagan's reflection because it is important to start considering that the ways in which things always happen may perhaps not be the best or most ethical or most useful ways. Have you ever had an experience like that? Maybe it was less obvious in that moment. Think back about times in your life when you have felt like your voice, your experiences, and your knowledge mattered less than those of others. Can you remember a time when you felt that your knowledge counted *more* than others'? Perhaps you were teaching a class or were positioned as an authority figure at work or at a community meeting. How did that feel to you at the time? How does it feel now? These questions about power dynamics and one's position in the world are important to reflect on before committing to CPI.

As we consider how or if we engage with communities in CPI toward positive social change, reconciliation, or peacebuilding, we urge you to think intentionally and often about how what we take for granted as normal or even desirable may run counter to commitments of social justice and change. To begin this reconsideration of whose knowledge counts, we need to establish a few foundational concepts that will appear throughout this book.

Positionality and Reflexivity

As you may have noticed in Meagan's story at the beginning of this chapter, she holds a particular identity and position within her family. Her identity, and yours, are not static concepts: Identity is complex, changes in different contexts and geographies, and is constantly evolving. As we mentioned before, we need to reflect on our identities to ethically engage in CPI. We understand **positionality** to be those intersecting, multiple, and evolving identities that involve both the totality and individuality of our experiences in this world, our socialization, our physical markers, our privileges, and the ways in which we are socially, politically, and economically targeted. More concretely, positionality can be thought of as our position in this world. Positionality is who we are. It is not a list of identities. It is not a statement like many we see in class papers or manuscripts: "I am a white, cisgender, educated, middle-class woman." While it includes the identities listed here, it is much more expansive than such a list. Grappling with our own positionality involves a process of **reflexivity**, which can include self-questioning and critically reflecting on our relationships to other individuals and groups as well as social, political, and economic structures and systems. Positionality statements provide an opportunity to reflect on our privileges while also understanding **intersectionality** (Collins, 2002; Crenshaw, 1989), or how an individual's various identities produce a competing and interconnected web of oppression and discrimination. By critically reflecting on our social categories, we can better understand our relationships to systems of power.

We believe that uncovering and questioning our own positionality as researchers or social inquirers is a necessary first step to engaging with communities. If we do not make explicit for ourselves who we are, what our interest or agenda is, where our expertise lies, what our personal and professional needs are, and what biases we may carry, how can we enter a community claiming to be open to or understanding of their identities, agendas, expertise, needs, or biases?

Ontology and Epistemology

As we start to reflect on our identities and positions in the world, the opportunity arises to question the research process and knowledge creation. The next two concepts work hand in hand and are often hard to discuss separately. **Ontology**, simply put, relates to what can be known. Each research tradition or paradigm holds ontological assumptions on the definition of reality:

Positivism, which is rooted in the scientific method, contends that there is an objective reality or truth that can be discovered through research and the search for knowledge. Constructivists assume relativism—there are multiple realities dependent on individuals' experiences, socialization, and cognition. Critical theorists posit that the nature of reality must be approached from historical realism—how knowledge and reality have been shaped by socioeconomic class, race, ethnicity, gender, and abilities. Participatory and postmodern researchers assume that reality is socially constructed but must be based on the recognition and participation of those with lived experience (Lincoln et al., 2011).

On the other hand, **epistemology** refers to how we know or how we come to know. Just as with ontology, each paradigm has its own epistemological assumptions. Since positivism evolved from the scientific method, its proponents see findings as true or objective. Although a positivist orientation is most often assumed in the life sciences, it has been endorsed by those in the social sciences as well. On the other hand, constructivist, critical, and participatory paradigms embrace the subjective, noting that much of what we know and how we come to know it can only be truly known by the knower (Lincoln et al., 2011). We can come to a fuller understanding of someone's reality through dialogue and study, and as we do so, we co-construct knowledge that is shaped by our own experiences and those of others (i.e., co-constructing knowledge and reality).

Thus, when we approach research from any paradigm—be it positivism or a critical and participatory paradigm—we must establish our ontological and epistemological bases, which are considered when we speak to the quality and commitments behind our work. As you can see, some of these paradigms are generally incommensurable. While you may find it difficult to combine ontological and epistemological assumptions from the positivist and the critical paradigms, many researchers are able to reconcile and justify the critical paradigm with constructivism or participatory/postmodern orientations. Before learning about CPI's ontological and epistemological roots, it is important to understand the assumptions about knowledge that we are carrying with us.

REFLEXIVITY QUESTION

How have you been socialized to think about what can be known and how we come to know?

For many of us, we have been brought up in a society that values knowledge of the tangible or concrete. I know because I *see*. I know because I *feel*. I know because I *touch*. In terms of how we come to know, many of us were taught the scientific method in school: State your hypothesis, test it, modify the hypothesis, test it again, and so on. This method, and so many of its derivatives, value what can be established or illustrated in tangible ways. How many times have you heard someone say, "Prove it," or "I'll know it when I see it," or some other version of that?

What do *you* think can be known? Consider, for a moment, how you know you are loved by someone. Or how you feel when you are sad or discouraged. We often give an example in our introductory research methods classes of the statement, "I love my children." You can, through something like the scientific method, verify that I have children, laying out definitions of what it means to "have" children, definitions of who is a "child," and more. Once you have determined those definitions, you could obtain "evidence" of my love for them (I provide for them financially, I feed them, I bandage their wounds, I take care of them emotionally), but you cannot ever *know* my love for them. Similarly, you can never *know* my pain or sadness when I am discriminated against because of my identities. You may be able to empathize, but your knowledge will never fully inhabit the same space as my knowledge. We will delve more deeply into other concepts related to what can be known and how we know, such as science, scientism, positivism, and postpositivism, in Chapter 3.

For now, it is important to understand that CPI is rooted in a critical tradition that privileges the knowledge and expertise of all individuals. It situates each person as the expert of their own lived experience. It is a form of inquiry that calls on us to question the status quo, to push against systems of oppression, and to build relationships based on respectful human interaction, all for the purpose of co-constructing knowledges and practices that aim for social transformation in solidarity.

Epistemologies That Inform CPI

Before we get more into the topic of why epistemology matters, we thought it would be valuable to pause and reflect on the epistemological roots of CPI. In this section, we highlight the importance of drawing from a multiplicity of systems (knowledge, language, and culture)—holding true to the concept of **knowledge democratization** and its role in CPI. While we briefly summarize a number of epistemologies here, you can look to Chapter 3 to learn more about these various traditions.

First, we place the work of several Indigenous[1] scholars and communities at the forefront of this summary, as throughout history, these ways of knowing were often invalidated through colonization, displacement, and historical erasure. In *Pulling Together: A Guide for Indigenization of Post-Secondary Institutions* (Antoine et al., 2018), Asma-na-hi Antoine, an Indigenous educator (Toquaht, Nuuchah-nulth), and her Indigenous and non-Indigenous co-authors note that across various Indigenous epistemologies, knowledge is a practice based in relationality (an interdependence among peoples, the environment, and the metaphysical), holism (learning through emotion, spirit, mind, and body), and spiritual development (understanding the interrelation between the sacred and secular). The concepts of interconnectedness and relationships are embedded within Indigenous epistemologies, demonstrating how these epistemologies can inform the principles of CPI.

Beyond Indigenous scholarship, it is imperative that we introduce the work of those across the Global South, as many of the fundamental principles of CPI are based in the work of notable scholar–activists such as Paulo Freire in Brazil, Orlando Fals-Borda in Colombia, and Mohammad Anisur Rahman in Bangladesh. In the 1970s, Finnish researcher Marja-Liisa Swantz should also be credited, as her collaboration with the University of Dar es Salaam in Tanzania and local community members was one of the first instances when these types of activities were termed "participatory research" (Swantz, 1982, 2008). In their work, they showed how participation, democracy, and pluralism are vital in promoting forms of inquiry that are anchored in and aim for equitable knowledge creation (or *knowledge democracy*) and social change.

In noting that social change (or action) is aligned with inquiry, these scholar--activists in the Global South drew on the work of Karl Marx and Max Weber. They demonstrate that it is not enough to simply theorize about social problems, but it is necessary to understand oppressive structures and seek change. This idea of inquiry as a critical activity toward transformative change was foundational to the work of the Frankfurt School. These scholars, many of whom escaped Nazi Germany, showed that action, without theory, could simply lead to the continuation of conformist thought and practices that perpetuate an oppressive status quo. Through the work of Jürgen Habermas, practitioners of CPI aim to understand how collective action can be achieved through committing to mutual understanding, reaching consensus, and creating space for dialogue and deliberation. While the work of these scholars, from Marx to the Frankfurt School, shaped the basis of much of what we see in critical inquiry, it should be noted that their perspectives were grounded and limited by their experiences as White, European men. Over time, feminist scholars such as Donna Haraway (1988) established the importance of situated or embodied knowledge, a notion inherent in CPI. That said, we must acknowledge that the feminist theorists most often cited in academic literature are those who identify as White, cisgender women; thus, it is necessary to consider whose ideas we are citing, the perspectives they bring to their work, and those we may be excluding or silencing. Figure 1.1 displays the various schools of thought that have contributed to critical forms of participatory inquiry and how these interdependent ideas provide the epistemological and ontological foundation for how one theorizes and practices CPI.

Although the idea of situating knowledge is essential to feminist theory and CPI as well, it is important to note the work of postcolonial and feminist literary critic Gayatri Chakravorty Spivak (1981), who suggests that critical theorists should not affix one epistemological view to all women (or any other social group). Similarly, Patricia Hill Collins (2002) describes in *Black Feminist Thought* how dominant research paradigms portray majoritarian views as neutral or objective, while minority views are often thought of as outliers or treated as less than. Collins and other critical race theorists (Crenshaw et al., 1995; Solórzano & Yosso, 2002) question why dominant research designs often portray communities of Color through a deficit lens rather than exploring how race and racism may shape the systems that affect these communities.

FIGURE 1.1 ■ Various Schools of Critical Thought Contributing to CPI Theory and Practice

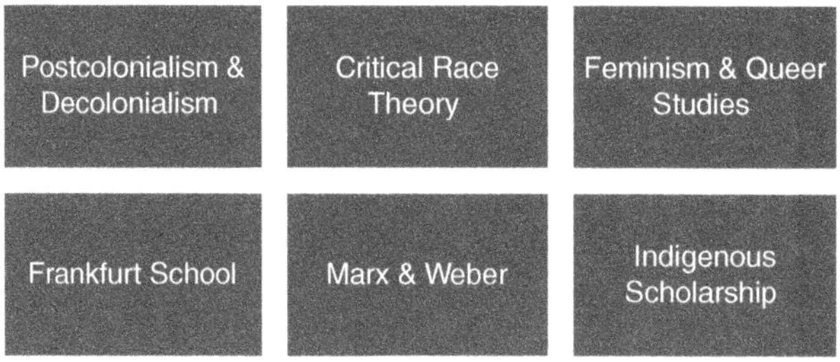

By exploring the work of various scholars and practitioners of critical theory, we see how these various strands can inform CPI. Remember, CPI is a form of inquiry that questions the status quo and oppressive systems, all for the purpose of co-constructing equitable knowledge systems and pushing for transformative change. Also, by understanding how various strands of critical theory inform CPI—from Indigenous to Global South to critical race theory—we intentionally counter acts of **epistemicide** (de Sousa Santos, 2008; Hall & Tandon, 2017), or efforts to erase the knowledge of subordinated cultures.

It is not our goal, nor is it desirable or helpful, to separate ontologies and epistemologies into tidy, dichotomous, or distinct categories or types. Ontological and epistemological beliefs and approaches are always blurred, always overlapping, and always contextualized. In addition, they are tied up with our own positionalities and often evolve over time. For example, we may believe in, value, and enact a Black feminist epistemology, but because we have been socialized in ways that do not value that approach, we may sometimes act in ways that are contrary to that epistemology. We may engage with a community that values or holds a different epistemology. As critical participatory inquirers, we seek to better understand, respect, and act in relation to that community's epistemology.

It is vital to question how our epistemological assumptions—how we (come to) know—influence (intentionally and unintentionally) the questions we ask, the methods we use, and how we interact with others. Use the scenario and questions in Box 1.1 to think through the relationship between positionality, epistemology, and methods.

BOX 1.1: CONSIDERING EPISTEMOLOGICAL MIS/ MATCH

Consider, for instance, a student in Canada who approaches a critical friend for assistance on her dissertation proposal. The study will be related to justice-oriented pedagogies in secondary schools in Uganda. The student-researcher identifies as White and claims a critical and participatory epistemology and an explicitly anti-racist agenda. The study she proposes will use interviews and focus groups of Black school teachers in Uganda to better understand how they employ justice-oriented pedagogies in their classrooms. What advice should the friend offer?

- How is the student positioning herself in relation to those with whom she will engage? (Is she positioning herself as Knower or the teachers as Knowers? Somewhere in between? How?)
- How does her stated epistemology (critical, participatory) align with her chosen methods? (Do her methods reinforce a CPI epistemological stance? Do her methods indicate she values and honors the teachers' expertise as knowledge? In what ways?)
- How might the methods she intends to use help or hinder her ability to better understand the participants' intentions and experiences? (Do her chosen methods allow the teachers the opportunity to be sincere, open, and honest about their experiences, or will the methods lean toward the extractive?)

- What are some other possibilities for engaging with this group of teachers or for better understanding justice-oriented pedagogies? (Could she consider other methods or approaches that would clearly connect with a CPI epistemology? Could she wait to decide on methods until after she engages dialogically with the teachers and builds authentic relationships?)

We note that the reflexive questions here are not simply meant to be answered as a check-box exercise, which could potentially lead to implicitly justifying and enacting hegemonic practices. Rather, as Pillow (2003) states, we must ask ourselves difficult questions to evoke discomfort, in an effort to improve the quality and ethics of our critical inquiry. We must also use these opportunities for reflexivity to think beyond the instrumental ("I should build relationships so I can get better data") and move toward the relational and ethical. We expand on this later in the book. For now it is important to work on pushing ourselves to explicitly link positionality with epistemology and methodology.

As you think through these questions, we encourage you to take a moment and add to the positionality inventory you started at the beginning of this chapter. You may choose to add some research questions or topics you are interested in pursuing. You may also list a few methods you would like to use or have learned about. Finally, write out the contexts in which you may begin your inquiry. Then, as you move forward in this chapter and beyond, perhaps you could add some visual components (like arrows, circles, etc.) to illustrate to yourself how your stated epistemology matches (or does not match) your goals, methods, and contexts. This is just a starting point. As we move on, we will help you clarify how or if your epistemological assumptions align with the methods you use.

Why Epistemology Matters

Epistemology and the goals, agendas, and commitments that stem from one's positionality determine and inform every step of the inquiry process, even if we do not make them explicit. Often as researchers we feel more comfortable pretending that we are detached from our research and the communities with which we work, that we have no agenda, that as long as we control for certain variables or enact multiple validity techniques, we do not need to consider our*selves*. This could not be further from the truth. We believe that strong inquiry is inherently connected to and enhanced by clarifying and foregrounding our own positionalities and epistemologies. Figure 1.2 may be helpful to clearly see how epistemology matters in the grand scheme of inquiry, guiding every step of the process.

THE LINEAGE OF KNOWLEDGE DEMOCRATIZATION

Moving on from the various epistemologies that inform CPI, in this section we further trace its development. We start with CPI's Indigenous roots through what is typically known as action research, including the related approach of participatory action research. We will establish the

FIGURE 1.2 ■ Cycle of Continuous Reflexivity

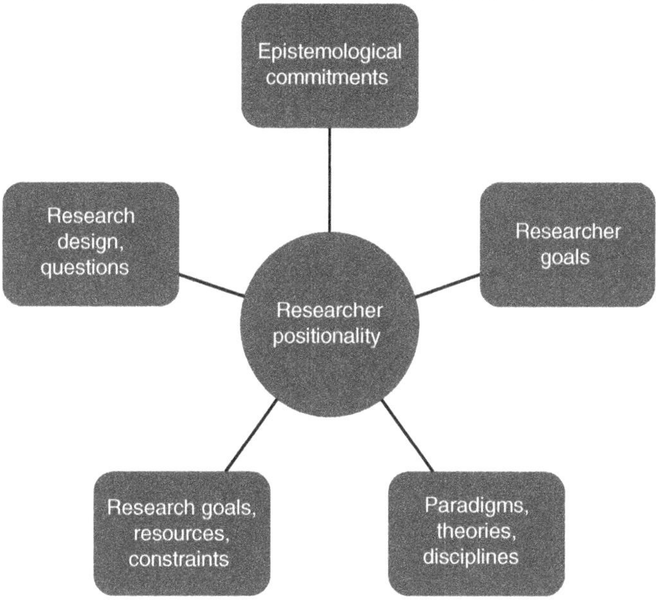

origins and epistemologies of this movement to democratize knowledge and then provide an overview of the current family tree of participatory inquiry.

Research as Inquiry Among Indigenous Peoples

Tracing the history of Indigenous inquiry is not as simple as combing through textbooks and journal articles to show how Indigenous ways of knowing were the first to contribute to methodological discussions. As previously mentioned, many forms of Indigenous knowledge around the world have been coopted, appropriated, displaced, or erased through colonialism (Smith et al., 2018).

REFLEXIVITY QUESTION

How have you seen colonialism enacted in or through research practices in your own field?

As Cook-Lynn (1997) shows in a history of Native American Studies (NAS) in North America, Indigenous scholars met in the 1970s to create networks and space where NAS could be seen as an autonomous discipline. The purpose of these discussions—and the development of courses, academic programs, and recruitment of Indigenous scholars—was not simply to create another academic discipline but to show how NAS was different. NAS would emerge as a discipline grounded in local knowledge systems (not simply the knowledge of academics), and it would be specific to the multiplicity of oral traditions, languages, and geographies across the First Nations.

Through the NAS project, Indigenous forms of inquiry were not established to further the reductionist views of the traditional scientific method; rather, the initial development of NAS was inherently based in an ethic of care, participation, and knowledge democracy. Prior to the development of NAS in the 1970s, these principles are evidenced as early as the 1940s, through what we would generally define as participatory methods, by Cree bureaucrats conducting land use studies in North America (Jackson, 1993).

Linda Tuhiwai Smith's groundbreaking book, *Decolonizing Methodologies: Research and Indigenous Peoples* (1999), is written from the author's perspective as a professor of Indigenous education in New Zealand who identifies as Indigenous Māori. In the book, Tuhiwai Smith critiques the heritage and harms of Western/Northern imperialist/colonialist research and provides guidance toward a "framework of self-determination, decolonization and social justice" for "those researchers who work with, alongside and for communities who have chosen to identify themselves as indigenous" (pp. 4–5). This framework shares many CPI values, particularly the emphasis on "cultural protocols, values and behaviors as an integral part of methodology" and the importance of sharing knowledge with "people in culturally appropriate ways" (Smith, 1999, p. 15) as well as a "long-term commitment" to communities. Much like CPI, Indigenous inquiry stresses that research must be contextualized according to local knowledge systems and cultures—it is not simply research about Indigenous peoples. Studies should be focused on Indigenous experience and conducted by Indigenous peoples (Smith, 1999). Although this summary focuses on an example of Indigenous inquiry across North America, the use of participatory methods is well documented by Indigenous scholars around the world, from New Zealand (Bishop & Glynn, 2003) to Botswana (Chilisa, 2020).

Research as Action in the Global North

Participatory methods also have a strong tradition in the Global North. One form, **action research** (AR), is typically traced to social psychologist Kurt Lewin's social change research in the 1940s (Feldman, 2017; McTaggart et al., 2017). Lewin, who had fled Nazi Germany in 1933, aimed to address prejudice and intergroup tensions in the United States by bringing community members into participatory, nonhierarchical dialogue. Informed by Lewin's (1943, 1951) field theory, this form of inquiry sought to surface and disrupt "entrenched habits of power" (Glassman et al., 2013, p. 274) in order to effect change in community relations. Unlike more traditional forms of social research, AR aims not just to document the status quo or conduct experiments in accordance with the scientific method but to *transform* reality through a reflective, democratic, and collective problem-solving process (Glassman et al., 2013).

AR comprises a continuous cycle of planning, acting, observing, and reflecting and positions participants and researchers as learners and actors who implement the solutions they devise (McTaggart et al., 2017). The approach has three distinct features (Glassman et al., 2013; Kemmis & McTaggart, 2005):

1. Shared ownership of research,

2. Community-based knowledge creation/analysis of social problems, and

3. Local, community-based actions to solve real-world problems.

The data provide evidence of the change process instead of simply the outcome. This sounds quite different from the traditional scientific method, doesn't it?

Lewin's AR approach gained ground, becoming a social movement influenced by other researchers, activists, and both governmental and nongovernmental organizations (Glassman et al., 2013). This movement also incorporated ideas from progressive educators of the era, including Dewey (1933), Piaget (1932), and Gardner's (1946) and Bradford's (1967) conception of adult education as a democratic quest for transformation (Glassman et al., 2013; McTaggart, 1991). A 1946 scholarly publication authored by Ronald Lippitt and Marian Radke called for social scientists to "understand, examine and challenge the dynamics of prejudice among social groups" (p. 167) through a cyclical nine-step process. Lippitt and Radke asserted that top-down efforts would not effectively diminish prejudice and that "the process of re-education is a spontaneous, voluntary acceptance of new values and behavioral patterns" (p. 172). They expressed a belief that the fledgling AR movement could help expose and ultimately reduce "conflict and misunderstanding between ethnic groups" (p. 172) evident in "both everyday and catastrophic problems" (Glassman et al., 2013, p. 276).

Other forms of AR also emerged around the same time, including one led by University of Chicago sociologist George Mead (Glassman et al., 2013). William Foote Whyte, a PhD graduate of this department, developed a form of participatory action research focused primarily on mapping community interactions and organizational structures with a view to changing behavioral patterns. Embracing a more traditional notion of the purpose of research, Whyte was openly critical of Lewin's approach, seemingly missing the democratic ethic around which it was designed (Glassman et al., 2013; Whyte, 1994). Chris Argyris, who studied under Whyte and founded a social research center at the Massachusetts Institute of Technology (Glassman et al., 2013), melded Whyte's practices with a more democratic, justice-focused ethic (Glassman et al., 2013, p. 282). In post–World War II England, Eric Trist, who was influenced by Lewin's work, cofounded the Tavistok Institute with an emphasis on psychotherapy; his approach to AR accounted for power dynamics in human behavior and organizational change (Glassman et al., 2013).

As you can see, the interpretations of Lewin's transformative AR were already starting to differentiate and drift from the original principles by the mid-20th century in North America and Europe. Now, we will look at how knowledge democratization developed in other parts of the world in the second half of the century in light of local contexts and concerns.

Research as Activism in the Global South

A more radical approach to inquiry emerged in Latin America and other parts of the Global South in the 1970s as a response to sociopolitical and intellectual domination from the Global North (Fals-Borda, 1987; Glassman & Erdem, 2014). As Fals-Borda, a leader of this movement in Colombia who coined the term "**participatory action research**" (Rahman, 2008) recounts, many intellectuals' ideas about "the relation between theory and practice" shifted drastically over the last three decades of the 20th century. These intellectuals were compelled by widespread "structural crises," "economic exploitation and human/cultural destruction," and everyday problems to take a stand against the dominance of "value-neutrality and aloofness" (Fals-Borda, 2001, p. 27) in scientific inquiry that propped up these injustices. Some adopted and adapted Lewin's AR as a promising framework for resisting positivist and colonial abuses (Fals-Borda, 2001).

Southern, participatory AR developed largely around Brazilian educator Paulo Freire's critical pedagogy, particularly the concept of ***conscientização***, or development of critical consciousness (Freire, 1970). Becoming aware or "conscientized" about oppression, Freire argued, is the first step in gaining liberation. Freire suggested that this occurs through critical reflection on and dialogue about one's lived experiences and circumstances and then taking action to challenge injustice: he called this marriage of reflection and action or theory and practice praxis. We cover this in more detail in Chapter 3. For now, it is important to understand that Freire's critical pedagogy has been key in the development of critical participatory inquiry.

Fals-Borda (2001) traces the development of this decentralized movement, spearheaded mainly by social scientists from anthropology, sociology, education, and theology who were deeply concerned by conditions in their communities, which they connected to capitalism and "universalistic modernization" (p. 27). They saw a need for "a radical critique and reorientation of social theory and practice" (Fals-Borda, 2001, p. 27) that broke with the practices and institutions of academia; in 1970, many even left their university jobs and established "alternative institutions and procedures for research and action" to solve real-world problems. This occurred through organizing and civil disobedience in India, Tanzania, Colombia, Brazil, and Mexico (Fals-Borda, 2001). Participatory action research (PAR) came to be seen as "a vivencia necessary for the achievement of progress and democracy . . . not only as a research methodology but also as a philosophy of life" (Fals-Borda, 2001, p. 31).

This philosophy grew into a truly global movement. The World Symposium of Action Research was held in Cartagena, Colombia, in 1977, bringing together speakers from Nicaragua, Germany, United States, Peru, Mexico, and Sweden (Fals-Borda, 2001). The 1997 meeting, again in Cartagena, included 2,000 delegates from 61 countries. Throughout this evolution of Northern and Southern (participatory) action research, a range of different approaches and research practices developed (Greenwood & Levin, 2007). Also, with this increased interest and use of AR in university courses and research projects, worries rose about straying from the foundational principles and epistemology of the approach: Would this lead to a new colonization of knowledge?

There are differing views on the relationship between Northern and Southern developments in AR. Some scholars, like Glassman and Erdem (2014) and Greenwood and Levin (2007), see Southern AR as evolving in parallel to Northern AR but within oppressive contexts from Latin America to Africa and South/Southeast Asia and expressly developed as a tool in the struggle for democracy and equality. Similarly, Fals-Borda (2006) "interprets the origins of PAR in the so-called Third World an endogenous proposal based on an examination of local social, cultural, historical, and environmental roots in order to explain, describe, systematize, and transform context and existing conditions" (Santos, 2015, p. 498). While acknowledging the role

FIGURE 1.3 ■ Lineage or Generations of PAR

First generation	Second generation	Third generation	Fourth generation
Action research J.L. Moreno (1910s) Kurt Lewin (1930s) Stephen Corey (educational action research) **Temporary decline due to positivistic ideology in the U.S.**	**British tradition** Tavistock Institute of Human Relations **following Lewin's theories** (starting in the 1940s) Ford Teaching Project (1970s)	**Critical + emancipatory** Appreciation for the practical character of the British tradition of action research Call for **more explicitly critical and emancipatory action research** (Carr & Kemmis, 1986)	**Participatory action research** Connect critical emancipatory AR and participation **Social movement theory:** Freire (1960s), Fals Borda **Adult education:** Budd Hall (1970s) **Development studies:** Robert Chambers (1980s)

Adapted from "Participatory Action Research: Communicative Action and the Public Sphere," by Stephen Kemmis and Robin McTaggart, in *Handbook of Qualitative Research* 3rd ed., by Norman K. Denzin and Yvonna S. Lincoln, eds. (Thousand Oaks, CA: SAGE), 559–604.

of international theoretical developments and cooperation like the congresses in Cartagena, Rahman (2008) shares Fals-Borda's assertion, pointing to rural development initiatives in South and Southeast Asia as origins of PAR practice (Santos, 2015).

On the other hand, as shown in Figure 1.3, Kemmis and McTaggart (2005) trace the lineage of PAR as the fourth generation of AR following the first generation of Lewin and company in the United States, a second generation in the United Kingdom, and then an international critical approach. Kemmis and McTaggart view Southern scholars as building on this foundation to inspire social movements and community development in Latin America, Africa, and South Asia. Regardless of the disputed lineage and fuzzy boundaries between AR and PAR, we agree with the likes of Fals-Borda and Mora-Osejo (2003), and Kemmis and McTaggart (2005), that a key, defining, and inalienable feature of participatory inquiry is its political nature.

It should be noted that Figure 1.3 is not meant to suggest a chronological order of what occurred or who enacted action research first or last. As previously mentioned in this chapter, knowledge and traditions from minoritized, colonized, and racialized communities have often been stolen, hidden, or disregarded within literature. Rather, Figure 1.3 denotes the major philosophical traditions surrounding various forms of action research and how they have been considered, acknowledged, and cited throughout history. Many of the scholars and communities who may identify within the third and fourth generation enacted their form of action research contemporaneously as those considered to be in the first and second generations.

REFLEXIVITY QUESTION

How do you view your own research through the lens of democracy, equality, and politics?

Calls emerged in the early 21st century for the development and use of an organic, localized paradigm suitable for each community's reality (***vivencia***) and needs (Fals-Borda & Mora-Osejo, 2003; Santos, 2015). Fals-Borda (2006) and Greenwood and Levin (2007) advocated for a convergence of Northern and Southern traditions in response to what they saw as the appropriation of AR's "radical ideas for social change" (Greenwood & Levin, 2007, p. 15) for creating more efficient organizational and industrial processes in North America and Western/Northern Europe, like Whyte and Trist's work. They also called out the "domestication" of AR for development purposes in forms like Rapid Rural Appraisal, Participatory Rural Appraisal, and Participatory Learning Analysis, which "unintentionally made participation into a commodity" (p. 15), which we will return to later.

Around the same time, however, action researchers seemed to incorporate participation into AR more generally, blurring the line between AR and PAR and the definition of participation itself (McTaggart, 1997; Santos, 2015). The approach was adopted into various disciplines, perhaps most notably education and public health, and strands such as critical and feminist PAR emerged in alignment with particular epistemological perspectives (Dick, 2009; Santos, 2015).

DEVELOPMENT INTO VARIOUS STRANDS AND THROUGH DIFFERENT DISCIPLINES

In this section, we briefly trace the adaptation of participatory inquiry into these strands and academic disciplines and call attention to some ways that it has drifted from its roots in the process. These varieties can be seen along a spectrum between PAR's critical ontoepistemological roots and more traditional ideas about research.

Strands

Although we cover several strands of participatory inquiry in this section, it is important to note that practitioners of these strands generally follow the core epistemological principles emphasized earlier in this chapter. For instance, researchers are not solely those affiliated with universities or academic institutions; there is an explicit acknowledgment that all community members can be involved in the knowledge creation and learning process. Rather than the researcher–scientist proposing a problem statement or hypothesis, issues are defined by community members, and community strengths and capacities are recognized in this process. Additionally, practitioners of these strands all follow the cyclical nature of action research and are interested in using research for action and beneficial social change.

CPAR

As you might guess, there is a strand of PAR that espouses an explicitly critical onto-epistemology and, given the title of this book, it might not surprise you that we most closely align with this strand. Critical participatory action research (CPAR) asserts that "people hold deep knowledge about their lives and experiences, and should help shape the questions, [and] frame the interpretations" of research (Torre & Fine, 2006, p. 458). The approach rejects the idea that objectivity is necessary or even possible and urges researchers to practice critical self-reflection throughout the process (Kemmis et al., 2014). As we will describe in Chapter 3, this strand views ethics as an ongoing practice rather than an institutional checklist or set of forms and as a way of ensuring the validity of the research (Lather, 1986). And most importantly, CPAR aims to illuminate, disrupt, and transform unjust conditions and practices alongside those affected by them (Kemmis et al., 2014; McTaggart et al., 2017; Sandwick et al., 2018). It is a "practice-changing practice" (Kemmis et al., 2014; McTaggart et al., 2017). CPAR is not always labeled as such, but a cursory examination of PAR studies will often reveal the researchers' epistemology.

CPAR is, in many ways, a reaction to the proliferation of AR approaches that developed during the second half of the 20th century and the cooptation of social action research (Kemmis et al., 2014). It is also a recommitment to Freire's critical pedagogy and PAR's origins in anticolonial movements in the Global South. CPAR has strong roots in the discipline of education; for example, in their influential 1986 book *Becoming Critical: Education, Knowledge, and Action Research*, Carr and Kemmis, educational researchers in the United Kingdom and Australia, respectively, critiqued both traditional approaches to research and the disconnect between theory and practice. They encouraged teachers to conduct their own inquiry, rejecting the idea that research should only be done by outside, university-based researchers, and outlining how they could use AR to reflect on, problematize, and ultimately transform their practice. Kemmis, McTaggart, and Nixon built on this in their 2014 guide for practitioners (primarily teachers but also health workers, organizational leaders, community groups, and others) planning CPAR projects. For example, CPAR has been used with and by youth in New York City to examine experiences of injustice and contest structures of privilege (Fox & Fine, 2015; Stoudt et al., 2012).

Feminist and Queer PAR

There is substantial overlap between critical, feminist, and queer ontoepistemology (Bain & Payne, 2016), but for the purposes of this chapter, we will highlight the unique aspects of each. These strands of PAR grew out of the belief that PAR could not be truly emancipatory without examining oppression and injustice (Maguire, 1996) for the purpose of disrupting cisgender, heterosexual, and patriarchal systems. For instance, feminist PAR can be defined as "a conceptual framework that enables a critical understanding of women's multiple perspectives and works towards inclusion and social change through participatory processes while exposing researchers' own biases and assumptions" (Reid & Gillberg, 2014, para. 1).

Patricia Maguire's 1987 book, *Doing Participatory Research: A Feminist Approach*, asserted that despite its focus on disrupting socioeconomic distinctions in research, PAR had continually marginalized women's perspectives. In line with feminist theories, Maguire's framework centers gender in the participatory inquiry process, acknowledging that gender is a socially constructed and oppressive system that forces women's knowledge and expertise to the periphery. In the years since, feminist PAR literature has expanded, incorporating feminist theory into the paradigm to more fully acknowledge and contest gendered forms of oppression (Reid & Gillberg, 2014). Reid and Frisby (2008) proposed a nine-part framework for feminist PAR that builds on Maguire's earlier work and incorporates the issues of intersectionality and representation. Feminist PAR has been used to document the experiences of adolescent South African girls after their parents' divorce (Botha & Hay, 2016) and to expose predatory lending practices of U.S. banks toward low-income people (Houh & Kalsem, 2015). Feminist PAR is not only concerned with women's experiences but seeks to highlight the role of gender in PAR more generally; for example, Singh et al. (2013) developed a set of strategies for feminist PAR with transgender communities.

Although Bain and Payne (2016) contend that "PAR and feminist and queer research are approaches to research that share similar values and practical concerns" (p. 332), they also illustrate how power dynamics in the co-creation of scholarly knowledge can lead to "dynamics of de-participation and exclusion that can erode the progressive, inclusive politics of feminist participatory methodologies" (p. 331). By reflecting on their experience of collaborating with participants from a queer youth program in Toronto, they detail how feminist participatory methodologies directed them toward more equitable power relations, but that their attempts at scholarly co-creation were met with queer de-participation during analysis, reporting, and publication. In reframing their research as queer PAR, they note the importance of work that originates in their own lived experiences and those of the participants in the queer youth program. Bain and Payne (2016) adeptly note that when they reframe feminist PAR through the term *queer*: "we do so to emphasize the disruptive potentialities of queerness as lived experience that subverts gender and sexual normative value systems and rationalities and allows us to consciously negotiate multiple situated positionalities" (p. 332).

These disruptive potentialities can be further seen in the "Restoring our Roots" PAR project, which sought to engage Indigenous youth who identify as Two-Spirit, non-binary, and/or LGBTQIA+ (2SLGBTQIA+) in land-based teaching (Fast et al., 2021). In this project, Elizabeth Fast, a Métis researcher, worked alongside graduate students and Indigenous members of their youth advisory committee to explore the impacts that land-based teaching and learning have for Indigenous youth, their families, Elders, and communities, especially those in urban settings who have been excluded from ritual. By working alongside 2SLGBTQIA+ Indigenous youth, Fast et al. (2021) show how their work has a disruptive potentiality in that colonial influences have led to violence, discrimination, and isolation for 2SLGBTQIA+ youth even though the oral histories of many Indigenous groups respect those who identify as Two-Spirit. Through this project, the documentation of 2SLGBTQIA+ Indigenous youths' experiences in land-based teaching and ritual, Fast et al. (2021) demonstrate that opportunities to disrupt through a praxis of inclusion, decolonization, and queering also lead to generative possibilities: "Decolonizing, queering, and creating non-binary inclusive spaces for land-based teaching where Indigenous 2SLGBTQIA+ youth feel safer are essential to the youths' overall self-esteem" (p. 134).

YPAR

As its name indicates, youth participatory action research engages youth as co-researchers in inquiry, enacting PAR epistemology that individuals of any background or status are experts on their lives (Schensul, 2014). The definition of participation ranges widely in such projects, from authentic involvement of youth in identification of a topic, selection of methods, collection and analysis of data, and sharing of findings to more tokenistic involvement (see Chapter 2 for more about types of participation). Because school is a significant part of youth lives, it is not surprising that much of YPAR occurs in schools or focuses on educational issues. For example, Cammarota (2011) uses PAR as a pedagogical model for urban youth, and Bertrand (2018) finds that YPAR can develop leadership skills among students of color. YPAR is used to document youth perspectives on educational barriers (Bhabha et al., 2017), teacher education (Brown & Rodríguez, 2017), and community life (Burke & Greene, 2015). YPAR also engages youth in inquiry on other issues that affect their lives, such as marginalization due to race, ethnicity, or migration status (Boutwell, 2015; Call-Cummings & Martinez, 2017). As we have found in our own YPAR work, this strand presents unique ethical quandaries and logistical challenges, particularly when done in school settings (Brion-Meisels & Alter, 2018).

CBPR

Community-based participatory research (CBPR or sometimes CBPAR) is often distinguished by partnerships between university researchers, organizations, and community members formed to tackle community-identified problems (Hacker, 2013; Vesely et al., 2019). As in PAR more generally, CBPR is typically rooted in Lewin's social action research and Freire's critical pedagogy, and community members are seen as holders of knowledge alongside professional practitioners and researchers (Hacker, 2013). CBPR epistemology emphasizes respectful relationships with participants, sharing of power over research objectives and methods, and an orientation toward action (Vesely et al., 2019). It is well established in the field of public health (Israel et al., 2005; Letiecq & Schmalzbauer, 2012; Minkler & Wallerstein, 2008). There are several handbooks and edited volumes illustrating CBPR in various disciplines. Our colleagues at George Mason University, Colleen Vesely, Bethany Letiecq, and Rachael Goodman, have used CBPR to understand resilience among immigrant families in the United States in light of structural and social barriers they face. The Appendix includes a more extended description of their work.

Disciplines

You might have noticed that these strands or epistemological perspectives intersect with multiple disciplines. Indeed, CPI is inherently interdisciplinary. Our attraction to the approach, given our varied interests and backgrounds in political science, public policy, international development, linguistics, human rights, conflict resolution, and migration might offer a useful illustration of this interdisciplinarity. But because we know it can be useful to see how it and its various strands have been adopted and adapted within specific disciplines, we offer here an overview of the use of participatory and action-oriented inquiry in various academic and professional disciplines, which might spark some ideas about how you could use it in the future. As you peruse this section, try to think about how or to what extent the ontology and epistemology behind some of these applications might align with the CPI perspective we outlined previously.

Education

It would probably be safe to say that participatory inquiry approaches have infiltrated the discipline of education more than others, and work in this field has in some ways encouraged adoption in other areas. Educational researchers seem to dominate many professional organizations and journals dedicated to AR/PAR. So, we will start our description of CPI's so-called family tree with education because of the influential role of this discipline in the spread of the approach and, arguably, in its shift away from some of its most foundational principles.

Critical participatory and action-oriented forms of inquiry have been used in a variety of ways within the field of education. For example, Cammarota and Fine (2008) have used PAR and YPAR as a form of emancipation for and with marginalized students. Silver-Pacuilla (2004) engaged feminist PAR with women with disabilities in an adult education program focused on literacy in the Southwestern United States. Torre (2009) engaged CPAR as a way of documenting unjust and unequal opportunity in New York City. Guerrero and Tinkler (2010) used participatory photography with refugee and displaced youth in the United States and Colombia as a socioemotional intervention. Brown and Rodríguez (2017), among many others, used PAR as a method of teacher education. Ní Sheanáin (2016) recruited her own primary school students in Ireland to help build an intercultural pedagogy among her teacher peers and to develop intercultural understandings among their students. We have used participatory inquiry in a variety of ways with students, teachers, school administrators, parents, and other educational stakeholders. Through those experiences we have noticed the difficulty—almost impossibility—of working within institutional structures of schooling, typically marked by hierarchical relationships among students, teachers, and administrators and rigid roles and procedures that make authentic power sharing extremely difficult. We will discuss these constraints and possible strategies later in the book.

Health

Perhaps surprisingly for a "hard" science, a number of scholars and practitioners in the health sciences have also embraced CBPR and PAR in recent years, for purposes ranging from nursing education to public health interventions. For example, Beatriz et al. (2018) engaged in YPAR to evaluate a healthy relationships workshop series for middle school students (11–14 years old) aimed at preventing teen dating violence in Boston, Massachusetts (U.S.). Peer researchers (14–18 years old) who had previously taken the workshops participated in all stages of the evaluation, including developing the pre- and postprogram survey and collecting and analyzing data. Also in Boston, Binet et al. (2019) conducted a longitudinal PAR study examining community health in relation to neighborhood conditions and change; 45 adult residents helped with the design of methods and instruments as well as carrying out data collection and collaborative analysis.

The health fields abound with examples of using participatory inquiry approaches, especially with Native, First Nations, and Indigenous populations in the United States, Canada, Australia, and beyond. For example, Cueva et al. (2018) used CBPAR to develop culturally relevant online cancer education modules about cancer for rural Alaska Native peoples with Community Health Aides and Practitioners, who were members of the target groups. The authors draw on Freire's popular education and Indigenous Ways of Knowing, which they describe incorporating into the modules through cultural values, teachings, and storytelling. Zubrzycki and colleagues (2017) explored cross-cultural collaboration between Aboriginal and non-Aboriginal health workers in rural Southeastern Australia by engaging 41 health workers in in participatory data collection and analysis around the issue of cancer services. The authors explicitly address the roles of colonialism, racism, and socioeconomic inequality in health outcomes among Indigenous Australians, the compatibility of PAR with an Indigenous paradigm, and their use of an Aboriginal theoretical framework and research protocols.

While examples of participatory inquiry abound in the United States, there are also numerous cases of participatory work being done all over the globe in the health fields. For example, Asirifi (2019) reports on her doctoral dissertation study using CBPR to build leadership capacity among undergraduate nursing students in Ghana through a collaborative, egalitarian problem-solving process based on power sharing with marginalized community members. Another example is from Devine et al. (2017), who report on a three-year PAR study to address barriers to sexual and reproductive health among women with disabilities in the Philippines, reporting positive outcomes like increased knowledge of and access to services. The process consisted of 10 meetings each of five Participatory Action Groups made up of women with disabilities and facilitated by co-researchers who were also women with disabilities, as well as interviews with group members. Lems et al. (2020) aimed to understand the perspectives of adolescent girls in Amsterdam from disadvantaged socioeconomic backgrounds on health behavior and to develop materials promoting healthy lifestyles using PAR. The authors portray an engaging, dialogic, collaborative, creative, and reflective process and describe participant contributions as "valuable" and "deep insights" (p. 206). Finally, Olumide et al. (2016) used photovoice (Wang & Burris, 1997), a photography-based PAR method that we describe in detail in Chapter 8, with 11 adolescents in Nigeria to define health and well-being and document threats in their community, part of an international project including sites in the United States, South Africa, India, and China.

Development

Participatory research has gained significant traction in the field of development as well, often crossing disciplinary boundaries with education, health, social work, human rights, migration, and so on. For example, Boedecker et al. (2019) integrated a CBPR approach with more traditional survey methods to improve food biodiversity and nutrition in Western Kenya and paired locations using CBPR with control locations receiving no intervention. One hundred eighty participants in the CBPR locations participated in a series of workshops to identify, plan, and implement farming procedures and educational activities to increase dietary diversity and nutrition in their communities while outside researchers measured effects of the intervention using baseline and end-line surveys and statistical analysis.

In rural Kenya, Beh and colleagues (2013) use a CBPAR approach to engage marginalized populations near conservation areas in photovoice (Wang & Burris, 1997) to elicit community input and strategize approaches for resource management. They emphasize the importance of community ownership, reciprocal knowledge creation, and change-focused outcomes in CBPAR. Campos et al. (2016) describe two PAR projects in Portugal in which community members participated in creating or implementing action plans for a local climate change-related problem. In India, Nix et al. (2019) used PAR to develop interdisciplinary solutions for sustainable low-income housing with local residents, who participated in problem identification, solution design, implementation, and evaluation. And in Haiti, Pyles (2015) reflects on ethical tensions in using PAR in development settings, focusing on earthquake recovery efforts with peasants, particularly the meaning of participation, power, race, class, and gender. She encourages practitioners to practice self-critique throughout the process.

Social Work

The field of social work has also historically led in its use of participatory methods and approaches. For example, Payne and Bryant (2018) report on their use of "street PAR," an explicitly critical, anti-racist "comprehensive research-activist program" (p. 450) that they designed, as part of a higher education intervention for incarcerated persons in Delaware (U.S.). Particularly in work with this population, the authors "advocate for the most aggressive definition of PAR" (p. 451) in terms of involving participants authentically in all aspects of the research. Another example comes from Johnston-Goodstar (2013), who worked with Native American youth to develop a definition of social justice for social work with Indigenous communities, drawing on Indigenous epistemologies and ontologies in a YPAR process.

Often, as you will see in later chapters, participatory methods include the use of arts-based inquiry approaches. For example, Van Katwyk and Seko (2019) take a critical, emancipatory stance toward YPAR, employing participatory arts-based methods with youth (ages 16--29) in both urban and rural locations in Ontario, Canada, to understand their definitions, perceptions, and experiences of resilience. Trained youth researchers planned and facilitated the arts workshops; artwork was displayed at a public gallery; and the authors conducted thematic data analysis of research memos, participant descriptions of their artwork, and group discussions.

Migration

Participatory inquiry has become prevalent in research about immigrants and refugees, who in many cases experience intersectional marginalization in terms of race and ethnicity, legal and socioeconomic status, cultural and linguistic knowledge, access to educational and healthcare services, and other factors. Some migration scholars tout participatory inquiry as a solution to logistical and ethical challenges, while others—us included—stress the need for increased attention to power relations and ethics in research with these populations (see Hauber-Özer & Call-Cummings, 2020 for a full discussion of ethics in visual participatory inquiry). Migration studies as a field is inherently interdisciplinary, so you will notice that the handful of examples we include here cross into other disciplines. Letiecq et al. (2014) use CBPR to document causes of high rates of depression among Mexican men working in

Montana (U.S.) and recommend mental health interventions for this population that take into account the stressors of family separation, economic and legal concerns, and discrimination. The authors note the need for increased caution due to the risk of deportation for undocumented participants. Baird et al. (2015) partnered with South Sudanese refugee women in Kansas (U.S.) to examine and develop action plans for health challenges experienced during resettlement.

Arts-based participatory methods, in particular, are seen as valuable means to facilitate expression for migrants who are not yet proficient in the dominant language of their society (Call-Cummings et al., 2019). Sloane and Wallin (2013) report on the potential of participatory theater to improve engagement of refugee families in Manitoba, Canada, in school planning at the local and national levels. The authors also tied theater-based participatory inquiry to the larger goal of transformative democracy. Photovoice (Wang & Burris, 1997; see Chapter 8) has become especially popular with migrant groups. In the field of social work, Kim et al. (2015) describe the use of photovoice as part of a study examining the experiences of 10 North Korean adolescent and young adult refugees living in South Korea. Despite the two countries' shared language and history and settlement support systems, participants expressed themes of loss, exclusion, and a mismatch of cultural values. During her ethnographic dissertation study, Miled (2020) employed the photovoice method with 10 refugee-background Muslim girls in a Canadian high school as an alternative to interviews. Miled reports that the girls found this multimedia method to be a valuable opportunity to overcome language and confidence barriers and express their identities and experiences of displacement and resettlement. Melissa also incorporated photovoice into her dissertation study as a means of challenging public perceptions of refugees in Turkey (see Chapter 8 for an example).

Conflict Resolution, Human Rights, and Peace Studies

Critical forms of inquiry, especially CPI, are a natural fit for studies focused on human rights, conflict resolution, and peace studies. Many of the same principles followed in CPI—inclusion, dialogue, participation—are espoused within frameworks focusing on rights, peace, and justice (Dazzo, 2016), such as the *Universal Declaration of Human Rights*. One instance of how participatory methods and emancipatory goals have been used is documented in the work of Arstein-Kerslake et al. (2019), to ensure that individuals with cognitive disabilities received a fair assessment of their fitness to stand trial in Australia's criminal justice system. The research team—comprised of academics, legal practitioners, and individuals with cognitive disabilities—blended principles from participatory research and the *Convention on the Rights of Persons with Disabilities* (CRPD) to guide their methodology; these principles included community participation, emancipation and reform, equal recognition and nondiscrimination, and community accessibility to research outputs. Through this participatory project, Arstein-Kerslake et al. (2019) were able to produce evidence and tangible change, showing that community legal centers were more effective in ensuring equality, fairness, and nondiscrimination than the status quo (i.e., court determination of unfitness).

CO-OPTATION AND APPROPRIATION OF PARTICIPATORY METHODS

We hope that this excursion through the use of participatory inquiry in various strands and disciplines has sparked inspiration and questions about how and why you could use the approach in your own work. The examples above illustrate that these academic disciplines are successfully developing and using participatory inquiry methods in many contexts and with diverse populations. However, in many instances, we see participatory methods used without grounding the entire project in a participatory ontology and epistemology. In fact, we note in too many instances that participatory methods are used in a depoliticized way that is completely divorced from CPI's critical, democratic, decolonial roots. Often due to deep-seated colonial, neoliberal, globalizing forces, habits, and assumptions, CPI and associated methodologies are used in ways that in fact reproduce the very inequities and injustices they supposedly seek to address. This is done in both subtle and overt ways. For example, often researchers that engage PAR, CBPR, CBPAR, or AR identify an area of concern to be studied, rather than allowing community members to do that. This takes away a community's power in exercising their judgment about what is important and what is necessary. They are told what is wrong and that they (or some aspect of their lives or experiences) are a problem and that the researchers have shown up to "help fix" the problem. This is the epitome of a deficit perspective and feeds into a colonial mentality.

Another concern we have is that some of the studies described above, while engaging "target" populations in data collection, may not have included these co-researchers in data analysis, often relying on more traditional statistical approaches rather than on local understandings. This amounts to essentially using community members to extract data from their friends, neighbors, or peers but then disregarding them as outside "experts" attempt to make sense of that same data. Analysis approaches are often described as thematic analysis or traditional approaches to coding. We have experienced this approach as particularly violent and deeply colonial.

In addition, while many of the authors cited above tout the potential for participatory approaches to encourage trust among university- and community-based co-researchers, they often do not explicitly grapple with power dynamics or issues of positionality. Readers are left to wonder how or if these were addressed. Failing to identify one's positionality can be an honest mistake on the part of university-based researchers, yet we see this failure as profoundly problematic, as it is often a White person who commits this mistake because they see themselves as the norm and the practice of naming one's identities as unnecessary. Indeed, we, the authors, have made this mistake previously and have learned that, while we may think of it as a "simple" oversight, in actuality it is an act of racist, colonial violence.

When distanced from its critical epistemological foundations, participatory inquiry can "reproduce traditional, taken-for-granted power structures that are meant to be challenged and disrupted" (Call-Cummings et al., 2019, p. 402; citing Call-Cummings & Martinez, 2016; Evans-Agnew & Rosemberg, 2016). These practices take away from the democratic approaches taught and used by early participatory inquirers like Freire and Fals-Borda and reduce a potentially powerful, emancipatory experience to another tool in a researcher's toolbox to be wielded when they want or need to claim that their work was somehow inclusive. We do not fault the researchers themselves, for the most part, because often participatory research is taught and understood as a method, as opposed to what we hope we you will start to see it as: an epistemological stance and a way of life.

RECOMMENDED PRACTICE 1.1: REVISITING REFLEXIVITY

Return to your responses for the introductory positionality activity, as part of the Focus Activity: Who Am I? at the start of this chapter. What might you add or change? As a critical participatory inquirer, it is important to continuously revisit these statements to understand how changes in your position and environment affect how and why you conduct CPI. Before you begin your own CPI project, make sure to revisit your positionality statement. Make sure you are doing more than just checking a box or employing a method. Be ready to engage in a reflexivity of discomfort (Pillow, 2003).

CONCLUSION

We have covered a lot of ground in this first chapter and hope this journey has sparked some reflection on the definition of knowledge, how it is created, and what the purpose of research is and should be. The fact that you are reading this book means you likely had some interest in "alternative" or collaborative methods of research, but by now you will have realized that what we are describing is more than an approach or method. We are describing an entirely different—but not new—paradigm about research, its purposes, and its practices. We are inviting you to join this global movement committed to democratizing and decolonizing knowledge.

In the following chapter we will get more into the "nuts and bolts" of CPI, including the meaning of participation, sharing ownership and decision making with community members, and what transformative outcomes can look like. However, we cannot overemphasize the importance of grounding any future use of CPI in an understanding of your positionality, ontology, epistemology as well as the radical, anti-oppressive paradigm out of which it was born.

SUMMARY OF KEY POINTS

- CPI requires a reconsideration of the definition of knowledge and whose knowledge counts.
- Positionality refers to an individual's relationships with the world resulting from identities, experiences, social, political, and economical positions, socialization, privilege,

biases, and so on. Understanding one's positionality is essential to doing critical inquiry with communities.

- Ontology is one's concept of reality or what can be known while epistemology is one's theory of knowledge or understanding of how we come to know. The traditional approach to research, often known as the scientific method, depends on tangible evidence, but CPI values other ways of knowing about reality. CPI draws on Indigenous knowledge(s), Marxist and feminist thought, and critical race theory and seeks to counter epistemicide—efforts to erase subordinated forms of knowledge—through knowledge democratization.
- CPI developed through Indigenous inquiry, action research, which originally aimed to solve social problems in the Global North, and participatory action research, a form of anti-colonial activism in the Global South.
- Participatory inquiry has evolved into various strands, most notably critical, feminist, youth, and community-based forms, and has been adopted into numerous academic disciplines, including education, health sciences, development, social work, migration, human rights, conflict resolution, and peace studies.
- This expansion of participatory inquiry has, in some cases, led to distancing from the critical, political nature of the approach and even cooptation of participation for a traditional research paradigm.

RECOMMENDED PRACTICE 1.2: REVISITING KNOWLEDGE

Journal about how you were socialized to think about knowledge. Think about your own (existing or future) CPI project and reflect on how the following questions would affect your project and how you engage with community members as co-researchers:

- What constitutes knowledge?
- How is knowledge created?
- Who creates knowledge?
- How do you know something is true?
- What counts as evidence?
- How are your ideas starting to change?

SUGGESTED ACTIVITIES

1. Draw a picture of a researcher or find one on the internet or in one of your textbooks. What does this person look like? What are they doing, and where? How does this image differ from what you might have drawn before reading this chapter?

2. Choose a study cited in the "Strands and Disciplines" section of this chapter that interested you. Read it and note how (if at all) the authors address their positionality, what they count as evidence, what kind of change (if any) they are working toward, and how they describe working with community members through the process.

3. Create your own cycle of reflexivity mind map. Notice where you get stuck. What needs more thought? Continue to add to this as you read more in the book.

KEY TERMS

action research
community-based participatory research
conscientização
epistemicide
epistemology
intersectionality
knowledge creation
knowledge democratization
ontology
participatory action research
positionality
reflexivity
vivencia

ENDNOTE

1. While we are aware that there are vastly different traditions seen or labeled as "Indigenous," it is generally accepted as the most common and inclusive term that encompasses First Nations, Aboriginal, and Native. Therefore, we use "Indigenous" throughout this text.

2 WHAT IS CRITICAL PARTICIPATORY INQUIRY?

LEARNING OBJECTIVES

By the end of this chapter, you will better understand

- How CPI is an epistemological stance, not a method or methodology.
- The messiness and flexibility of the CPI process.
- Major critiques of CPI.
- How CPI can play a role in advancing the people's knowledge for liberation and transformation in this historical moment.

FOCUS ACTIVITY 2.1: THE PURPOSE AND PRACTICE OF RESEARCH

Before you start reading this chapter, consider the following questions. You may answer them to yourself or record your answers and thoughts in your researcher journal:

1. What is research for?
2. Who is research for?
3. What is the difference between inquiry and research?

In every one of the research methodology courses we teach, we start by delving deep into ourselves, our positionalities (as we discussed in Chapter 1), and what our relationship is to the practice of research and to those with whom we will engage. By the second or third week of classes, inevitably, one or two or more students will ask something like, "I know that reflexivity is important and all, but I'm really interested in adding tools to my toolbox. How do I *do* this type of research?" We completely understand. However, without this reflexive work as grounding, those "tools in your toolbox" may be used incorrectly, or you may not be aware of some of the tools at your disposal.

In Chapter 1, we took a deep dive into the concepts of positionality and reflexivity to better understand who we are in relation to critical participatory inquiry (CPI). The goal of this chapter is to now move to what CPI actually is and what it is not. We will also begin to introduce the why and how of it all. This will set us up for future chapters that get into all those tools (methods) in your methodological toolbox.

CONCEPTS AND DEFINITIONS

As you discovered in Chapter 1, CPI grew out of a decentralized, multinational movement to rethink what research is and is for (i.e., to transform rather than just document or explain the status quo). In other words, CPI embraces a new paradigm about research which claims that knowledge creation cannot be separated from the identities of the researcher(s) and participants and the unique contexts in which it occurs. Here, we will clarify some foundational concepts that drove the development of this movement and continue to guide the CPI process.

Method vs. Methodology vs. Stance

You may have learned about research in terms of the scientific method, a standardized procedure leading neatly from a well-defined question to a hypothesis, an experiment designed to test the accuracy of the hypothesis and, ultimately, to a conclusion that either proves or disproves the hypothesis. CPI, however, is not a tidy set of steps or techniques; in fact, it is not a **method** at all in the traditional sense. We argue that it is not even a **methodology**, a broader approach or philosophy about research that guides the selection of a method and design of procedures. In contrast, CPI is an epistemology or a stance toward knowledge that influences a researcher's choices about how to enact it and what the desired outcome is. This stance is characterized by the goal of transforming attitudes, behaviors, or even entire systems.

Emancipation

As we discussed in Chapter 1, CPI is rooted in emancipatory pedagogy (Freire, 1970), which challenges dominant paradigms about knowledge and research. Originators interrogated the positivist assumption that "truth" is "a cumulative, linear complex of confirmed rules and absolute laws" (Fals-Borda, 2001, p. 28), recognizing that "science is socially constructed" and interpreted. Participatory epistemology claims that research has "democratic potential" at the grassroots level and thus needs to be *democratized* or opened up to the ordinary citizen (Appadurai, 2006, p. 167). In fact, Fals-Borda (2001) calls for a new scientific paradigm that privileges the knowledge of "the rebel, the heretical, the indigenous, and the common folk" (p. 28).

This can look like neighborhood council members debating a proposal to build a new shopping center, or students working alongside their instructor to co-construct a classroom agreement. This stance declares that community members, often individuals who have been historically pushed to the margins of society or who have been mistreated or violated by the research process itself, are experts on their worlds and must be meaningfully included in decisions that affect them. In other words, those closest to an issue know it best because of their lived experience, or *vivencia*, to use the original term in Spanish from Orlando Fals-Borda (Fals-Borda, 1987; Fals-Borda & Rahman, 1991; Ochocka et al., 2010).

As a result, "ordinary people" can and should be included as co-creators of knowledge and retain ownership of this knowledge. In fact, Arjun Appadurai (2006), an Indian American anthropologist, asserts that everyone has a *right* to research and that it should not be thought of as a "high-end, technical activity" (p. 167) requiring advanced formal education but as "the capacity to make disciplined inquiries into those things we need to know, but do not know yet" (p. 167).

Higher education in most countries across the world today is dominated by two competing interests: the ideal of a democratic learning environment and the neoliberal, capitalist ideology of market competition, with students positioned as consumers purchasing credentials to gain access to the job market (Giroux, 2002; Mirra & Rodgers, 2016). In the neoliberal university, the goal is sometimes seen as efficiently training a workforce rather than developing human beings to contribute to building a more just, equitable society, and knowledge becomes a commodity to be owned rather than a public good to be created. This ideology trickles down to PK–12 schooling, which features ever-narrowing definitions of knowledge and success evaluated by standardized assessments and enforced by accountability measures. Beyond concerns about critical thinking, these approaches to schooling divorce learning from real-world contexts and punish marginalized communities for their presumed failures to measure up. This logic presumes that success is based on merit but fails to recognize inequity in access to learning and measurement tools that are intentionally created to maintain the status quo and power structures that reproduce injustice.

Before moving on to the concept of resistance, it is important to extend the notion of emancipatory research to that of abolition. Abolitionism, with its origins in the movement to end slavery around the world and later the prison-industrial complex in the United States, has found a natural place in education and research. As noted by Mariam Kaba (2021), abolitionism is not simply about deconstruction; it is an intentional practice of critiquing harmful and violent practices with the aim to collectively imagine and create something new. Abolition, then, is a generative process that requires collective responsibility and accountability, rather than "delegating it to a third party—one that has been built to hide away social and political failures" (p. 4), such as prisons, harmful and violent educational practices (e.g., high-stakes testing, gendered-racialized disciplinary actions), and even, relating specifically to the research process, institutional review boards. Rather, an abolitionist theory toward research is one that resists the habit of solely critiquing and deconstructing, and one that imagines how researchers and communities can push beyond the traditional researcher-researched hierarchy to collectively imagine how relationships and respect are ingrained in research. In practice, this can be considered across the entire research process: the ways in which researchers and communities negotiate how data are collected, analyzed, written, and shared; reducing harm and violence by objecting to the use of race and ethnicity in defining research problem statements; forming partnerships based on reciprocity; and openly discussing monetary or in-kind compensation when community knowledge and expertise are shared. Based on Kaba's (2021) definitions of abolitionist theory and practice, then, abolitionist approaches to research must be rooted in transformative forms of justice, seeking to co-create processes that reduce harm and violence in research while imagining new futures based on relationality, respect, responsibility, and resistance.

Resistance

Although CPI extends far beyond the realm of education, one of its primary goals is to resist these narrow definitions of knowledge, and its potential is perhaps best illustrated by work with youth. For example, the Council of Youth Research[1], a YPAR collective of Los Angeles high school students, pushes back against representations of their school as "a dropout factory" through media production and other forms of civic engagement (Garcia et al., 2015). Youth researchers have presented their findings at Los Angeles City Hall and the American Educational Research Association (AERA) annual meeting, disrupting the typical delineation between researcher and researched. Mirra and Rogers's (2016) study of U.S. university faculty who engaged in YPAR revealed that they saw it as a way to build youth's skills both for succeeding in formal schooling and critiquing power structures governing education. In other words, it offers a way to both work within existing systems and work to change them. In Guatemala, Giovanni has worked alongside nonprofit staff and Indigenous community members to explore how community co-researchers would recommend improving systems of justice and memorialization, given the episodes of violence that community members witnessed and experienced during the country's internal armed conflict as well as current socioeconomic manifestations of systemic oppression. As a knowledge democratization project, this work starts with known methods (i.e., those that co-researchers already use in their daily lives) rather than assuming that Giovanni, as the researcher, should immediately train others. Community co-researchers have used methods known to them (e.g., sharing circles), as well as other collaborative methods that Giovanni has facilitated (e.g., democratic card sorting, Ripples of Change). We describe and provide examples of these methods in later chapters, but for now, it is important to note that the purpose of this work is to counter deficit stories by showcasing community knowledge and resiliency.

By creating knowledge about their lives and the forces that constrain them, individuals can then assert their rights to economic, social, and racial justice (Appadurai, 2006), wielding this knowledge as "creative and transforming leverage" for meaningful community change and sociopolitical action (Fals-Borda, 1991, p. 4). Participating in research is connected to "the social and cultural capacity to plan, hope, desire, and achieve socially valuable goals" (Appadurai, 2006, p. 176). This is especially true for those most marginalized by today's global socioeconomic and political hierarchies who have the most to gain by claiming their rights to knowledge and knowledge creation (Appadurai, 2006).

Humanism

A CPI stance also asserts that research needs to be holistic, infusing science with "a moral conscience" that brings together reason and personal ethics or "head and heart" for a "balanced handling of the ideal and the possible" (Fals-Borda, 2001, p. 29). Take, for example, a CPI project by C. Susanna Caxaj (2015), where communities across Mexico, Honduras, and Guatemala shared their stories of how mining operations affected their health and livelihoods, as well exchanging their strategies of resistance toward a multinational corporation. As Caxaj worked alongside a Maya Mam community in Guatemala, community co-researchers proposed holding a community-led tribunal—much like those held in international criminal courts—where they could share personal *testimonios*, highlighting how mining operations often led to health issues, ranging from the psychological and emotional to physical. During this tribunal, "jury members" throughout the Americas listened to these testimonies and found the mining corporation to be guilty of not only contributing to health issues but also to environmental and human rights violations. While this tribunal and the verdict received widespread coverage, it should be noted how Caxaj and community co-researchers addressed the moral conscience as conceptualized by Fals-Borda. For instance, before beginning the tribunal, Maya Mam spiritual leaders decolonized the room, arranging chairs in a circle, rather than what was considered to be a more colonial orientation of chairs organized in straight lines and connoting some sort of hierarchy of importance. Community leaders then prepared an altar in the middle of this circle and performed a ceremony. As Caxaj (2015) notes, this led the health tribunal to be "grounded in a Maya Mam place of meaning" (p. 5). Here, we can see even how the preparation of our collaborative activities, and how we share power and meaning with co-researchers, can lead us to better balance the ideal and the possible (Box 2.1).

BOX 2.1: PUSHING BACK AGAINST DEFICIT REPRESENTATIONS OF REFUGEE YOUTH

In designing her PhD dissertation research with Syrian young adults under temporary protection in Turkey, Melissa felt strongly that she needed to balance protecting participants (and herself) from potential negative repercussions while resisting deficit representations of refugees that dominate scholarly literature and public discourse worldwide. She selected an ethnographic design infused with CPI epistemology, which Smyth and McInerney (2013) call "advocacy ethnography." Instead of focusing on the barriers to higher education that refugees face, she used questionnaires, in-depth, semi-structured interviews, and photovoice (Wang & Burris, 1997) to collect rich, multimodal, multilingual data about how participants have overcome challenges—learning Turkish, passing entrance exams, navigating unfamiliar systems, covering living expenses—in their own words. Through narrative analysis methods, she crafted portraits that highlight the personal characteristics, strategies, and supports which enable academic success within an unstable, adverse environment; the portraits can be shared through social media to challenge misconceptions and misrepresentations of refugees in Turkey and beyond. This design was intended to account for the constraints of the sociopolitical context, which precludes criticism of government policies and institutions, while centering the knowledge and experiences of a marginalized group.

THE CPI PROCESS

At this point, you might be thinking, "That's all well and good, but how do you *do* it?" Although you might wish for a flow chart with a clear timeline, like other forms of research sometimes offer, CPI is a fluid, messy cycle of planning, action, observation, reflection, and responsive adjustments based on preliminary findings—or hunches, even mistakes (Fals-Borda, 1987; Kemmis & McTaggart, 2005; McTaggart et al., 2017). Like the epistemology underlying it, the CPI process challenges dominant research paradigms by approaching knowledge creation as a collaborative, democratic, action-focused inquiry practice distinct from the scientific method or other traditional, rigid methods. It is **dialogical**, meaning it depends on two-way communication, which requires an equal relationship between those who would traditionally play the roles of researcher and researched.

Who is involved in this process? In contrast with traditional approaches to research, CPI involves both internal and external "agents of change" (Fals-Borda, 1987, 1991), typically university researchers or practitioners and community members. These change agents "contribute their own knowledge, techniques and experiences to the transformation process" (Fals-Borda, 1987, p. 332), combining insider and outsider forms of knowledge (i.e., practical and academic) to produce "a much more accurate and correct picture of the reality that is being transformed." For example, outside researchers with formal training in data collection methods might provide guidance on developing a survey about childcare options in a low-income urban neighborhood, but insider researchers from the community should be the ones determining the relevant questions, conducting the survey, and analyzing the data.

Mutual Recognition

This collaboration, usually between individuals with very different positions in the sociopolitical hierarchy—think of an undocumented Latina single mother and a White, male, tenured professor working together in the project mentioned above—often results in tension or awkwardness. Fine and Torre (2004) apply Pratt's (1991) concept of *contact zones* to describe these interactions between people with very different cultural backgrounds, personal identities, and socioeconomic status, which requires explicit negotiation of power relationships within the research collective. They present this as an advantage of CPI, enabling the creation of knowledge that none of the co-researchers could have accomplished on their own. The goal is to move from an us/them mentality to a one of a team working together toward the same goal(s). Based on their work with youth, Call-Cummings and Dennis (2019) introduce the term "entangled self-assertion" to describe this kind of inquiry-oriented participation as "a collective reclaiming of power and dignity" (para. 39).

This process of reclaiming power can be tricky, complicated, messy, and confusing. Often, especially as people who are comfortable in our spaces and identities of relative power, we are pushed into positions and spaces of reflexive discomfort where we may, perhaps for the first time, come to see ourselves as colonizers of knowledge, complicit perpetrators of violence, or blissfully ignorant racists. Yet, it is within these contact zones that we form relationships of trust and respect and that we learn about our mutual implication in the work of social transformation. That is, we can better understand how our lives, experiences, and futures are tied up with one another. Paulo Freire (1970) framed this mutual implication as a relationship between the oppressor and the oppressed that must be broken from both sides in order to move toward social change. CPI enacts this through inquiry.

REFLEXIVITY QUESTION

Have you ever been a part of a contact zone? How did it feel? How did you respond to the experience physically, emotionally, or otherwise?

In order for this relationship of mutual implication to work, members of an inquiry collective need to explicitly—and often repeatedly—redefine the traditional, asymmetrical roles in research of subject (active researcher) and object (passive/submissive "sample") into an equitable, democratic subject–subject relationship (Fals-Borda, 1987). Fals-Borda (1991) declares that this type of participation is a democratic, altruistic core value "rooted in cultural traditions of the common people and in their real history" (p. 5) but damaged by "conquests, violence and all kinds of foreign invasions." In other words, CPI requires the decolonization of relationships and the creation of sustainable local practices that can continue without dependence on external "experts" (Fals-Borda, 1991). This is messy, hard work that requires flexibility and ongoing negotiation of roles (Call-Cummings, Hauber-Özer et al., 2019; Kemmis & McTaggart, 2005); it demands genuine commitment from all involved and long-term engagement (Fals-Borda, 1991, p. 4).

Considering the idea of **animators**—those who can breathe life into a CPI project—helps us to unpack the concept of sustainability more concretely. Sustainability, however, is a tricky concept, as it is more than simply ensuring a project can continue or obtain external funding. As Deeb-Sossa (2019) notes, the responsible inquirer should be warned that sustainability is difficult, as building trust and comradery with communities is necessary before we can start to think about sustainability. As Sri Lankan economist and participatory researcher Sirisena Tilakaratna (1991) described, sustainability does not happen by chance; there are several vital interrelated factors:

1. the emergence of a group of internal animators,
2. the practice of self-review by people's organizations,
3. the ability to move from micro groups to larger groupings, and finally
4. an expansion of the action agenda to move toward a total/comprehensive development effort.

In Box 2.2, we will cover these factors through a classic example by Muhammad Anisur Rahman.

BOX 2.2: SEEKING SUSTAINABILITY WITHOUT OUTSIDE EXPERTISE

Through an example of a community development project in the 1970s that sought to mitigate the socioeconomic risks of drought in Senegal, Fals-Borda and Rahman (1991) describes a process where a group of internal animators (Sustainability Factor 1) emerged and engaged with an outside expert working on a donor-sponsored project. These internal animators already had their own questions based on reviewing and evaluating their own experiences and challenges (Factor 2). Through collaboration with an external animator, they systematized this process of self-review and formed their first subcommittee for collective action. As their surveys and analysis continued, other villages in the zone of Bamba-Thialene heard about their work, which led to intervillage reflection sessions and the formation of fifteen other subcommittees (Factor 3). These subcommittees consolidated and created a Committee for Development Action. Through this organization, the committee was able to develop curriculum to train more internal animators, continue reflection sessions, self-finance activities, and obtain external funding. The last factor in Tilakaratna's list was also achieved, which meant the committee began forming what was considered a comprehensive development effort—or one that took a systemic view of issues, activities, and outcomes—rather than solely looking at the most immediate problem.

Participation

What counts as participation? In an essay published by UNICEF in 1992, Hart defines participation as "the process of sharing decisions which affect one's life and the life of the community in which one lives" (p. 5). This corresponds to the redefinition of knowledge or expertise, which in CPI epistemology comes from everyday lived experiences of ordinary people rather than from the ivory tower.

This redefinition of participation becomes more complex in work with children. Because of the inherent power differences between adults and children in most societies, children's views are not typically taken into account in decision making (Call-Cummings, Hauber-Özer et al., 2019; Dennis & Huf, 2016; Hart, 1992; Mayall, 2000). In research, children are seen as unreliable, so methods and analysis are tightly controlled by adult researchers (Hart, 1992). However, Hart asserts that children have a right to voice their opinions and need to learn active citizenship from an early age, which will increase both motivation for involvement and competence.

In practical terms, participation occurs along a continuum from symbolic involvement to initiation of the project and full engagement in decision making. There are various useful models of participation which represent the levels of participation as steps on a ladder: Arnstein's (1969, 2019) model for adults comes from the discipline of urban planning and community development while Hart's (1992), which is built on Arnstein's, was created for an international development context. We present them here side by side; note the similarities and differences between the levels of participation for adults and children.

Hart (1992) notes that the highest level of participation is not always necessary or appropriate, and that children might choose different levels of involvement. We have found this to be true with participants and co-researchers of all ages, as we recognize the need to respect that everyone has other interests, priorities, and responsibilities. Participation might also look different depending on the circumstances. For example, refugees working in a factory in Turkey without work permits might choose not to present their findings about unsafe working conditions to local government due to potential repercussions and might instead ask a university-based researcher to do so on their behalf. At the same time, we want to underscore that many people who have been routinely excluded from knowledge creation processes, have had their own knowledges extracted, colonized, or erased, or have been treated as less than, may choose a form of nonparticipation out of habit. Recognizing and addressing this is tricky and can only be understood through respectful, relational dialogue. This is why building relationships of trust is so important, and we will get into that in a later chapter. For now, the important thing is that participants, or co-researchers, should be the ones to determine their level of responsibility and should not be shut out of or tokenistically included in decision making (Box 2.3).

BOX 2.3: CLARIFYING LEVELS OF PARTICIPATION

In order to clarify the different levels of participation, here we offer a few scenarios for you to consider. Read each scenario and assign the corresponding number from Table 2.1. After you have assigned a number, think about how you might adjust the scenario, based on CPI epistemology, to allow for greater, more equitable participation. You may consider debriefing with a colleague or peer.

Scenario 1: A young adult with intellectual disabilities advocates for a work placement program through his public high school in Pennsylvania.

Scenario 2: Indigenous community members receive funding from a local nonprofit organization to create public works of art to commemorate those who "disappeared" during the Maya genocide.

Scenario 3: White parents in a gentrifying London neighborhood create an arts program and a fundraising group outside of the school-supported parent–teacher association.

Scenario 4: Black Lives Matter activists get police arrested and charged with murder for killing unarmed Black people.

Scenario 5: Community members organize in partnership with local university professors in Kampala, Uganda, to create a faith-based nonprofit organization to address unmet healthcare and educational needs for orphaned children, get funding, and establish a successful health center and private school.

Scenario 6: A local hospital conducts focus groups with former cancer patients and their family members to better understand patient care.

Negotiating participation is by no means easy. In reflecting on a recent school-based photovoice project with middle school English language learners that we assisted with, Meagan and Melissa realized that the university-based team running the project had not asked the youth for their input on the focus of the study (see Call-Cummings, Hauber-Özer et al., 2019, 2020). We also encountered tensions throughout the project because of the mismatch between our epistemological commitments to sharing power and the hierarchical structures and curricular requirements of the school, to which the project conformed to a certain degree. CPI should challenge, not acquiesce to, power structures that govern schooling, but is it ethical to encourage children—some of whom were undocumented immigrants—to speak out? To push a teacher to veer from the state-mandated learning outcomes? We will examine ethics as an ongoing practice in Chapter 3, but you can see that this relates to the basic building blocks of CPI.

REFLEXIVITY QUESTION

When might different approaches to participation be appropriate? What are some reasons that high levels of involvement might not be ideal or practical in a given situation?

Shared Ownership

We have seen firsthand how participation has been coopted in the international aid and development industry. The term *participation* is often used, but critiques have emerged that little time and few resources are actually devoted to it—even though communities often see it as a necessary component for a development project (Anderson et al., 2012). Without sufficient time or proper resourcing, though, it is easy to see how the term simply becomes a way for institutions to appear like they are doing the hard work of learning and creating new knowledge *with* communities. However, it cannot really be seen as authentic participation (Fals-Borda, 1991) if we are simply writing about participatory projects in funding proposals and assuming that community members will flock to join our sponsored project when we arrive without ever having met us or heard about our plans. This process needs to take into account the realities of local situations and power structures in communities and those brought in by nongovernmental organizations, official state actors, university research teams, and other outside entities.

We also need to think about the negative implications that participation can bring, such as the time it can take away from community members earning a livelihood (or that they may need to work in addition to their normal hours). This is a particular concern if they are not compensated for their role in participatory projects. Additionally, there are ethical considerations as we think about practical engagement, such as *who* to involve from the community and *how* throughout the participatory inquiry process, from recruitment and selection to data collection and analysis. And, to further complicate this, we need to consider the assumption that participation leads to authentic understanding of community concerns and demands. For example, in a review of women's participation in development projects around the world, Cornwall (2003) shows how "voice" does not necessarily translate to influence when decisions are made by male community leaders. For participation to occur, researchers must share ownership and control over each step of the process with those traditionally positioned as objects of research. This democratic, dialogical inquiry practice comprises community members identifying an area of concern, developing research questions, designing data collection methods, analyzing data, and deciding on how, where, and with whom to share findings (Cahill, 2007; Kilroy, 2011; Pittaway et al., 2010). That is to say, this process happens *with* community members, not *for* them (Freire, 1970). This requires long-term engagement in the community, understanding of local conditions, trust building, numerous formal and informal meetings with co-researchers, ongoing negotiation of goals, research design, and procedures, and discussion of findings (Dodson & Schmalzbauer, 2005; Kilroy, 2011). As an example, Wagaman and Sanchez (2017) speak to their experiences working with lesbian, gay, bisexual, transgender, and queer-identifying young adults, and how sharing ownership and control is not only a negotiation of power but also requires co-researchers to share the burden of vulnerability as they navigate the CPI process. Community members are equal partners—co-researchers—in this inquiry process with university-based researchers or practitioners.

In our own CPI experiences, we have seen how this type of engagement, or partnership, looks different in various contexts and with various people. Also, participation may look different at different times. For example, recall from the introduction that Meagan was a co-researcher on a CPI project with high school students and their teacher in a racially, ethnically, and socioeconomically diverse suburban area outside of Washington D.C. For the first year of their work together, the research team held formal meetings inside the students' school every week. Time was allotted for various projects, and in between meetings, Meagan and the teacher co-researcher would correspond via email. In the second year of the project, the group had developed stronger relationships, so conversations and planning started happening between meetings and in much more informal ways. The research collective created a group chat to be able to carry on conversations on their phones and in ways that were much more authentic for the student co-researchers involved. In addition, a few of the students that had been leaders in the collective took on fewer research responsibilities because they had other work and school commitments. Other students took more visible leadership roles and began making data collection and analysis decisions. This simple example shows that as group dynamics and needs evolve, so will levels, types, and modes of participation (Box 2.4).

BOX 2.4: ANALYZING PARTICIPATION

Choose one of the case studies in the Appendix and consider the following questions:

1. How were the research focus and questions chosen?
2. Who designed the data collection methods? Who carried them out?
3. Who analyzed the data and how?
4. Who decided how findings would be shared? Whose name was included on any resulting publications?

Let's pause here to consider a crucial point: Who knows more about a local issue? A person who comes from the outside to study it, or a person who has a lifetime of experience with it? The person who has lived and breathed this issue their whole life might take it for granted, or think it is normal or even useful. It takes a democratic, dialogic inquiry partnership to leverage both insider and outsider sets of expertise and knowledge to learn something new and transform reality into something better. With a little planning and meaningful participation, community members become co-researchers with equal power over the process and ownership of the knowledge created (Ponic et al., 2010).

For example, consider a major budget grocery chain looking for a location to build a new store in Philadelphia, Pennsylvania (U.S.). The grocery chain's needs analysis identifies a low-income residential area known as a food desert because grocery stores are few and far between, and many residents rely on corner stores, which carry mostly overpriced, shelf-stable foods full of sugar and preservatives. Management finds a commercial lot in a shopping center on a major street bordering the neighborhood and begins construction. The store stocks lots of affordable fresh fruits and vegetables, even more "exotic" items like plantains and papayas that would be in demand in this primarily Hispanic, Black Caribbean, and Southeast Asian neighborhood. After the grand opening, the store manager notices that many customers are White and that taxis start hanging around in the parking lot, picking up customers of Color with large purchases of mostly non-perishable frozen and canned foods. What's going on?

You might have guessed that the store is inaccessible by foot and public transit to local residential areas, so residents have to stock up when they can get transportation while White customers drive in from nearby lower middle-class neighborhoods to take advantage of the good prices. Buying fresh produce is not practical for local residents in this situation, and consumption habits are based largely on what has been available at corner stores. If the grocery chain's needs analysis had engaged local community participants, they likely would have recommended building the store inside the neighborhood where they could frequently stop by. They might have suggested partnering with the neighborhood's public library, adult education classes, houses of worship, and business association to create a public awareness campaign—or even hiring local residents to teach a cooking class focused on making traditional Puerto Rican, Dominican, Haitian, Palestinian, and Cambodian foods with ingredients available at the new store. The neighborhood mosque might have organized weekly carpools to the store following Friday afternoon prayers. Meaningful solutions to local problems require local expertise, but they often benefit from outside perspectives too.

Ownership is closely related to participation. Take another look at Table 2.1 and consider which levels of participation might lead to community members feeling more ownership of the project. Building trust and determining priorities with communities are essential for ownership and success of the project. For example, Kilroy (2011) traces the limited success of reintegration programs for ex-combatants in Sierra Leone to a lack of ownership in the development process. Salsberg et al. (2017) identify aspects that helped to shift ownership of a diabetes prevention project in an Indigenous community in Quebec, Canada, from university to community partners: strong leadership from both groups, "refreshing and stimulating" outside ideas, alignment of project and stakeholder goals, and trust building (p. 338). Sprague et al. (2019) assert that bidirectional trust and communication in participatory health research can lead to increased

TABLE 2.1 ■ Models of Participation

		Adults (Arnstein, 1969)	Children (Hart, 1992)
Participation	8	Citizen control: community members taking complete decision-making power over an initiative (e.g., a school or non-profit board)	Child-initiated, shared decisions with adults: adults offering insights and guidance based on children's ideas; more common among youth/ teenagers
	7	Delegated power: citizens getting dominant decision-making power over a specific issue or program, either through delegation from above or organizing and getting funding to start an initiative	Child-initiated and directed: children deciding on a project and taking action; happens commonly in play
	6	Partnership: community members taking actual decision-making power, usually due to an existing power base	Adult initiated, shared decisions with children: even though the project is conceived by adults, engaging children in making decisions; purposely including voices that may typically be ignored, like those with disabilities
	5	Placation: including community representatives on committees/boards in an advisory role with little power; powerholders still make decisions or have the majority of the votes	Consulted and informed: informing children fully about the project and genuinely consulting them for their ideas
	4	Consultation: collecting community members' views with no guarantee that they will impact decision making and little chance of meaningful change (e.g., opinion surveys, community meetings)	Assigned but informed: while adults initiated the project, ensuring that involved children understand the purpose of the project and their involvement, have a meaningful role, and willingly participate
Nonparticipation	3	Informing: teaching community members about their "rights, responsibilities, and options" (p. 27), often later in the process and without opportunities for feedback or negotiation (e.g., informational meetings, pamphlets)	Tokenism: including children in surface way without a choice of subject or style; assuming them to represent other children's opinions
	2	Therapy: attempting to "cure" community members of their problems by imposing majority values instead of changing oppressive conditions	Decoration: using children to support a cause without claiming participation (e.g., photos in fundraising materials)
	1	Manipulation: inviting community members as representatives on committees/boards to get their support or "educate" them; presenting the illusion of participation as a PR strategy	Manipulation: inviting children to represent a cause without truly understanding it or their ability to understand being recognized; children being consulted but not given feedback or included in discussion/analysis of their ideas

ownership of interventions, improved programming, and reduced marginalization of individuals with stigmatized health conditions such as HIV.

REFLEXIVITY QUESTION

Think about experiences you have had in your own life. How have you seen insiders and outsiders, or community members and outside experts, partner in an equitable, respectful way, to share ownership of a knowledge creation process?

Ownership of an inquiry process is closely tied to decision making. As we have described, this starts with lived experience. Internal and external change agents (Fals-Borda, 1987) engage in mutual education: in other words, community members and researchers learn from each other about the issue of concern and possibilities for transformation (Lind, 2008; Mirra & Rogers, 2016; Ochocka et al., 2010). Consider what would have gone differently in the budget grocery store example if the business would have first taken the time for mutual education.

Humility

In PAR, CBPR, and AR literature, we have seen that community members are often afforded the opportunity to participate in designing and carrying out data collection, drawing on their intimate knowledge of the context and issues being investigated and their networks. It is less common, but we argue crucial, for community co-researchers to have a meaningful role in analyzing data, developing findings, and sharing research. Often, this is because analysis is seen as a highly technical or specialized skill reserved for those who have been trained "properly." This view is in total and complete contrast to CPI's epistemological stance that experience is expertise. It is our view that everyone conducts data analysis everyday—whether we call it analysis or not. We are constantly making meaning out of our experiences. As we open our eyes in the morning (or whenever we wake up given our varied circumstances), we cast our eyes around the room, perhaps listening for sounds to indicate who else is awake, who has already gone to work, who has left for school, and what children are doing. We instantly make decisions for our own actions based on the analysis we have just conducted. Reserving the right to conduct data analysis for those who have some particular certification is to give in to—or uphold and reproduce—power dynamics that are both deeply entrenched and highly inequitable and unjust.

At the same time, we hesitate to teach analysis methods to community members to impart a kind of community certification to these co-researchers. This common approach is anchored in what Freire (1970) described as the banking model of education, whereby supposed knowers or experts deposit knowledge into non-experts, or community members, as if they are empty vessels, void of any useful knowledge. This type of practice runs the risk of reproducing an ontology and epistemology that deems a certain type of knowledge as superior and experiential knowledge as less valuable or valid. That said, balancing divergent knowledges and sets of expertise can be tricky and requires careful thought. Fine and Torre (2004) make a good point in this regard: "As political theorist Nancy Fraser (1990) would argue, we believe it is disingenuous to invite co-researchers to the table without equipping them (and us) with shared skills, knowledge and language for full participation" (p. 19).

We would suggest that as you consider how you might approach this balance, you rely heavily on the "and us" in Fine and Torre's point above; that is, that not only are "we" equipping "them" with requisite skills, knowledge, and language, but "they" are also equipping "us" so that we can better understand contextual factors as well as the ways in which they already engage in inquiry on a daily basis. At the same time, we urge you to remain vigilant and guard against any practices that instantiate an "us" and "them" mentality. The goal is to *share* ownership, *share* knowledge, *share* practices. To move toward a collaborative, collective "we" (Call-Cummings & Dennis, 2019). With all that said, when you review literature that claims a critical, participatory stance, we strongly encourage you not to take practices at face value. Really examine how a claimed CPI approach is being wielded. All too often we know that just because an author lays claim to one epistemology or another does not mean they (or we) actually live up to it.

We will offer a few examples to help clarify how critical participatory inquirers can live up to a CPI epistemology throughout the inquiry process. One of our favorite examples is from Dodson and Schmalzbauer (2005), who engaged community members who had not taken part in data collection in a series of collaborative co-analysis focus groups. This process did not seek to confirm the accuracy of data, as in typical member checking procedures, but to interpret it based on community members' intimate knowledge of the context and conditions. Another example comes from Pittaway et al. (2010), who describe their reciprocal approach to research that is responsive to participants' priorities and needs at each stage, for example, providing training so refugee women could document human rights abuses and advocate for increased protection. In this approach, the participants made most decisions about how to share the findings, which can reduce researchers' "outputs" but increase participant ownership (Pittaway et al., 2010). In another example, Gibbs et al. (2018) describe a large, multisite study examining the psychosocial impacts of bushfires in Victoria, Australia. The authors describe making repeated visits to each site to meet with community members and incorporating their comments and suggestions into the study design, research questions, survey contents, recruitment methods, analysis, and sharing findings. They note that while this multisite design precluded each community's control over the process, it enabled researchers to build trust and gain deeper insights.

Dialogue

As you can see, practitioners of CPI will not always do everything perfectly. That is, while we are experts in one way, we are likely not experts in every way. We may be awkward in our interactions. We may unintentionally create misunderstandings. We may make decisions only to realize that we should have included community members in the process. We will make mistakes; there is no way around it. But if we can anchor our CPI work in trust, openness, and dialogue, we will avoid many of the pitfalls that often beset us. This requires ongoing negotiation of collaborative relationships through humble dialogue. Note: the goal of such dialogue may not always be consensus. There may very well be disagreement and even conflict. In fact, disagreement and conflict, in many instances, may signal strong, democratic participation. The goal of inquiry-oriented dialogue is not to minimize disagreement or discomfort, rather, it should be mutual education and understanding. I can understand you, your perspectives, and your experiences, even if or when I do not agree with you.

In one of Meagan's CPI projects, she worked with several of her extended family members to grapple with their own whiteness and their responsibilities as White women in the context of racial injustice in the United States. During a virtual discussion, one of her co-researcher family members indicated she wanted to be able to stand up in a nonconfrontational way to her neighbors who may say racist things or act in racist ways in passing. Meagan suggested that she engage by offering simple, humble counter-experiences: "You might say something like, 'Huh. Interesting. That hasn't been my experience.' Or 'I've never experienced it that way. Can you tell me more about your experience?'" This type of response encourages dialogue, communicates humility, and seeks for greater understanding. The goal of CPI is to facilitate the humble, open, democratic, dialogic communication and action most of us hope for in our everyday experiences and interactions.

The Goal or Outcome

When we think about forms of CPI, like participatory action research, we often hear students ask about the type of action or impact that their research will result in. When we think about impact, of course, we tend to think at the highest levels. This does not mean your CPI project needs to result in some type of sweeping policy reform. The goal or outcome of each CPI project will differ, based on what co-researchers need and what they determine to be important. That said, it is important to talk about the goals of a project with all those involved. As you think reflexively about your own CPI project, here are a few questions to ask about the type of outcomes that might be of interest: Are co-researchers interested in some type of *personal* transformation, like being able to critically examine their own situations? Do co-researchers want to see a *social* transformation, like changing a discriminatory practice at a social service organization in their neighborhood? These questions bring up potential forms of action or impact, but each CPI project will differ when it comes to the particular kind of personal or social transformation.

Transformation is an important topic when it comes to CPI, but there is a lot in the scholarly literature where researchers assume that those engaged will be transformed or empowered. This is understandable, though, as the foundational works call for this type of inquiry to do just that: transform or empower (Fals-Borda, 1987; Fals-Borda & Rahman, 1991; Freire, 1972). Consider *personal* transformation: critically examining one's situation. This is not typically the type of outcome that a participant may think about because it does not feel very tangible. However, we have seen through our own CPI projects that it is actually the most likely kind of transformation to take place and is often highly valued by research collectives and co-researchers. Being able to reflect and critically understand one's own social situation—for example, understanding an incidence of racism, or breaking down why a certain policy is discriminatory and how it affects you—is a type of change or action. As Freire (1970) notes, participants must first "unveil the world of oppression and through praxis commit themselves to its transformation" (p. 54). We will talk more about this concept of praxis in Chapter 3, but at this moment, just remember that it is a cyclical process of reflection and action.

Moving from the *personal*, consider *social* transformation: changing a discriminatory practice or policy. How can a CPI project work toward other forms of change, even through advocacy or direct action? As Fine and Torre (2004) have demonstrated in their CPI project with women in prison, they have undertaken "policy-in-practice" analyses with co-researchers to dissect how certain social policies (e.g., parole practices, housing policies) affect who is imprisoned and how for long. In this project, the group not only produced reports but also met with government officials and collaborated with community-based organizations to conduct advocacy. Policy change—such as reforming the prison system in the United States—would, of course, take years and is not something one CPI project could accomplish, although it can be a contributing force. In other circumstances, policy changes can be tied directly to a CPI project's goals. Take, for instance, the example mentioned in Chapter 1, where Arstein-Kerslake et al. (2019) were able to show the Australian Government that community legal centers were far more effective than courts when it came to ensuring that individuals with cognitive disabilities were properly assessed as being legally fit to stand trial.

As you can see, transformation can take many forms in a CPI project, but when it comes to pushing for action, we need to recall the role of the animator. In a CPI project, this requires internal and external animators (Fals Borda, 1991). Those internal to a particular struggle will bring their own knowledge and methods as well as expertise gained from living through experiences, practices, and policies, whereas others (such as academics and practitioners) may bring other types of knowledge, methods, and experiences. As we have discussed before, in order to be successful, the responsible inquirer needs to value all forms of knowledge and understand that *commitment* is another basic ingredient.

That said, transformation can often be seen as a loaded term in CPI. If you are conducting CPI, many scholars will ask what type of action you are seeking to create, or they just may assume that you and your co-researchers are experiencing high levels of cognitive transformation or critical consciousness. However, rather than seeing transformation as a given, we need to think about *what* action means and *how* it is achieved. When we assume it will happen, we run the risk of tokenizing co-researchers as marginalized individuals who need to be empowered.

The purpose of CPI is "investigating reality in order to transform it" (Fals Borda, 1979). The goal is to transform the conditions of participants' lives, which often occurs in indirect ways "mediated through systems of influence" and in connection with social movements (Fals-Borda, 2001; McTaggart et al., 2017). The process itself can also be personally transformative or emancipatory for all involved (Fals-Borda, 1987; Fals-Borda & Rahman, 1991; Freire, 1970). In fact, researchers often aim to effect change in "three [interconnected] things: practitioners' practices, their understandings of their practices, and the conditions in which they practice" (McTaggart et al., 2017, p. 27) through "individual and collective self-transformation" (p. 28).

Individual transformation can be understood as the conscientization process that Freire (1970) described, developing critical consciousness of oppression and inequity through collectively investigating shared personal concerns (Cahill, 2007). In other words, investigating personal experiences and contexts can lead to awareness of how marginalized communities are perceived, represented, and exploited by outsiders (Cahill, 2007; Freire, 1970). This, in turn, can help individuals envision different pathways for themselves. Reflecting on her dissertation project with young women of Color in New York City, Cahill (2007) adopts the feminist poststructuralist concept of subjectivity or "other possibilities of being in the world" (p. 269, citing Cameron & Gibson, 2005). Unlike a stable, defined notion of identity, subjectivity can be "multiple, contradictory, and in process" (Cahill, 2007, p. 269), continually shaped by experience, social and cultural practices, and, in this case, research. This echoes Freire's (1970) assertion that we are "beings in the process of *becoming*" (p. 65). As Cahill (2007) demonstrates, this process of conscientization—confronting racism, discrimination, and dehumanization—can be fueled by anger but can also have a therapeutic quality as a way to make sense of experience and redefine oneself.

Returning for a moment to Meagan's CPI project, we can see how this process of becoming—or conscientization—can sometimes play out for mutual understanding. Meagan invited her extended family members who identified as women to participate with her in a dialogue group that would be focused on race and anti-racism. Their idea was to dig into the history of structural, institutional, and interpersonal racism in the United States and talk through their responsibilities as White women in social movements for racial justice. After their first meeting, which turned out to be a difficult, awkward, and uncomfortable conversation about the roots of racism, Meagan started to feel uneasiness in the pit of her stomach, wondering if the group was doomed because the work of growing into anti-racism was perhaps too hard. As she grappled with these thoughts, she reached out to her cousin, who shared similar life experiences and political views. Her cousin suggested that at the next meeting they start with a round of "re-introductions about who we are and why we are doing this work." At the next meeting, each person in attendance re-introduced themselves. They had assumed they knew each other—there were mothers and daughters, cousins who were best friends, sisters and sisters-in-law—but they soon realized they had been operating for years on a level of blissful ignorance and superficial understandings of the others' lived experiences. Inviting those simple re-introductions made a difference in being able to reach toward mutual understanding and education.

This simple experience can illustrate that CPI is deeply personal and almost necessitates a redefinition—or reintroduction—of oneself, to oneself. We started thinking through this concept of positionality in Chapter 1, considering questions like *Who am I?* and *Why am I here?* We would add that, perhaps after engaging oneself in a process of explicit self-re-introduction, critical participatory inquirers also find ways to enact this with co-researchers to interrupt the assumptions we make, the understandings we think we already have, and the misunderstandings we are sure to come across. Allowing each person in the inquiry collective to take their own path of becoming is a necessary and crucial component of the CPI process that is anchored in CPI's holistic, relational epistemology that puts a premium on emotional or spiritual development and interconnectedness. In addition, CPI collectives must also allow for, even invite, individual members of the group to be unsure about who they are, to be unable to articulate their reasons for participation, and to evolve and change. Remaining open to the many possibilities of being and becoming allows the process to be freeing—or emancipatory—to those involved in it.

This process is often referred to as empowerment, but this word has problematic connotations of powerless people being given power by those who have it. In addition, it takes for granted, or neglects to question, how those who supposedly have power received it in the first place (most often they or we benefitted from the oppression of those who we now seek to "empower"). In light of her CPI work, Meagan defines critical empowerment as "the process of gaining control over knowledge creation as well as the process of coming to see one's own authentically created knowledge as valuable and useful to society" (Call-Cummings, 2018, p. 400). Through CPI, participants can discover the power that they already have and use it to challenge marginalization and injustice (Call-Cummings & James, 2015). This is also true for the university-based researcher or practitioner. Kennedy (2018), for example, presents a model of personal transformation experienced by adult YPAR facilitators, moving from feeling overwhelmed to practicing critical self-reflection, releasing expectations, learning to share power with youth, establishing a collective identity, and gaining a new approach to work with youth.

Individual awareness can then propel collective transformation. That is, the personal becomes political (Cahill, 2007; citing Fine et al., 2001; hooks, 1995). This often takes the form of concrete local action to increase understanding, challenge injustice, and change conditions in the community or its institutions by and for those most directly affected. This "revolutionary" action through "countervailing power" (Fals-Borda, 1987, p. 6) can take different forms. Erel et al. (2017), for example, describe the use of participatory theater methods[2] (see Chapter 7) with low-income migrant mothers in London to articulate and develop shared understandings of their experiences with marginalization and public discourse that defines them as drains on social welfare and "threats to social and cultural cohesion" (p. 303). Through the theater workshops, the mothers developed strategies to deal with social problems, like being refused a doctor's appointment, and gained confidence for taking action in real-life situations. Another example comes from The Mestizo Arts & Activism collective in Salt Lake City, Utah (U.S.). This project demonstrates the potential of arts-based critical participatory inquiry with undocumented Latinx youth in the western United States to build solidarity, expose racialized, xenophobic social exclusion and labor exploitation, challenge public perceptions, and resist increasingly anti-immigrant rhetoric and policies (Cahill et al., 2019; Quijada Cerecer et al., 2013).

Participatory action can also take on a political dimension as it "moves from the micro to the macro level" (Fals-Borda, 1987, p. 334). External partners might, for example, link local community members to regional, national, or even international movements working on a similar issue (Fals-Borda, 1991). Thus, CPI is intended to mobilize grassroots movements for justice and equity (Fals-Borda, 1991) (Box 2.5).

BOX 2.5: MOVING FROM MICRO TO MACRO WITH KAQCHIKEL MAYA COMMUNITIES IN GUATEMALA

In his work in Guatemala, Giovanni has taken an explicit political stance, exploring the micro- and macro-level, as well as how exploitations create barriers to participation (Dazzo, 2020). For instance, at the micro-level, he found that while community members were interested and willing to participate in collaborative data collection and analysis sessions, some participants were quite unfamiliar with the idea. During lunch one day, an Indigenous co-researcher, Carmencita, stated, "When you are asked to participate, but no one has ever asked you before, you're afraid." This example highlights how inquirers must see participatory action as a philosophy at the micro-level, noting how inquiry can confront barriers to participation and self-realization, and promote empowerment through sustained dialogue. At the macro-level, he has also thought about how this work can translate to a larger scale. Through working with community members and nonprofit staff, there has been an element of activating others in the process. These animators have breathed life into the project, coordinating and conducting their own data gathering and analysis activities without his facilitation. This has been an exciting part of the work, seeing how small collaborative moments can multiply and turn into a larger movement. However, as we mentioned above, sustainability is something that needs to be fostered rather than assumed.

Despite its perceived potential for transformation, CPI is not a panacea to the pitfalls of traditional research. Particularly in hierarchical, institutional settings like schools, hospitals, multinational organizations, and governments, CPI requires "explicit, collaborative, critical, and continuous exploration of power dynamics and relationships" (Call-Cummings, Dennis et al., 2019, p. 410). In addition to not being a panacea, it is also, in our experience, not a choice. Rather, it is a way of life that is rooted in our convictions and is connected to who we are and who we want to be. As Fals-Borda and Rahman (1991) remind us "at this challenging moment that a rather permanent existential choice is made when one decides to live and work with PAR" (p. 29). This is not a blueprint for research but a way of life, "an ethical stand," and a persistent commitment toward the "an overall, structural transformation of society and culture" (Fals-Borda & Rahman, 1991, p. 29).

CRITIQUES OF CPI

While we are committed to a critical, participatory inquiry stance, we do want to acknowledge that CPI is not without critique. Because CPI by design engages marginalized and oppressed people in documenting and transforming the conditions of oppression, it carries significant risks for these participants. In such situations, researchers' goals of leveling power relationships with participants may conflict with their ethical and moral obligation to protect vulnerable populations (Call-Cummings et al., 2020). In addition, we are also aware that asking people who have been pushed to the margins of society to take ownership of a process that works toward the dismantling of that oppression is patently unfair. We are hopeful that as you learn more about CPI you will work against this possibility and engage both those who experience oppression as well as those who perpetrate it in the transformation process. We often fall into both roles simultaneously. Remaining cognizant of our ever-evolving positionalities can help us maintain a reflexive stance and push back on this possibility.

In addition, we also note a potential for CPI to expose already vulnerable individuals and groups to greater risk, whether physical, emotional, or psychological. For example, in their work with "poor mothers," Dodson and Schmalzbauer (2005) address logistical and ethical complications of participatory inquiry with marginalized people, particularly the role of silence as a strategy for coping with unjust authority. They note the difficulty of "seeking to build knowledge with people who live the conditions under study without disrupting their ways of protecting themselves and their families" (p. 952). Melissa's dissertation (Box 2.1) is another example of taking structural constraints into consideration in work with marginalized participants.

Visual participatory methods such as photovoice (Wang & Burris, 1997; see Chapter 7 in this volume) and digital storytelling (Greene et al., 2018; Gubrium et al., 2014) are often touted as empowering because of their potential to facilitate expression/voice and self-representation (e.g., Guerrero & Tinkler, 2010; Harper, 2016, 2017; Marquez-Zenkov et al., 2007; Wang & Burris, 1994), but they also present ethical dilemmas about privacy and confidentiality (Burles & Thomas, 2014; Hannes & Parylo, 2014; Hauber-Özer & Call-Cummings, 2020; Teti, 2019; Wang & Redwood-Jones, 2001). This is particularly true for marginalized groups; for example, breach of confidentiality in CPI with undocumented migrants or refugees could lead to deportation (Pittaway et al., 2010; Sahay et al., 2016; Tuck & Del Vecchio, 2018).

There are also concerns around the tensions and difficulties of sharing power in research with children, especially children of Color who are already experiencing complex and layered oppressions (Call-Cummings et al., 2020). Particularly in contexts like schools, where hierarchy is rigid and power dynamics often unquestioned, we have seen a greater need for reflexivity as we negotiate roles (Call-Cummings, 2017). Take, for example, Meagan's experience during her dissertation work. She was engaging in CPI with a group of undocumented Latinx high school students in rural USA. They had clearly articulated to Meagan the ways in which they experienced oppression through practices of silencing at their school and within their local community through formal policies and informal practices. They did not feel comfortable conducting one-on-one interviews with their White teachers or school administrators, so they asked Meagan to do those interviews because she was less vulnerable to risk than they were. Of course, this choice did not fix the vulnerabilities they felt. As they displayed pictures and accompanying narratives of their lives in their school library, they were exposed to the reactions of other students, teachers, community members, and policymakers. They could have experienced increased levels of bullying, greater disciplinary actions, or other subtler responses to their self-exposure. It is of vital concern to remain aware of and be open about how CPI can expose those who are already vulnerable.

CONCLUSION

In this chapter, we have provided numerous examples of what CPI is and how it can take shape in varied contexts. We have emphasized how everyone involved in CPI should seek to share ownership and responsibility in the process, and we have also offered a few words of caution related to the potential for CPI to re-oppress and expose those who are already vulnerable.

In 1991, Fals-Borda and Rahman urged scholars, practitioners, educators, and activists to recognize the ongoing and even increased need for PAR compared to its emergence in 1970. As they stated, "the world is still passing through the same era of confusion and conflict in which PAR was born" (p. 30). Half a century after the approach developed in the slums of Brazil, we are experiencing a dizzying level of conflict, violence, displacement, division, and suffering and a widening gap between the powerful and the oppressed. We urge you to commit to this way of life and to seek out your roles in advancing the people's knowledge for liberation and transformation.

RECOMMENDED PRACTICE 2.1: ANIMATORS AND SUSTAINABILITY

Think back to Tilakaratna's (1991) description of sustainability and the four interrelated factors:

(1) the emergence of a group of internal animators, (2) practice of self-review by people's organizations, (3) the ability to move from micro groups to larger groupings, and finally (4) an expansion of the action agenda to move toward a total/comprehensive development effort. Think about these interrelated factors in relation to your own CPI project. Consider these questions (and consult co-researchers if your collective is already established): Who are internal animators and how might they emerge? How could you and your co-researchers enact the practice of self-review? How would your collective move from micro to macro groupings? How might your agenda for action adapt or expand? Write out your responses or create a conceptual map that plots out these actors and factors. Considering these from the beginning provides an opportunity to think through sustainability and how your engagement and partnerships can move toward this goal.

SUMMARY OF KEY POINTS

- Rather than a research method or methodology, CPI is an epistemology or stance toward knowledge and knowledge creation that guides choices about research procedures and goals.
- This epistemology values the experiences of ordinary and marginalized people as expertise, which contrasts with dominant ideas about research and higher education.
- CPI involves internal and external agents of change who work together to produce an accurate picture of the issue of concern and to work for change. This often requires negotiation of roles and power relations between people with very different backgrounds and experiences.
- Participation can be seen along a spectrum from manipulative or tokenistic inclusion of community members to full decision-making power and leadership.
- Genuinely sharing ownership with community members throughout the inquiry process is crucial but difficult, requiring long-term engagement, understanding of the local context, trust building, and ongoing discussion.
- CPI's transformative goal can take many forms, from increased personal awareness to social and political change.

- There are many important critiques of CPI, including the potential to expose participants to risk and tensions related to institutional and interpersonal power relations, which require careful consideration.

SUGGESTED ACTIVITIES

1. Journal about the idea of expertise. What do you have expertise about, and how did you gain that knowledge (experience, formal education, informal learning from a family member, etc.)? How have your ideas about expertise started to change, if at all, after reading this chapter?
2. Think of a problem in your community that would not typically be a subject for traditional research (like the scenarios above). Brainstorm how you might approach documenting and trying to solve it using CPI. Which internal and external agents of change might be involved? What challenges (e.g., roles, ethical dilemmas, structural constraints) might you face along the way? What kind of information would you gather? What steps might you take to try to develop and implement solutions?
3. In a pair or small group, choose a current or recent activist movement (e.g., racial justice, women's reproductive rights, or climate change) and analyze the approach taken. In what ways does it resemble CPI? Where would it fall on the ladder of participation? Does the affected population seem to have ownership of the process, or is participation tokenistic or even manipulative? How are roles and decisions negotiated? How could a CPI approach be beneficial? Present your ideas to the class and gather their feedback.

KEY TERMS

animators
dialogical
method
methodology

ENDNOTES

1. https://idea.gseis.ucla.edu/projects/the-council-of-youth-research
2. You can watch sample scenes from this project at http://www.open.ac.uk/socialsciences/migrant-mothers/participatory-theatre/

3 ETHICS AND VALIDITY IN PARTICIPATORY INQUIRY

LEARNING OBJECTIVES

By the end of this chapter, you will better understand

- The intersections between ethics and validity in the context of CPI.
- The core concepts of praxis, objectivity, subjectivity, bias, and access and how they play a major role in CPI.
- What theories and philosophies anchor CPI's conceptualization of validity.

FOCUS ACTIVITY 3.1: WHAT IS VALID AND ETHICAL RESEARCH?

Grappling with intersecting theories and philosophies can be difficult. As we discuss questions of ethics and validity in this chapter, some reflection at the outset will be useful. Take a moment to talk through these questions with a friend or colleague, or record any thoughts you have in a research journal:

1. Forgetting for a moment the lists and theories you have been taught, what makes research "good"?
2. Think back to the earliest memory you have of thinking something (perhaps an argument or an opinion) was "valid." At the time, what did that mean to you?
3. Think back to a moment in which you thought someone or something was *un*ethical. Why did you think so? What could have changed your thinking?
4. Have you ever had the experience of thinking one thing about a person—or their work—and then, after you got to know them better, your opinion changed? Think about that (typical) experience in relation to research. Might it be possible for research to be made better—more valid—the more we know our participants, our research sites, and the communities with whom we work? Consider this as you move into this chapter.

BOX 3.1: A NOTE ON WHY WE USE THE TERM *VALIDITY*

Within qualitative methodology, it is important to recognize that some find the word *validity* to be off-putting. This is due to some associating the term with traditional forms of research (i.e., [post]positivist orientations), which was seen to perpetuate violence and harm on minoritized and racialized communities (e.g., the Tuskegee Syphilis Study). In some cases, qualitative researchers have instead chosen to utilize words such as quality and trustworthiness (Lincoln & Guba, 1985). For instance, Lincoln & Guba (1985) offer four criteria for trustworthiness: credibility (i.e., confidence in whether findings are congruent with reality or truth, broadly defined), transferability (i.e., whether lessons can be applied somewhere else), dependability (i.e., demonstrating that findings are consistent, often through peer review and feedback), and confirmability (i.e., ensuring the researcher attends to their biases, often approached by checking interpretations with participants and utilizing multiple methods, data sources, and checks). We encourage readers to explore these terms so they can make an informed decision in their own work. However, while these criteria can be helpful, we argue that it is not the term validity that has perpetuated harm and violence, but the individuals who have conducted research. This is not solely a question of (post)positivist or quantitative researchers subjecting communities to harm and violence, but one where qualitative and critical theorists can do so through the use of conceptual frameworks (e.g., grit, color blindness) and biases (e.g., neoliberalism, institutional racism). Just as Tuhiwai Smith (2012) details how the "collective memory of imperialism has been perpetuated through the ways in which knowledge about indigenous peoples was collected" (p. 1), she also speaks of the necessity to establish the "validity of Māori knowledge" (p. 172). This latter point is made to establish Māori knowledge as legitimate when presented against the work of non-Indigenous researchers and government policies. As we use the term *validity* throughout this chapter and this book, we see it as a form of "talking back" to or "daring to disagree" (hooks, 1999) with what is seen as the authoritative figure of (post)positivist interpretations of validity observed in both quantitative and qualitative research. For these reasons, we believe that validity is a term that should be taken back for the benefit of the entire research enterprise. It should be considered according to the quantitative or qualitative methods and approaches that the researcher uses rather than being co-opted by or attached to one epistemological or methodological tradition.

As we were writing the outline for this book, we had a number of discussions on how exactly the concepts and practices surrounding ethics and validity should be presented in our chapters. In many of the methodology textbooks that we have reviewed or used, we noticed that validity frameworks are often addressed first; then, in a shorter subsection within a chapter on research design (usually at the end), there are a few paragraphs on ethical issues. The word *issues* is often attached to ethics, connoting the negative implications that could occur if not adhered to by the researcher, rather than any positive implication that could benefit participants of the study. As you reviewed the table of contents or opened your book to this chapter, you likely noticed that we felt that ethics and validity could not be presented separately. We also did not want to include a chapter that privileged this notion that the researcher should first think about validity and only consider ethics after they have understood whether their study follows the usual frameworks for quality, credibility, and trustworthiness (Lincoln & Guba, 1985).

From our stance on critical participatory inquiry, ethics and validity cannot be viewed or practiced as two distinct concepts. We believe that each topic is so mired in the other that it would be a disservice to our research—and the communities with whom we work—to ever think of them as separate. This may be an odd pairing as many scholars and practitioners will devise separate lectures, modules, or chapters on ethics and validity. In combining these topics, however, we do not want to diminish the importance of one or the other. Rather, we emphasize that to be seen as valid, critical participatory inquiry must be relational, and as relationships require respectful human interaction, ethics must be constantly considered and ingrained within our practice.

In addition, we want to note that while this chapter may at first glance appear theoretically dense, that is the opposite of our intention. Instead, we hope to sift through the many theoretical debates around validity to present clear articulations of how critical participatory inquiry can and should be practiced—by academic researchers, practitioners across disciplines, organizational leaders, activists, and all others. Our goal is to carefully reflect on and, frankly, disassemble the mechanisms most often used to establish validity in order to illustrate how critical participatory inquiry relies on ethics and ethical decisions to be counted as valid.

DIFFICULTY OF SEPARATING ETHICS AND VALIDITY IN PARTICIPATORY INQUIRY

For the critical participatory inquirer, options abound regarding guidelines for validity (Kemmis & McTaggart, 2005; Lincoln & Guba, 1985; Lincoln et al., 2011). To start, most researchers are introduced to concepts of validity in their introductory research methods courses, which often focus heavily on statistical concepts. From this perspective, researchers begin to associate validity with quantitative measurement or with terms such as *construct validity* (Cronbach & Meehl, 1955), which values the degree that evidence supports an argument and its intended purpose (Messick, 1995). If we are to think about validity for the purpose of critical participatory inquiry, however, the researcher needs to discard the idea that validity is synonymous with statistics.

See the note within Box 3.1 at the beginning of this chapter. We recognize that the term *validity* is contested across methodological and epistemological orientations, especially in the context of critical inquiry. Because of this and the reasons outlined in Box 3.1, we dig back into the etymology of the terms *validity* and *ethics* in order to understand the history of these words and contextualize how the two cannot be separated if one is to truly practice critical participatory inquiry. Consider the key points below, which might clarify why we chose to meld validity and ethics and to start with the roots of these terms.

Key Considerations for Melding Ethics and Validity for Critical Participatory Inquiry

- *Knowledge democracy*: By questioning and understanding the history behind language and societal practices (including research), the critical participatory inquirer can increase the likelihood that a project is valid and ethical according to various knowledge systems and cultures (de Sousa Santos, 2008; Fricker, 2007; Hall & Tandon, 2017).

- *Humility in practice*: In becoming students of the communities they seek to work alongside, the critical participatory inquirer can note how their epistemology (ways of knowing), ontology (reality or how we consider truth), axiology (values and ethics), and methodologies (approaches and methods) converge or diverge with what communities may consider valid and ethical. In this section, we recognize conceptualizations of humility as a prominent feature across decolonizing methodologies (Gaztambide-Fernández, 2012; Tuhiwai Smith, 2012) and critical race theory (Bell, 1987; Collins, 2010).
- *Questioning oppressive systems*: As we explore the history and philosophy of science and the terminology we use, we can come to understand how research has maintained a limited understanding of objectivity, validity, and institutional ethics, which have preserved systems of oppression. As noted by Indigenous scholars, these systems have not only stolen land, life, and labor but also knowledge, without much benefit to the communities involved in research (Chilisa, 2012; Kovach, 2009; Tuck & Yang, 2012).

We briefly explored the etymology of the research terms we are socialized to accept and how our interpretations of these terms may deviate from their original connotations. To start, validity derives from the Latin term *validus*, meaning strong. As previously mentioned, researchers are often taught to think about validity by defaulting to notions of whether they are measuring what they initially intended to measure. Unfortunately, this socialization inhibits thinking more broadly about how *strong* our interpretations may be, not only from our own viewpoints but also from the those of communities who hold different knowledge systems or definitions of validity.

In addition to the limited interpretation of how researchers understand the word *validity*, we also see this in how the word *ethics* is applied in research. Ethics originates from the Greek *ethos*, meaning how a community's values and beliefs are manifested through its culture, moral character, or nature. Yet some may conflate the term with the technocratic process of applying for and obtaining approval from an institutional review board (IRB), which is tasked with reviewing research protocols to ensure that the rights of human subjects are protected. However, the question "Is your research ethical?" is not synonymous with "Did you obtain IRB approval?" In this chapter, we will explore various conceptualizations of ethics, from procedural elements such as an IRB and micro-ethics or ethics in practice, which relate to the quandaries that arise during personal interactions and practical research considerations (Guillemin & Gillam, 2004). In addition to procedural and micro-ethics, we question why ethics—if we are to understand the word from its root—are generally only considered from the value and belief systems that the researcher's community holds, rather than the value and belief systems of where the research is being conducted. In this case, let's think about an example that spans procedural and micro-ethics: If you, as the critical participatory inquirer, are conducting research with Aboriginal researchers in Australia, have you considered what the community would consider valid and ethical inquiry? Or have you only approached validity and ethics from the perspective of the IRB and other Eurocentric ideas of research? For some, these concepts and questions may be familiar, while for others, they may seem radical. That said, although the term *radical* is generally associated with words such as *revolutionary* or *progressive*, in reality, it refers to the root of something (from the Latin term *radix*). Given this definition, we start our discussion by considering what it means to think about the radical (or root) nature of valid (or strong) and ethical (or moral) inquiry.

Moving from theory to practice, we want to pose a few questions to spur your thinking about ethics and validity in critical participatory inquiry. As you continue through this chapter, consider *how* you will take up ethics and validity in your own research projects. As an exercise, we have included a few questions (see Box 3.2) that we think about when we conduct our own projects. The questions provide an opportunity to reflect on ethics and validity before you start your own research. Since participatory inquiry requires flexibility (because you are making decisions with others), it also requires you to consider these questions as you work through the process. These questions can be useful reminders of how ethics and validity are intertwined within critical participatory inquiry.

BOX 3.2: REFLEXIVE QUESTIONS SURROUNDING VALIDITY AND ETHICS IN PRACTICE

- Did the research project improve relationships, dialogue, or critical consciousness?
- Did it lead to the outcomes that community members sought to achieve?
- Will communities feel that the project is transformative?
- If I entered a community, did its members feel that the research was worth their time?
- Did community members get as much out of the research process as I did?
- If community members did not perceive the project to be transformative or inclusive, is it no longer valid or ethical?

CONCEPTS AND DEFINITIONAL ISSUES

By looking back at the root of the terms that we learn in other research courses, it becomes clearer how some may take for granted the meanings behind these words. If we think about the context in which we use them in the modern research enterprise, you can also see where history diverges with our current understanding or practice or how these terms have been coopted to benefit a positivist or postpositivist view of research, which narrowly defines what counts as valid knowledge, accepting only observable evidence as scientific.

Praxis

Before we get too far into these concepts of validity, we approach the question of research from the conceptual and definitional views of ethics that are in line with critical participatory inquiry. In beginning with the *Nicomachean Ethics* (Aristotle, 1999), we show how

Aristotelian logic was concerned with the concept of *praxis* or how a theory or skills are practiced or embodied by an individual. According to Aristotle, in order to lead a good or moral life, an individual must first develop virtue of character (an ethical or moral nature). Through ethical practice or a moral life, it is possible to move from the theory and creation of knowledge to what Aristotle sees as a form of knowledge in action: praxis. Even from these early discussions of inquiry, this idea of praxis demonstrates the emphasis on how knowledge, in order to be valid, must be rooted in ethics and lead to action. While much of the literature on participatory research came much later, this term aids us in understanding the rationale for critical forms of participatory inquiry, especially as it has been reconceptualized and redefined by various scholars and practitioners.

Later conceptualizations of praxis emerge in the work of Marx (Simon, 1994), which were rooted in his reading of another German philosopher, Ludwig Feuerbach. As Marx proclaimed in his eleventh thesis on Feuerbach's work, "The philosophers have only interpreted the world, in various ways; the point, however, is to change it" (Simon, 1994, p. 101). This call for change featured prominently in Marx's interpretation of praxis, as he asserted that theory and action must be unified in an effort to change the world. Marx's interpretation of praxis showed the necessity of a *practical-critical activity*, in which individuals should not simply theorize about societal problems; rather, society, as a whole, needs to understand its problems and seek change from within. It was this emphasis on the practical-critical that led two Italian philosophers, Antonio Labriola (in the 19th century) and Antonio Gramsci (in the 20th century) to describe Marx's ideology as a *philosophy of praxis* (Gramsci, 1978).

This concept of a critical praxis toward transformative change, at both an individual and societal level, became a foundational characteristic of critical theory for the scholars of the Institute of Social Research at the University of Frankfurt, commonly referred to as the Frankfurt School. Through the work of Max Horkheimer and Theodor Adorno (1947/2002), the Institute's scholars established the notion of correct or true praxis, demonstrating the vital role of theory guiding action. The importance of theory in the critical theoretical equation, however, was not to reproduce the distanced observer from empiricism; rather, the Frankfurt School critical theorists were careful in illustrating "true *praxis* as a collective endeavor" (Jay, 1973, p. 64). In its earliest conceptions, the Frankfurt School scholars sought to disassociate themselves from pragmatism, which they saw as promoting action for action's sake. As you recall from Chapter 1, action research and critical participatory inquiry share a history. However, action research can generally be associated with pragmatism, whereas CPI uses critical theory as a theoretical framework. In proposing the concept of true praxis, Horkheimer and Adorno sought to show how action without theory could simply lead to the continuation of conformist thought and practices that perpetuate an oppressive status quo.

This philosophy of praxis—or an interaction where theory and action are continuously informed and refined by the other (Kincheloe et al., 2017)—is present in the work of Paulo Freire, a Brazilian educator who saw the transformative nature of critical pedagogical practices. In one of Freire's (1972) best known works, *The Pedagogy of the Oppressed*, he makes the case for a critical approach to praxis. There is an assumption that the oppressed, through the process of *conscientizaçao* (i.e., a process of critical consciousness borne out of mutual respect), will come to understand (1) their own history and place in society (i.e., self-actualization), (2) the role of power and the oppressor (i.e., mutual understanding), and (3) how to resolve systems of oppression (i.e., action, but more specifically, social transformation). The goal then becomes to engage both oppressor and oppressed in making changes to break the cycle of oppression. Influenced by the works of Marx and the Frankfurt School, Freire's conceptualization of praxis is rooted in the practice of ethics: Critical inquiry is considered valid when it creates space for reflection and dialogue and empowers the oppressed toward emancipatory action. At its core, critical participatory inquiry is relational, dialogic, and emancipatory (Fals-Borda & Rahman, 1991).

REFLEXIVITY QUESTION

What does praxis look like for your own critical participatory inquiry project?

As participatory inquiry is a social process (Kemmis & McTaggart, 2005), it is necessary to see the connection between individual and societal change, as mentioned in the works of Paulo Freire (1972) and Jürgen Habermas (1984, 1996), another Frankfurt School theorist. For instance, as an individual tries to understand their own situation and actions in an effort to change, they can then collectively work with others to more effectively understand societal situations and practices that need to be reformed. This relational cycle then continues through to collective action; we then see improved understanding and action by the individual, and so forth.

Understanding praxis can often be an abstract exercise, especially if we do not think about (1) how critical participatory inquiry is a social process and (2) the relationship between the individual and social spheres (Kemmis & McTaggart, 2005). In the reflection activity below (Box 3.3), think about how your critical participatory inquiry project could preempt change at both individual and societal levels.

BOX 3.3: REFLECTION ACTIVITY: EXPLORING PRAXIS IN CRITICAL PARTICIPATORY INQUIRY

In this activity, think about the theories and actions that would need to be explored at each individual and societal level in order to bring about transformation. For each question below, it is helpful to think about how each individual and social transformation takes place and shapes the next, as well as how it affects the entire participatory inquiry process. *Note*: Change can start anywhere in this chain; it is not necessary to start with social media.

Societal Transformation

Social media: How do power dynamics, language, and work interact to affect how people describe, work, and relate to one another?

Social structures: How do cultural, economic, and sociopolitical structures support or hinder transformation?

Social media... [change continues]

Societal Transformation

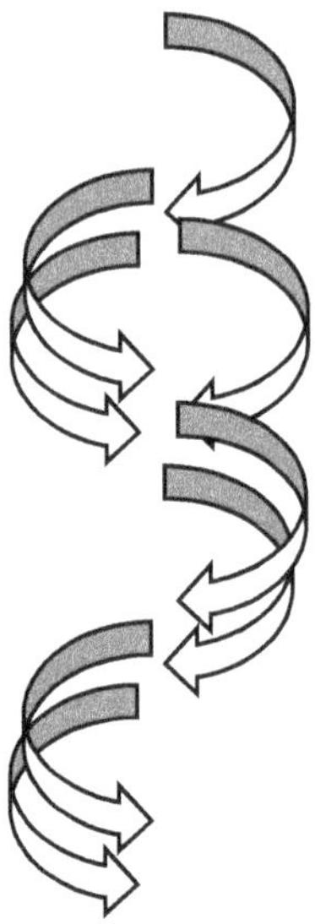

Individual Transformation

Social practices: How can individuals explore and (re)construct modes of communication, production, and social interactions so they are more rational, productive, and just?

Forms of knowledge: How can systems of knowledge, skills, and social integration be (re) constructed to produce beneficial interactions?

Social practices... [change continues]

Adapted from Kemmis & McTaggart (2005, p. 566)

Since critical participatory inquiry is a social process (Kemmis & McTaggart, 2005), students often ask whether this messy, relational, dialogic, and action-oriented process is objective. If research participants are involved in the inquiry process as co-researchers creating research questions, constructing data, and interpreting findings, is the process too subjective (and, in turn, invalid)? How do I obtain a sufficient sample size to make the research representative and arrive at the "truth" (i.e., unbiased and objective findings)? Will co-researchers just tell us what we want to hear? In this next section, we address these questions as we cover the topics of **objectivity** and subjectivity in the inquiry process.

Objectivity and Subjectivity

The previously posed questions are all relevant, but they take for granted, or make assumptions about, definitions of objectivity and subjectivity. Often, we treat objectivity as synonymous with validity or truth and subjectivity as synonymous with a lack of validity or truth: These definitions are inaccurate and misleading. Indeed, much like quantitative researchers, we also need to define what objectivity and subjectivity mean when it comes to critical participatory inquiry. Earlier in this chapter, we noted the Latin root of the word *valid*, which means strong, but what makes a strong or valid argument from a critical theoretical perspective? According to Carspecken (1996), the critical epistemology formulated by Jürgen Habermas (1984), which draws from the ontological viewpoint of pragmatist philosophers such as Dewey, Mead, Pierce, and James, shows how the concept of truth depends on whether there is cultural consensus. Locating truth within this realm of cultural understanding (i.e., whether a community agrees or reaches consensus on a certain claim) shows that critical researchers believe that what is agreed on as truth today may not be the case tomorrow. There are truth claims that can be agreed on by those who share a common culture, language, and worldview, but those truth claims may not be accepted a century later. In other words, the truth is fallible. We will briefly cover how we define objectivity and subjectivity, but for a comprehensive overview, we encourage readers to take a look at Carspecken's (1996) *Critical Ethnography in Educational Research.*

From a criticalist perspective, truth claims are assessed according to a series of **validity claims** based on human interaction, such as reaching consensus (Carspecken, 1996; Habermas, 1984). Unlike the concepts often taught in introductory research methods courses, we do not approach objectivity from the view that the researcher must be removed from or invisible in the research process. Rather, from a criticalist view, there are several types of validity claims: objective claims, subjective claims, and value claims (which include normative claims).

Bias and Access

To interpret whether a statement is based in objective, subjective, or value claims, it becomes part of our job to assess the type of **access** needed to understand the truth claim within each statement. In critical inquiry, access is an important concept because it allows us to understand researcher **bias**. Are we observing, hearing, or interpreting something based on our own understanding and what we want to find? Or are we open to exploring the knowledge, language, and cultural systems needed to understand the objective, subjective, and value claims made by others?

Before we get more into the type of access needed to understand various validity claims, let's briefly talk about bias in qualitative research. Generally speaking, we are taught about bias in introductory research or statistics courses, usually in relation to finding results that we wanted to find rather than what is there. We also learn that researchers should remove themselves as much as possible from the research process to prevent "tainting" the process or findings. However, understanding bias in this way is not possible in critical participatory inquiry because the process is relational; community engagement and dialogue are essential. Instead, when we think about bias in critical participatory inquiry (and qualitative inquiry as a whole) we address it through a process known as reflexivity. We will talk about this concept more in Chapter 4, but at this point, it is important to note that reflexivity is the "process of reflecting critically on the self as researcher" (Lincoln et al., 2011, p. 124). As inquirers, why do we need to reflect critically about ourselves? Because we bring our own views and multiple identities (i.e., from identifying with a certain ethnicity, working as instructors and researchers, associating with a particular socioeconomic group or political ideology) to the inquiry process. It is important to understand these views and identities and how they come into play as we approach the inquiry process, from whom we engage with to how we craft questions and interpret findings. Exploring our multiple identities through critical self-reflection, however, helps us see how the complexities of our own identities are involved in the inquiry process as well as in how we interpret validity claims.

When thinking about validity claims, we usually start with objectivity. Although many of the methods mentioned in this book are qualitative and subjective in nature, we include terms such as objectivity because, in some cases, communities may want to engage with quantitative methods or debates on the objectivity of their findings. This could be due to their interests in collecting quantitative data (e.g., community demographics, data on community finances) as well as utilizing these data when presenting claims to decision makers. For objective claims, which relate to concepts that are objectivist or concrete in nature (e.g., gravity), we can consider this to be a question of the world (Carspecken, 1996). Questions of the world demonstrate that many individuals have access to the knowledge, culture, and language needed to understand a concept. Take for instance this statement: "If I drop this rock, it will fall to the ground." If someone does not believe us, we can demonstrate that a rock will fall to the ground, and they can observe how it falls to the ground; thus, there are ways to observe or measure our statement. In demonstrating how the rock falls to the ground, we are negotiating consensus and moving toward sharing the same knowledge. We refer to this as having *direct access* and *multiple access*.

Unlike objective claims, which demonstrate an understanding of objectivist concepts—or *the world*—we see **subjective claims** as explaining "my world," "your world," "her world" (Carspecken, 1996). While we assessed objective statements from the idea of multiple access (the world), we assess subjective statements based on the idea of *privileged access* (my world, your world, her world). Take for example this statement: "I'm a good parent." From this statement, you can see that this statement represents an individual's reality—"their world"—rather than "the world." You would need privileged access to understand this statement, as it depends on their feelings and intentions and whether they are being honest or not. While you can agree ("They're a good parent.") or make a counterclaim to disagree ("They're not a good parent."), these statements do not necessarily validate or negate that person's feelings or intentions. So, we can see that the subjective realm is dictated by self-knowledge (i.e., what the person knows or perceives about their feelings, desires, intentions), your knowledge, (i.e., what you know about the other person), and their performance (i.e., what the person wants to present to others).

At this point, you may be questioning the subjective nature of the previous statement ("I'm a good parent."), and saying that we can, of course, determine whether someone is a good parent based on societal expectations. But expectations around what a parent should and ought to do in one society or culture may not be the same in another (there are likely similarities, though). When we start to bring in explanations of what makes something good, bad, right, or wrong, we move into our third category: value claims. Arriving at consensus on value statements is difficult as the properties of the argument are not wholly supported by multiple access or privileged access. Rather, the argument can move endlessly between objective and subjective statements made by two opposing views (two opposing individuals, political parties, etc.). In Table 3.1, we present examples of the three claims often made when attempting to understand the validity claims behind a statement. We

TABLE 3.1 ■ Assessing Validity Claims

Statement	What type of claim is this?	What type of access is needed to understand the validity behind this claim?
"If I drop this rock, it will fall to the ground."	Objective	This claim is accessible to multiple observers (*direct* and *multiple access*). Multiple individuals can see this phenomenon. If there is a disagreement, individuals can observe or measure that if I drop a rock, it will fall. We can arrive at a common definition of what qualifies as a rock, falling, and the concept of gravity.
"Barbara is frustrated because she doesn't understand the assignment."	Subjective	This claim requires us to know what Barbara is feeling, but only Barbara can honestly indicate what she is feeling (*privileged access*).
"Teachers should help all students to the best of their ability, no matter their background."	Normative (values)	*Shared* or *mutually agreed-upon values* are demonstrated in that most individuals in society agree that teachers should help all students, regardless of their backgrounds.

Adapted from Carspecken 1996, p. 62–84.

present a statement, indicate the type of claim, and then show what type of access is needed to understand that claim.

In talking about objectivity and subjectivity, we wanted to show how these two terms can be approached from the viewpoint of a criticalist. Now, return to the questions posed at the start of this section. As a quick exercise, think about how we have defined *objectivity* and *subjectivity*. Think about the type of critical participatory inquiry project that you would like to facilitate and consider how objectivity and subjectivity help or hinder the CPI process. As you think, we hope it will be helpful to see how defining objectivity and subjectivity could be understood in terms of the access needed to make sense of (or validate) the nature of the statements we are attempting to explore or understand through our inquiry. More specifically, we should not equate validity with objectivity.

ENGAGING VALIDITY FRAMEWORKS

As previously mentioned, we are often socialized to think about validity in terms of data collection and measurement: Are we using the correct instruments to measure what we want and to then infer something from it? As Messick (1989) defined it, *validity* in quantitative studies is seen as the ability to arrive at appropriate interpretations, inferences (i.e., conclusions), and actions based on the data that is collected. However, if we remove a few keywords here such as statistics and inference, we can see that there is not much difference, at face value, in what we would like to achieve through any type of inquiry, even critical participatory inquiry. From a logic standpoint, we would, of course, want to arrive at interpretations, conclusions, and actions that are based on what we have co-constructed with our community of co-researchers.

Understanding Validity: From Positivism to Critical Inquiry

To understand validity, however, it is important to learn about it from a historical perspective so we can see how others may define it and how it has become a contested term. Unlike researchers subscribing to positivism, in critical participatory inquiry, we do not dissect validity according to terms such as *internal validity* (i.e., inferring that a causal relationship exists between two variables or establishing cause and effect) or *external validity* (i.e., whether results can be generalized across populations, settings, times, and outcomes) (Campbell & Stanley, 1963; Cook & Campbell, 1979). In a positivist paradigm, it is important to understand validity from this viewpoint because it serves the aims of prediction and control. Prediction and control, in turn, serve the purpose of proving the one true reality of the phenomenon being studied and then replicating subsequent studies to ensure that the same results are obtained (Lincoln et al., 2011). In critical participatory inquiry, however, validity isn't derived from controlling variables and predicting phenomena, but from the aim of understanding communities' complex and multifaceted realities (Kilgore, 2001). Acknowledging the fluid nature of realties and democratically engaging with communities (Heron & Reason, 1997) serve the purpose of co-constructing knowledge and using it for transformative or emancipatory purposes. Examples of this can be seen across field and disciplines, including teacher research in education, a form of action research where teachers conduct inquiry, based on their learned and tacit knowledges, to transform their teaching practices and improve classroom environments and students' progress (Cochran-Smith & Lytle, 1990); and community-engaged research in health settings, which privileges multiple perspectives to ensure that clinical research and the associated interventions and outcomes are relevant to patients (Sprague Martinez et al., 2018). In a sense, validity can be assessed from the commitment to praxis and social change (Erickson, 2011).

From these examples, you can see the differences in how we interpret validity based on the purpose of the inquiry process. Lincoln et al.'s (2011) work on paradigms illustrates "how questions in one framework make little, if any, sense in another": Are we asking, "Catholic questions directed to a Methodist audience" or "Hindu questions to a Muslim" (p. 118)? Unfortunately, the term *validity* has often been co-opted by those conducting research associated with the epistemological paradigm of positivism. As a result, inquiry that does not closely align with a positivist view of validity is seen as somehow illegitimate. Then again, from a positivist view, how are data validated? In essence, validation is seen from the viewpoint that the researcher is representing and measuring a particular construct, which can include abstract or latent variables (e.g., satisfaction, self-esteem) or concrete variables (e.g., age, height). When we define validity from a positivist paradigm, we see that measurement is often the *purpose* behind the research, and to arrive at a valid (strong) argument, the positivist researcher must be able to show that they arrived at a sound conclusion for their stated purpose (measurement).

What if our intended purpose does not include measuring latent variables but understanding the lived experiences of marginalized groups, constructing new knowledge with them as co-researchers, and pushing for social change? What if our intended purpose is to use evidence to inform action, whether that action includes raising critical consciousness, improving relationships, or reforming practices and policies? Box 3.4 discusses the concept and practice of epistemological consistency, which is a way to consider how the intended purpose of your inquiry process determines how you interpret and define validity. In the next sections, we address several variations of validity, showing how the term has been debated and contested.

BOX 3.4: EPISTEMOLOGICAL CONSISTENCY

We encourage you to reflect on why the intended *purpose* of your inquiry process determines how you interpret and define validity. Just as you would assess the validity or logic behind a claim, you would also need to justify the logic of how you interpret and define validity. This is called **epistemological consistency**. Consider that you are approaching your participatory inquiry from a criticalist viewpoint, in which you are seeking to (1) understand the lived experiences in a community, (2) co-construct knowledge with them, and (3) push for individual and societal transformation. If this were the case, then it would not make much sense to judge the quality of this project on (1) your sole reliance on observable data (i.e., surveys over interviews), (2) maintaining distance between community members, and (3) your ability to obtain one verifiable *truth*. Rather, if you state that you are taking a criticalist view, then other readers and researchers expect to judge your project on its ability to reach criticalist aims. If you claim to approach your inquiry through one paradigm while using the language and methods of another, others may not actually understand the purpose of your research—this is one reason why it is important to maintain epistemological consistency. It is also important to show a clear line from your epistemological paradigm to the language and methods that you use so that you are able to show that you are maintaining consistent and coherent values in your work.

Indigenous and Global South Paradigms

Rather than moving through the chronological order of various conceptualizations of validity, we made an intentional decision to present this concept from the perspective of several Indigenous and Global South scholars and communities. We are not simply nodding to Indigenous and Global South researchers here; rather, we are saying that these frameworks are crucial to understanding how to approach validity in critical participatory inquiry. We show several versions, as it is important to not consider Indigenous and Global South scholars and communities as a monolith but to note the distinctions behind various views, just as we would note them between positivist and critical paradigms. As we mentioned earlier, the critical participatory inquirer should often ask if they are respecting and considering ethics and validity from a multiplicity of knowledge, language, and culture systems. In the case of Indigenous and Global South systems around the world, many have been forgotten due to epistemicide, the killing of knowledge systems (de Sousa Santos, 2008; Hall & Tandon, 2017). Because knowledge systems have been displaced and destroyed, many Indigenous conceptualizations of ethics and validity cannot be placed within the tidy timelines that we often see referenced in European literature (e.g., Aristotle → St. Augustine → Cieszkowski → Kant → Kierkegaard → Hess → Marx → Gramsci → Lukacs → Arendt).

First, let's start by moving away from the typical peer-reviewed scholarly literature we may cover in our courses to show how Indigenous communities have documented ethics and validity in their own community-engaged research protocols. The Akwesasne of the Mohawk Nation—located across the provinces of Ontario and Quebec in present-day Canada and the state of New York in the present-day United States—are among a growing number of Indigenous peoples to create their own research protocols rooted in their knowledge systems and culture. In 1996, the Akwesasne Task Force on the Environment (ATFE), and its associated Research Advisory Committee (RAC) outlined several guiding principles and criteria to improve the research agreements that researchers proposed to the Akwesasne community as well as to foster respectful and mutually beneficial community–researcher relationships. Research projects, in order to be considered valid and ethical, should follow the Akwesasne's guiding principles of *skennen* (peace), *kariwiio* (good word), and *kasastensera* (strength) and the associated criteria of reason, righteousness, respect, equity, and empowerment. In these guiding principles, validity is not divorced from ethics, which is similar to the concepts proposed by Aristotle. Rather, in order for a research project to be considered valid or *kasastensera* (remember, valid means strong), a proposed project should seek to create opportunities where researchers' and community members' thinking and practices are respected, power and decision making are shared, resources and material benefits are clearly outlined and reciprocal, and harm is not done to the communities and land involved in research.

As Linda Tuhiwai Smith (2012) notes in *Decolonizing Methodologies: Research and Indigenous Peoples*, the Waitangi Tribunal in New Zealand in 1975 provided a space for Māori people to raise issue with the dispossession and occupation of land that had occurred through British colonialism since 1840. Following the Waitangi Tribunal, the Treaty of Waitangi Amendment Act of 1985 led to the creation of research programs by Māori researchers and communities. According to Tuhiwai Smith (2012), the concept of Kaupapa Māori explicitly elucidates the inherent knowledge systems, values, and practices from the basis of Māori culture and language. As first theorized by Graham Hingangaroa Smith (1992), Kaupapa Māori is based on six principles: *tino rangatiratanga* (sovereignty, autonomy, or self-determination), *taonga tuku iho* (cultural aspiration), ako Māori (culturally preferred pedagogy), *kia piki ake i ngā raruraru o te kainga* (socioeconomic mediation or positive benefit), *whānau* (acknowledging responsibility and obligation to extended family), and *kaupapa* (collective vision). Following the Waitangi Tribunal and Treaty of Waitangi, Graham Hingangaroa Smith not only demonstrates the concepts of validity and ethics tied to Kaupapa Māori research but also in how they are situated as a site of resistance and intervention against the colonial mission that subjugated Māori knowledge, language, and culture as less than Western traditions. Tuhiwai Smith (2012) expands on these six principles, showing how Māori researchers can think about validity and ethics through cultural terms, including concepts such as respect, generosity, caution, and humility.

As Graham Hingangaroa Smith (1992) notes, one interpretation of Kaupapa Māori research is grounded in Giroux's (1983) notion that research and education can have an emancipatory effect.

Showing how Kaupapa Māori stems from local values of collectivism and cultural aspiration creates a counter-narrative and a site of resistance to Western conceptualizations of validity and ethics that are rooted in individualism and the distanced, objective observer. Similar to much of Giroux's (1982, 1983, 2011) work, Hingangaroa Smith shows that local and contextualized knowledge can be seen as an avenue for social change. Rather than inquiry that may reproduce the deficits portrayed by the distanced and "objective" observer, local and contextualized knowledge is seen as a way to validly and ethically focus on what local communities have gotten right, what they would like to change, and what they would like to focus on and improve going forward.

REFLEXIVITY QUESTION

In reading through these Indigenous frameworks of validity, how do they resonate with your own research goals and plans? Do you have concerns or questions about engaging these frameworks, given your own positionality?

You may question why ethnic or race-based frameworks of validity and ethics are needed; however, it becomes clear that what many scholars have defined as scientific and objective research has actually had catastrophic effects on those relegated to the status of "subjects" to be observed and tested. In many cases, extreme versions of positivism in the social sciences and Western educational systems have deprived entire communities from seeing their knowledge and views as valid (Pihama, 2015). This criticism, however, extends not only to postpositivist research but also to the critical and emancipatory forms of inquiry theorized by Western scholars.

In addition to these frameworks, it is absolutely necessary to mention that many of the fundamental principles of critical participatory inquiry are based in the work done by those in the Global South. This is not to say that the Global North does not have its own tradition of critical participatory inquiry (Budd Hall in Canada, Robert Chambers in England, and John Gaventa in the United States are prominent examples), but much of the work from the Global South has been so integral that you may have noticed many names cited throughout various sections of this chapter already, for example, Freire's concept of *conscientizaçao* (i.e., critical consciousness-raising).

As noted in Chapter 1, Global South scholars have asserted that critical participatory inquiry should promote a collective praxis (Rahman & Fals-Borda, 1991), showing how the theoretical notions of participation, democracy, and pluralism can be used to inform a valid and ethical form of inquiry that seeks equitable knowledge creation and social transformation (Fals-Borda & Rahman, 1991; Freire, 1982; Kassam & Mustafa, 1982; Nyoni, 1991; Tandon, 1989). The work done by the critical participatory inquirers cited throughout this book is epistemologically consistent, regardless of whether they were born in the Global South or Global North. Thus, the history and tradition of critical participatory inquiry is not something that can be said to be uniquely Eurocentric or secured in a tidy timeline of progress and modernity. Rather, there is ample evidence that critical researchers around the world have been working alongside communities, each in their own epistemologically consistent ways, to question the status quo and promote emancipatory aims through modes of pluralistic thinking and inquiry. In addition to the frameworks offered by Indigenous and Global South scholars and communities, we outline several validity frameworks established by scholars from various schools of critical theory in the next section.

Critical Approaches to Validity

As critical scholars sought to demonstrate that their work was epistemologically consistent with criticalist aims, there was an evolution and proliferation of guidelines, leading to an assortment of terms describing quality and validity in nonpositivist forms of inquiry. As students of critical participatory inquiry, it is important to understand the history of these guidelines and terms. First, before the advent of these terms, many critical inquirers lacked the language they needed to show that their work was legitimate or to justify it. It was also much easier for readers to delegitimize critical work on the grounds of not holding to positivist views of validity, objectivity, and distanced research that sought to find the truth. In Box 3.5, we provide a brief overview of several critical interpretations of validity from academic literature. This is not meant to be an exhaustive or comprehensive guide but an introduction to these scholars and their ideas. We encourage you to delve deeper into these topics by accessing the articles referenced here.

BOX 3.5: CRITICAL INTERPRETATIONS OF VALIDITY

Authenticity (Guba & Lincoln, 1989): Guba and Lincoln encouraged researchers to search for authenticity in research, including five elements that outline adequacy and ethics: fairness (or balance), ontological authenticity, educative authenticity, catalytic authenticity, and tactical authenticity.

Catalytic validity (Lather, 1986): Lather's reconceptualization of validity called on critical theorists to pursue "rigor as well as relevance" (p. 67), by contemplating the credibility and trustworthiness of their data while also reflecting on how research creates space for participants' societal transformation and critical consciousness.

Ethic of caring and personal accountability (Collins, 2010): In her foundational work on critical race theory, *Black Feminist Thought*, Collins shows how many Black women present an *ethic of caring*, demonstrating how personal expressiveness, emotion, and empathy are "central to the knowledge validation process" (p. 263). Additionally, an ethic of personal accountability is not solely a capacity but requires unlearning the dominant roles we adopt to dismantle "structural, disciplinary, hegemonic, and interpersonal domains" (p. 18).

Transformational validity (Cho & Trent, 2006): Cho and Trent outline transactional validity or *how* we conduct inquiry (e.g., member checking) as well as the notion of *transformational validity*, which goes back to the importance of action in critical inquiry and *why* we conduct research: Does our research make a difference in the lives of the individuals and communities with whom we work?

Psychopolitical validity (Prilleltensky, 2003, 2008): Examining power is central to the idea of psychopolitical validity, which requires that researchers account for how power differentials affect what we study. Inequalities must also be challenged to counteract oppression and encourage emancipatory processes that promote personal, group, and community well-being.

Communicative validity (Carspecken, 1996; Call-Cummings, 2017; Kvale, 1994): Utilizing Habermas' theories of communicative action (1984), scholars have critically reflected on how our roles must be negotiated to further contribute to processes that open space for dialogue and mutual understanding between groups.

REFLEXIVITY QUESTION

As you think about your own critical inquiry project, how would you maintain transactional validity (rigor) while also pushing for transformational validity (relevance)?

Here, we provide a brief summary of the evolution of the term in critical validity. While concerns over validity were traditionally centered around topics of quality, trustworthiness, and reliability (Atkinson et al., 2003; Creswell, 2007; Guba, 1981; Lincoln et al., 2011), for several decades, theorists developed frameworks and criteria that called for critical inquiry to be increasingly judged by its emancipatory and action-oriented qualities (Cho & Trent, 2006; Harding, 1992; Lather, 1986; Massey & Barreras, 2013). In moving toward "the ameliorative aspects of the research" (Cho & Trent, 2006, p. 324), validity is not an act achieved as a result of certain techniques but is "determined by the resultant actions prompted by the research endeavor" (p. 324). As you move into the next section, keep thinking about how ethics and validity guide your critical participatory work. For this reason, we highlight the importance of several foundational ideas that form the basis for validity in CPI.

Deliberative Democratic Dialogue and Communicative Validity

As we see with the previously discussed forms of validity, the early critical theorists (e.g., Freire) that we mentioned are referenced throughout this section. It is no different when we talk about deliberative democratic dialogue and communicative validity, as these ideas are rooted in the work of Jürgen Habermas (1984). Here, it is important to think back to the history of action research and participatory inquiry recounted in Chapter 1 (Kemmis & McTaggart, 2005). In their review, Kemmis and McTaggart stress critical emancipatory action research and participatory inquiry draw heavily from the theories of communicative space and communicative action (Habermas, 1996; Kemmis & McTaggart, 2005). Through the concepts of deliberative democratic dialogue and his theory of communicative action, Habermas speaks to the importance of working with three primary orientations: a commitment to mutual understanding, reaching consensus in a way that is not forced, and creating communicative space (Mertens, 2009).

These ideas become central for the critical participatory process as a democratic and dialogic form of inquiry, a critical form of reflection and action that is potentially empowering or transformative. Thus, for the critical participatory inquirer, the act of detaching oneself from the democratic and dialogic process disregards Habermas's (1984, 1996) theory of communicative action, which "*opens communicative space* between people" to achieve or move toward mutual understanding (Kemmis & McTaggart, 2005, p. 576, emphasis in original). Regarding the methodological implications for critical participatory inquiry, Kemmis and McTaggart (2005) note, validity can be stimulated through the social practice of this type of research. As co-researchers, we seek to attain intersubjective agreement and to ensure that consensus is democratically achieved rather than forced. When we think about our processes of data collection and analysis, validity can be strengthened by deliberating on the questions to be asked with community co-researchers. The process of adapting methods to local epistemologies, however, demonstrates how validity and ethics become further intertwined if the inquirer is interested in co-designing culturally responsive processes.

As Meagan demonstrated in her own project with high school students in Idaho, United States, "ethics coincide with validity on the level of calling into question how we participate with one another" (Call-Cummings, 2017, p. 199). Utilizing Habermas' theories of communicative action, she critically reflects on three moments of role negotiation: (1) as an outsider to the high school establishing her role in the collective, (2) training students in the collective on methods, and (3) unanticipated role decisions as her role as the "university-based researcher" is further established. In exploring these moments of role negotiation within the collective, she demonstrates how communicative validity can be developed, lost, or gained throughout the inquiry process. This raises a number of questions for those interested in critical participatory inquiry. While the participatory process is often seen as methodologically adaptive, this flexibility can and often does manifest itself in the form of ethical quandaries of how to negotiate relationships, nurture communicative space, and push for action with co-researchers. However, through this process of formulating questions and processes with community members, there is potential to lead to "critical knowledge production and democratic possibilities, about inquiry tied to action for justice and recognition" (Fine, 2018, p. 77).

Validity as Self/Praxis. The idea of recognition is an important concept if we consider validity as a form of self or as contextualizing one's knowledge and experiences as legitimate. As we have mentioned in this chapter and throughout this book, research can often be seen as extractive (Pittaway et al., 2010) or engaging in epistemicide (de Sousa Santos, 2008; Hall & Tandon, 2017). Critical race theory (Crenshaw et al., 1995; Delgado Bernal, 2002) and critical race methodology (Solórzano & Yosso, 2002) offer ways to demonstrate how those in the majority often present their own knowledge as "neutral" and "objective" rather than recognizing this as possibly detrimental to those in the minority. Through their work on LatCrit theory, Solórzano and Yosso confront the fact that research conducted in and on communities of Color tends to be deficit oriented, focusing primarily on how students of Color do not meet educational standards. Through LatCrit, scholars challenge these deficit stories and flip the script: Is it Latinx students who do not meet educational standards, or is it race and racism that dictate how educational systems affect and portray people of color (LatCrit Primer, 2002)?

How race and racism shape the systems in which people of Color live and how White communities may implicitly or explicitly dominate others are addressed in Patricia Hill Collins' *matrix of domination*, which displays how various domains in society (e.g., interpersonal, disciplinary) can be understood to work against populations of Color. This domination extends to how dominant research paradigms generally portray majoritarian views as neutral, while minority views are treated as less than. As mentioned in Box 3.5, Collins (2010) shows how personal expressiveness, emotion, and empathy are "central to the knowledge validation process" (p. 263) for many Black women (i.e., an ethic of caring); in turn, challenging the Eurocentric interpretations of validity that dominate university settings, which stipulate that knowledge creation be distanced, expressionless, and emotionless (i.e., neutral and objective).

If we look at these criteria—expressiveness, emotion, and empathy—we see that this is not only present in Collins' ethic of caring but also in Barbara Dennis' (2018) concept of *validity as praxis*. In a study where she spoke with religious practitioners about their beliefs, Dennis shows how praxis can be interpreted as the inquirer's intention, personal interest, and ability to listen past the facts. Whereas in postpositivist validity frameworks we are told to maintain our distance and neutrality, Dennis demonstrates how the inquirer can create a typology of "interest markers" (e.g., nonverbal encouragement, eye contact) to show her participants that she is intentional and interested in what they have to say. Now, imagine if you were being interviewed and the researcher showed absolutely no interest in what you were saying. Would you want to say more? Would you feel that your knowledge was valid? By showing personal interest and emotion, the inquirer opens up communicative space (Habermas, 1996; Tanner, 2019; Wicks & Reason, 2009), and the participant feels that their knowledge is validated and possibly feels comfortable sharing more. Additionally, as the inquirer listens past the facts, they are able to begin making explicit what is implicit. Recall Carspecken's ideas of validity claims (earlier in this chapter): In critical inquiry, we are not simply interested in objective, factual claims but the objective, subjective, and normative claims in the statements that individuals make. Validity as praxis demonstrates how validity is an ethical and interrelational act of mutual understanding between inquirer and participant. How can we ensure that "validity is the praxis of potential" (Dennis, 2013, p. 115)? Before concluding, we suggest working through the Recommended Practice activity to articulate how you may frame the validity of your own critical participatory inquiry in order to reach toward epistemological consistency.

RECOMMENDED PRACTICE 3.1: CRITICAL SELF-REFLECTION—HOW CAN YOU FACILITATE CRITICAL PARTICIPATORY INQUIRY?

Before we move into the next chapter, critically reflect on these variants of validity. Question how they can help or hinder your own critical participatory inquiry process as you get started:

- How can these frameworks help you to establish valid and ethical inquiry projects that democratically engage a community of co-researchers?
- How can you use these frameworks to question the power dynamics behind various systems (knowledge, language, and culture) and push for forms of inquiry that advance social change?
- What does it mean for you to approach the co-construction of method and findings validly and ethically?

- If or when you frame your research within a particular validity framework, what are the positive and negative implications on your critical participatory inquiry process? Whose views are you un/intentionally hiding? Whose voices are you un/intentionally muting? Are you invalidating other ways of knowing?

CONCLUSION

In this chapter we have covered various concepts and definitions of validity. These range from the Eurocentric models that tend to be practiced in university settings to the frameworks established by Indigenous, Global South, and critical race scholars and communities, which push for more equitable forms of knowledge creation. We show how critical inquiry challenges the dominant notion that objectivity is equated with validity. To counter this, we demonstrate theoretical models for understanding bias and access. These models require the critical participatory inquirer to understanding the complexity of claims, or the objective, subjective, and normative (value) claims within statements.

We have intentionally chosen to not include lots of details about the institutional review board in an effort to practice what we preach. We have clarified that critical participatory ethics takes a positive, proactive approach to ethics. That is, we move beyond an institutional, procedural approach that relies heavily on a negative "do no harm" standard. Critical participatory inquiry relies on a positive, "do good" approach to ethics, and we have offered suggestions and examples for how this is tied up in establishing validity. In addition, we have emphasized the concept of epistemological consistency, which is a crucial aspect of social inquiry in general and should be considered prior to beginning a project.

SUMMARY OF KEY POINTS

- Within critical participatory inquiry, ethics and validity are entangled and difficult to separate. To be seen as valid, critical participatory inquiry must be relational, and as relationships require respectful human interaction, ethics must be constantly considered and ingrained within our practice.
- Knowledge democracy is an important concept when talking about validity and ethics in critical participatory inquiry. From this view, inquiry is valid and ethical when it privileges various knowledge systems, languages, and cultures.
- Critical participatory inquirers use reflexivity (critical self-reflection) to reflect on our positions as researchers. We bring our own views and multiple identities to the inquiry process, and it can affect the questions we ask (or do not ask), what we hear (or do not hear), and how we interpret others' words. This becomes an important technique in understanding researcher bias.

- For inquiry to be valid, it must be epistemologically consistent. That is, the intended purpose of our inquiry process should determine how we interpret and define validity. Validity, as defined by one paradigm, should not be used to justify, rationalize, or judge inquiry that is produced by another paradigm.
- It is vital that the critical participatory inquirer understand various validity frameworks, from Indigenous and Global South frameworks to critical race and LatCrit to more Eurocentric models of critical theory. This not only improves the validity of our inquiry but also helps to ensure that we respect knowledge democracy.

SUGGESTED ACTIVITIES

1. Create a mind map or process cycle of how you consider ethics and validity to be interrelated or dependent on one another. You might first try this theoretically and then overlay details related to your own critical participatory inquiry to see if your project fits your intended approach.
2. Start a reflexivity journal. Even before you enter a community or apply for IRB approval, start journaling about your intentions and goals as well as questions and concerns.

KEY TERMS

access
bias
catalytic validity
epistemological consistency
objectivity
subjective claims
validity claims

4 BUILDING (ON) RELATIONSHIPS

LEARNING OBJECTIVES

By the end of this chapter, you will be able to

- Analyze your own insider–outsider status within communities of which you are a part.
- Describe the reflexivity process.
- Discuss how relationships among co-researchers look different in CPI.
- Explain major ethical considerations for CPI.
- Enact strategies to build equitable inquiry relationships.

FOCUS ACTIVITY 4.1: REFLECTING ON RELATIONSHIPS

Before you start reading this chapter, consider the following questions. You may answer them to yourself or record your answers and thoughts in your researcher journal. This will form the basis of a research relationship "matrix" that will help you make decisions about how and with whom to conduct inquiry. Right now, though, just brainstorm:

1. Whom do I know or associate with? (Groups? Individuals?)
2. What are the problems, issues, and interests I see or hold right now?
3. What are the problem, issues, and interests that those with whom I interact see or hold right now? How might these be different from the ones I see or hold?
4. How do my relationships and these issues intersect? What are the possibilities for inquiry?

Have you ever been in a situation when you felt called to action but you were not quite sure how to do it? Perhaps you were hanging out with a group of friends or family members, maybe talking about an issue or current event and you or someone said something like, "We should do something about this!" What did you do? For many of us, that desire to "do something" often stops there—or maybe after a few more minutes of dreaming about protesting or writing letters or making calls. But for critical participatory inquirers, that can be the beginning of something exciting. When we have that thought to "do something," that is the birth—the spark—of a new project. This chapter will provide some food for thought around how we as social inquirers can engage with existing and potential relationships and use critical participatory inquiry as a tool for social change.

CONCEPTS AND DEFINITIONS

In Chapter 1, we discussed the importance of maintaining epistemological consistency or congruency—matching our ways of knowing to the methods we use. When we understand what we are committed to as inherently epistemological—grounded in our personal knowledge, experience, and convictions about the world—we can make inquiry decisions that will match those commitments. This means that if I believe that understanding someone else's lived experience is best arrived at through equitable dialogue with that person, I should engage in inquiry that foregrounds or privileges that person's voice and experiences. One of the great things about CPI is that we can investigate issues and problems and questions as we are. critical participatory inquiry (CPI) allows us to be ourselves and to work with the people closest to us for social change. We can free ourselves from the fallacy of neutrality (see Chapter 3) and anchor our work in our own epistemological commitments. This joining of positionalities can feel mentally and emotionally liberating and can give us exciting inquiry opportunities. At the same time, though, it can be fraught with challenges we may not expect. In the next section, we discuss some of the challenges and opportunities of engaging in inquiry as insiders, outsiders, and everything in between.

Insider–Outsider Status

As critical participatory inquirers, we often find ourselves in an in-between position, navigating the tensions and power dynamics that arise from insider and outsider positionalities (Collins, 2010). Melissa felt this as she engaged in CPI with young adults who had migrated from Syria to Turkey. Having migrated from the United States to Turkey herself, she felt similarly out of place navigating a complex and deeply nuanced culture, trying to learn a new language, and attempting to make friends and fit in in a country that was not her own. She could connect well with her Syrian co-inquirers in many ways; yet, of course, she did not share their experiences of war and forced migration. She came from a place of privilege as she had chosen to migrate in order to be with her Turkish partner, and as an American and a native-speaking English teacher, "her kind" was much more welcome in Turkey. In this way, she was most decidedly an outsider.

Many social science researchers would probably identify with this in-betweenness. For example, a male nurse practitioner might be interested in researching COVID-19 burnout among nurses (who are mostly female) in the hospital where he works, or a Black professor of psychology might want to document posttraumatic stress and community resilience in relation to police brutality in their childhood community in Ferguson, Missouri. These hypothetical researchers share professional or personal ties with potential participants, which would provide unique opportunities for inquiry, but they may also encounter resistance or exclusion because of socioeconomic distinctions, gender, or other power dynamics.

This range of positions from insider to outsider is sometimes described as a "continuum of positionality" (Herr & Anderson, 2005; see Figure 4.1), but it is important to note that this is complex and dynamic, as Ghaffar-Kucher (2015) terms it, the "ever-shifting sands of insider and outsider statuses" (p. 1188).

REFLEXIVITY QUESTION

When have you felt the in-betweenness of being both an insider and an outsider? Perhaps this has occurred in a social context, or in a professional setting. How did it feel to exist and move in that space? What choices did you make, when, and with whom? When did you feel at ease and when did you feel discomfort? How did you make sense of those feelings? What was your inner dialogue?

Insider–outsider positionality (Collins, 1989, 2010) is also rooted in epistemology and often requires intentional choices. For example, Melissa identifies as a migrant rather than the more common "expat" designation that most privileged North American or European foreign residents in Turkey adopt. She does so to push back against social stratification based on national origin and native language in Turkish society and to indicate her commitment both to her adopted country and to advocating for other, less "desirable" migrants. Her positionality offers her access to both Turkish and migrant communities, but she also has to navigate constraints in both. As illustrated in Figure 4.1, researchers must acknowledge their multiple identities to address the complexities behind their insider and outsider statuses. For instance, Collins (1989) defines researchers who conduct studies on or with their own social group as outsiders-within, as they may still identify with a particular group based on identities (e.g., race, ethnicity, gender), but their position as a researcher moves them more to an outsider status. In Melissa's example, there were instances where her identities were situated from more of an insider status, and at other points in time as more of an outsider. As you reflect on your multiple positions when working alongside community members in a CPI project, it helps to think about your insider–outsider positions on a continuum, as well as the extent of community participation. For instance, will you be studying others from afar, which can be done through surveys or observation, without engaging with them much or at all (top-left position in Figure 4.1)? Or, if you are working alongside others, will your engagement move between collaboration with other insiders (bottom-right position), as an outsider invited by another group to offer support (top-middle position), and/or through a reciprocal collaboration that includes joint decision making and co-learning (top-right position)? Even

FIGURE 4.1 ■ Continuum of Researcher Positionality (positions adapted from Herr & Anderson, 2005)

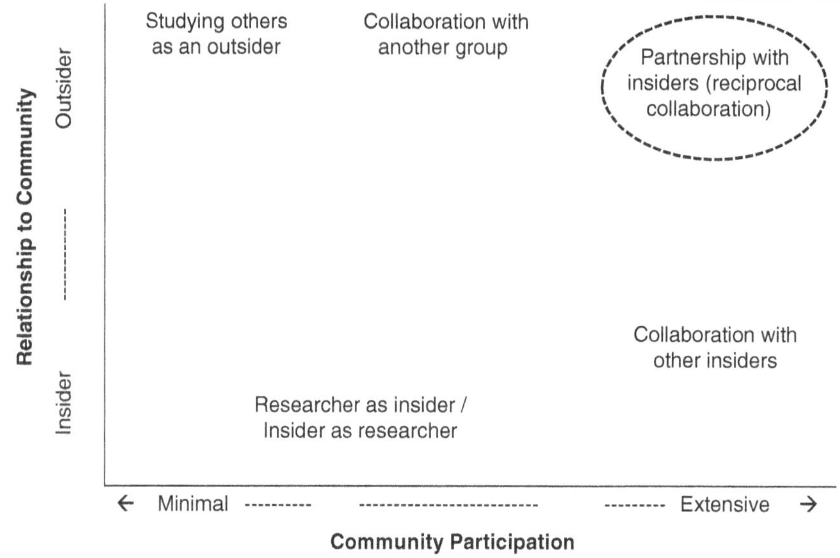

within one project, we can move along a continuum that comprises several of these positions, or a combination of them. Moreover, as these statuses are not static, this process calls on us to continually reflect on our positionality, how others may see us as researchers, and how these positions may morph or (d)evolve.

Insider–outsider status can present ethical and methodological dilemmas; it requires ongoing critical reflexivity to anticipate potential pitfalls and respond appropriately to unexpected tensions. Miled (2019) describes several incidents during her fieldwork with Muslim-identifying refugee youth in Canada that caused her to see her own "Muslim identity as a space of multiple negotiations that can cross participants' Muslim identities at just one intersection" (p. 9). As a Pakistani researcher, Ghaffar-Kucher (2015) recalls encountering assumptions that her work with Pakistani American youth in New York City was biased and therefore less valid (a problematic critique from positivist concepts of research that we address elsewhere) while also feeling a "burden of representation" (p. 1187) or the expectation that she would speak for her entire community. She asserts that the insider researcher needs to carefully consider "how one positions oneself and how one is positioned by others" (p. 1187). We recommend spending some time considering this before jumping into CPI, regardless of how close or far you feel from your potential co-researchers or participants. For example, in preparation for her dissertation research with Syrian refugees in Turkey, Melissa reflected on her insider–outsider status as a fellow migrant and Turkish language learner with social, legal, and economic advantages her participants would not have and how this should inform her research design (Hauber-Özer, 2019). She also reflected on interactions and relationships throughout her data collection, for instance, intentionally positioning herself as a fellow migrant and language learner during interviews (see Box 4.1).

BOX 4.1: INSIDER–OUTSIDER POSITIONING

Melissa carefully structured her dissertation study to build trust and rapport with her participants through a series of meetings and to incorporate their feedback and priorities into data collection and analysis. However, the COVID-19 pandemic reached Turkey just as she planned to start recruitment, forcing her to shift to an entirely remote and much more linear process, meaning that the first time she met most of her participants was during an in-depth, semistructured interview following an online background questionnaire. In the following excerpt (translated from Turkish by Melissa) from the beginning of her interview with Aynur (pseudonym), we see her efforts to build rapport and position herself as a fellow migrant who had experienced similar challenges. This also helped to increase intersubjective understanding as they had shared knowledge of the procedures and barriers foreigners in Turkey face.

Melissa: Okay, what's your major?
Aynur: Civil engineering.
Melissa: How did you choose this major?
Aynur: I didn't choose it; it chose me. It happened like this . . . actually I lost two years. I mean, I didn't lose them; I started university late. I studied the language for a year. The second year I was doing . . . do you know the YÖS [foreign student exam]?
Melissa: Yes.
Aynur: There's an exam for foreigners. I was preparing for that. Also, um, doing my high school diploma equivalency. Do you know what that means?
Melissa: Mmhm.
Aynur: I tried to get my equivalency certificate; I tried to study medicine like my mom and dad wanted . . . but later I chose civil engineering. Later I was accepted into civil [engineering].
Melissa: Well, engineering is a really nice profession. That's really good.
Aynur: Well . . .
Melissa: I hope you like it.
Aynur: Actually, getting accepted was easy, but studying it is hard. But I'm doing it.
Melissa: There's nothing you can do; it's like that in Turkey. I'm a foreigner too: I'm American. I worked hard to learn Turkish too, and I want to get my equivalency certificate. I mean, I started, but yeah, it's difficult.
Aynur: [Getting] equivalency is really difficult.
Melissa: It's difficult, it's expensive, and it's a lot of work. I mean, it takes a long time. Going to Ankara [the capital] and so on.
Aynur: Exactly.

Reflexivity

As we discussed in Chapter 3, reflexivity is the "process of reflecting critically on the self as researcher" (Lincoln et al., 2011, p. 124), and it is related to both ethics (Guillemin & Gillam, 2004; see Chapter 3) and positionality (see Chapter 1). You've practiced reflexivity several times in each chapter to examine your identities, worldview, experiences, knowledge, and potential research interests. That is, you have critically reflected on your viewpoints and identities and how these might affect what and how you research and the conclusions you draw from the data. Miled (2019) explains, "As researchers, our multiple locations (social, political, cultural) infiltrate into and impact our research, from the moment we express our research interests to the moment we present our findings and we celebrate our accomplishments" (p. 5). We agree that our experiences and worldviews will always have some effect on the decisions we make in our inquiry. However, too often the default view is to be concerned about the supposed negative effects they might have. Too little attention is paid to the complexity of how our positionalities can both resource and constrain our inquiry. Engaging in reflexive practice can help us grapple with that complexity and tease out what are often simultaneously affordances and challenges for our inquiry.

We will discuss practical approaches to the *doing* of reflexivity later in the chapter. For now, it is important to consider how reflexivity applies to relationships with others and with the systems and structures within which we conduct participatory inquiry in a broad sense. In her research on the experiences of Bosnian refugee youth, Mosselson (2010) found that reflexivity was crucial to navigating interactions with participants, ongoing research decisions, and data analysis, and we have concluded the same in our own work (e.g., Call-Cummings et al., 2019, 2020). However, in reflecting on mistakes and unresolved questions about her completed dissertation research, Meagan illustrates how reflexivity is a messy process (Call-Cummings et al., 2019). It does not provide tidy answers and may, in fact, bring up more questions about us and our relationships to others and to systems and structures of power and oppression. Milner (2007) offers a helpful framework for considering how one might go about practicing critical self-reflexivity. He suggests a process of researching the self, the self in relation to others, and the self in relation to the system. One important aspect of practicing reflexivity is to not get caught up in what some refer to as "naval gazing." We can get so focused on ourselves, on who we are as researchers, that we lose sight of—or totally miss—how we are positioned in relation to others and to systems of which we are a part.

ETHICAL CONSIDERATIONS

Because CPI is anchored in creating or building on authentic relationships, it is necessary to think through the ethical (and intertwined validity) implications of those relationships. As we discussed in Chapter 3, ethics and validity are best enacted throughout the project as *ethics in practice* (Guillemin & Gillam, 2004). Although we often associate validity with data, we can't separate these data from the ethics of equitable relationships in participatory inquiry. So, before we even start to gather data, we need to ask if we have adequately reflected on issues around power and authority when establishing relationships with co-researchers and if we will act with ethical urgency when co-researchers raise questions about who owns and controls data (Luttrell & Chalfen, 2010).

Here, we want to provide some guidance based on our experiences (and mistakes) and other researchers' insights on important considerations for inquiry with different types of populations. Of course, each community and participant will be unique, but these considerations might help you to prepare for and conduct research that more fully reflects your values and facilitates positive and productive relationships with participants. You will see that we pay particular attention to potential power dynamics in the research collective and encourage you to do the same. In fact, we have wrestled with whether it is even possible to build equitable relationships within hierarchical institutions and systems such as schools or the criminal legal system, but we hope that our transparency here will help you to avoid some of the pitfalls and blind spots that we have grappled with.

What Are Research Relationships in CPI?

So, what do research relationships look like in the context of critical participatory inquiry? Research or inquiry relationships can look as different as the relationships we form in our everyday lives. Some research relationships may be more oriented toward a professional or formal approach, while other research relationships might be more informal. This would most likely depend on who is involved, the setting in which the inquiry is taking place, and the goals of the inquiry itself. Most research relationships—like most everyday relationships—go through a kind of evolution that may start out more formal—and sometimes, uncomfortable or awkward—but may, with time, collaboration, and mutual education, evolve into closer relationships characterized by high levels of trust and even deep friendship (Box 4.2).

BOX 4.2: CPI AND RELATIONSHIPS—BY SHARRELL HASSELL-GOODMAN

Sharrell's Black feminist participatory action research (PAR) dissertation project prioritized relationship building among a collective group of 22 first-generation undergraduate and graduate women of the African diaspora (Black, African American, African, Afro-Caribbean, Afro-Cuban, Afro-Latina). The research project originated with a cohort of six women Sharrell was familiar with and in proximity of campus; however, after the pandemic began, the collective recruited additional co-researchers through affinity social media spaces to make a second cohort. Each of the cohorts' relationships evolved as co-researchers engaged in group interview sessions after describing their experiences as college students. In slight contrast to the first cohort, the second cohort developed affinity space during a time of racial injustice within a pandemic. This meant building relationships on Zoom while mothers in the cohort were on camera with children in the background. For several members in both cohorts, however, relationships developed outside the space of the research project, with co-researchers exchanging contact information and seeking professional advice from one another.

While each cohort developed its own unique dynamic and ethos, the relationships in both were liberatory in part because of co-researchers' shared experiences as *First-Generation Women of the African Diaspora* (FGWAD) navigating systems and structures of power and oppression. The first cohort, for example, developed deeper relationships more quickly, sharing and discussing issues of trauma; this kind of reciprocity appeared more intense with co-researchers' physical affirmations and sharing of the same space. While the second cohort also shared very personal convictions and philosophies, their dynamic began as though it were operating within the scope of respectability politics, but as it progressed, it became more spiritual in nature. As one co-researcher put it, leaving a group meeting sometimes felt like leaving a church service. Both cohorts maintained a familiarity around sharing stories where they felt seen and heard, with co-researchers' verbal and physical affirmations ("me too," "mmhmm," etc.) creating a liberatory and yet intimate experience for the collective.

The PAR process allowed the collective to move beyond the research project as an end goal and instead become a space wherein co-researchers developed deep friendships and equitable relationships in counter to the surveilled spaces of the academy. While co-researchers were initially hesitant to take up explicit leadership roles, they gradually came to take full ownership of the project, making decisions about data collection methods, analysis techniques, and social action projects. These leadership roles then shifted and opened up the idea of expertise in relation to the ways the collective showed up in the academy; as co-researchers navigated power-sharing with each other, they facilitated each other's liberation. For example, undergraduates in their 20s were initially intimidated by being in a collective with women in their 40s and 50s in the middle of their careers, while the women with more established careers reveled in the undergraduates' clarity surrounding their racial identities so early in their college careers. These collective, communal spaces created a circumstance for these women to coalesce and develop these deep, equitable relationships where they shared career, family, and personal advice, long after the research portion ended.

As illustrated by Sharrell's dissertation inquiry collective, relationships can look very different than what some who are more used to "traditional" research would expect. This can pose problems—or at least prompt questions—among dissertation committees, funding organizations, and institutional review boards (IRBs). All of these groups are in positions to "approve" research before it begins. Institutional ethics review boards, which set guidelines and policies related to the ethical practice of research, as well as other bodies that seek to understand a person's research plans prior to them being enacted, most often frame ethics according to a medical model of avoiding harm to participants. As we discussed in Chapter 3, this model does not match CPI's underlying epistemology. Rather, the ethical guidelines or rules these boards and committees understand speak to a specific type of acceptable research relationship where research is done *on* people rather than *with* them. Researchers who are used to these guidelines may be surprised by the idea that research relationships may (or should) be quite friendly, informal, and ongoing beyond the life of the study itself. As we said in Chapter 3, we believe that only through equitable and authentic relationships can truly ethical and valid inquiry be done. As you consider your own research and inquiry plans, keep in mind that you will most likely need some level of permission from a dissertation, thesis, or advisory committee, funding organization, or institutional review board. You will need to make sure to clearly articulate the relational nature of CPI, and you may need to think about how you will frame your future research in terms that members of those committees will understand and appreciate. Often this means more work for you: more explanation, more evidence of "successful" CPI, more time, and more writing.

Relationships With Youth

As you know by now, Meagan, Giovanni, and Melissa have been involved in CPI with children and youth in various contexts. Although institutional review boards are typically quite stringent about guidelines for ethical research with minors (under 18 in the United States), we have found that they often stop short of addressing the less tangible but very real power dynamics operating in many research settings. This is not limited to the discipline of education, but much inquiry with children does take place in either formal or nonformal educational settings, which are often structured—whether consciously or otherwise—by a distinct binary between children and adults (Dennis & Huf, 2017). Even the common claims of youth PAR being "empowering" or "giving voice" position adults as imparting power to powerless youth (Cook-Sather, 2006).

In Chapter 2, we mentioned some tensions that emerged while assisting with a photovoice project with middle school English language learners. In particular, we were concerned by the mismatch between our critical, democratic participatory approach to inquiry and the authority structures and curricular rigidity typical of U.S. schools (see Call-Cummings et al., 2019, 2020). While it used the participatory approach of photovoice, the project was designed as an educational intervention to help students develop their English literacy in line with the school curriculum and learning objectives. We were positioned as adult "Knowers" who initiated the project, identified the topic, and trained child participants in the proper procedures. Over about three months, the lead researcher and a few graduate students provided age-appropriate instruction on the photovoice method and explained the focus (challenges in the school, community, or world), and additional graduate student facilitators worked with small groups of middle school students to take and select photographs in line with the topic and then draft and edit short narratives to accompany the photographs. On the ladder of participation, this project would best be described as tokenistic (Hart, 1992, see Table 2.1).

This is not to say that we did *harm*, exactly; the project was likely enjoyable for the student participants, and the host teacher deemed it a useful way to improve students' English writing skills. However, in hindsight, it did not align with our epistemological commitments to sharing power and decision making with youth co-researchers. If anything, it likely reproduced the adult–child power binary (Gallacher & Gallagher, 2008) rather than facilitating equitable relationships. Other participatory researchers have documented similar challenges (e.g., Kohfeldt et al., 2011; Phillips et al., 2010).

Relationships With Marginalized Populations

There are similar concerns about relationships in participatory inquiry with minoritized populations. For instance, power relations between the researcher and participants call into question to what extent participation is voluntary (Hannes & Parylo, 2014). Does more distance (as in traditional, positivist approaches) prevent coercion, or does an established relationship set up certain expectations? In inquiry with people seeking asylum, might participants volunteer in hopes that researchers—who presumably have more power and resources—will help them obtain humanitarian assistance or refugee status (Hugman et al., 2011)? Might participants feel exploited by researchers "stealing" their stories without giving anything in return (Pittaway et al., 2010)? Such issues may not be typically addressed in IRB procedures and must be considered throughout the life of a project, not just during the planning stage.

As MacKenzie et al. (2007) point out, informed consent procedures are based on the "assumption that participants are autonomous, understand the implications of giving consent and are in relatively equal positions of power with researchers" (p. 302). In situations of unequal power, true consent requires earning participants' trust, ensuring that they have decision-making power over what information about them is shared, and sharing reports and publications created from their data (Hugman et al., 2011; MacKenzie et al., 2007). For researchers working with young children, English language learners, nonliterate adults, or people with intellectual or visual disabilities, a written consent form may be seen as inappropriate; the process must occur in a form of communication suitable for participants (see Boxall & Ralph, 2009). Within any CPI project, we must understand our responsibilities to our institutions and to the communities we work alongside. In some cases, university-affiliated researchers may need to complete IRB-approved consent forms, while also considering whether a separate co-created community agreement is needed. In the Appendix, you can see an example of Sascha Reed's work and how she theoretically problematized and practically approached consent forms in her *Everyday Friends Research* group, which included co-researchers with intellectual and developmental disabilities (IDD).

Furthermore, rather than signing a single form, consent (like research more generally) should be an ongoing, iterative process, re-negotiating agreements and plans in partnership with participants in response to evolving circumstances or concerns (Hugman et al., 2011; MacKenzie et al., 2007). While there may be exceptions, this may not align with typical IRB requirements, which demand a linear description of planned research activities and precisely worded consent documents prior to data collection and may require modifications to the IRB application as the project progresses. For example, Melissa obtained consent from participants at each of her three stages of data collection and submitted several modifications to her IRB application during the 6-month process to reflect changes made in response to pandemic conditions and participant needs. The concept of **reciprocity** (discussed in more depth in Chapter 10) is also valuable here: instead of thinking only about how to avoid harm to participants, we encourage you to consider how the research could benefit participants in meaningful ways (MacKenzie et al., 2007). In fact, this is the whole idea of CPI: the goal(s), questions, design, data collection, analysis, and process of sharing findings should be centered on community concerns and priorities rather than solely on an outside researcher's agenda.

In addition, researchers need to carefully consider ethical issues regarding privacy and confidentiality, particularly in research that involves vulnerable groups like refugees, undocumented immigrants, people with intellectual disabilities, and LGBTQ+ youth (Boxall & Ralph, 2009; Hannes & Parylo, 2014; Hauber-Özer & Call-Cummings, 2020; Sahay et al., 2016). After all, these individuals can face very real risks if confidentiality is breached. In visual methods like photovoice, for example, co-researchers must be aware of and follow ethical procedures for obtaining consent from individuals depicted in photographs (Hannes & Parylo, 2014). On the other hand, ethics requirements can stifle or silence individuals, for example, by requiring the use of pseudonyms when participants wish to be identified. In other words, every stage of research must be built on relationships of trust and reciprocity.

Decolonizing Relationships

As Wendy Luttrell (2010) notes, "negotiating research relationships" (p. 13) is at the core of qualitative research, and we believe this is an important step in decolonizing our relationships in CPI. *Negotiation* frames the process of nurturing inquiry relationships as a reciprocal act where all co-researchers have the agency to make decisions in contrast to the authoritarian trap we can fall into where we, as the researchers, feel the need to control all steps of the processes. While it is important to negotiate and manage good relationships with co-researchers, we first need to realize that research relationships have often caused harm to communities.

When it comes to decolonizing relationships—more specifically, dismantling the power imbalances and prevalence of Western approaches in relationship building—it helps to start from an *ethic of humility* (Limes-Taylor Henderson & Esposito, 2017). Limes-Taylor Henderson and Esposito (2017) have conducted inquiry as outsiders-within (Collins, 1989) in locations where they could identify as part of the community but also as outsiders (i.e., academics), yet they still call on researchers to err on the side of ignorance and claim it. We cannot know everything, and we should be open to learning from the communities we work alongside. Erring on the side of ignorance allows us to put aside our own ideologies and to remain accountable as co-learners. Similarly, Martiniquais psychologist and critical theorist, Frantz Fanon (1963/2014) referred to this as *decolonizing our minds*: What would it take to rid ourselves of the colonial vestiges of the scientific method, where we claim a supremacy of knowledge in order to prove things as we study and experiment on others?

We should also be clear that—as scholars Eve Tuck and Wayne Yang (2012) affirm—*decolonization is not a metaphor*. Rather, in our practice, we should understand how we may be complicit in perpetuating coloniality through our relationships. In our research relationships, do we preserve a status quo that privileges Western knowledge systems and practices? That said, this demands more than inward reflection. It requires strategies to address the repatriation of resources to historically oppressed communities. Will we pay participants for their time, and if so, how (Surmiak, 2020)? If they share meals with us, will we return this hospitality? Through a decolonial framework, it becomes necessary to ask how we plan to work alongside others to support their struggle. Being partners in this struggle, however, does not absolve us of colonial tendencies. Rather, in decolonizing our relationships, we start by asking how we can first decolonize the self by pushing against Eurocentricity (Popova, 2016). Additionally, it requires us to question individualistic tendencies, asking what solidarity actually looks like if we are to remain in a collective relationship and struggle that dismantles oppressive systems (Boudreau Morris, 2016). We discuss the topic of solidarity in CPI more in Chapter 10. Additionally, for an example of what this may practically look like in a CPI project, you can learn more from the *Amigas de la Comunidad* case study in the Appendix.

As we think about decolonizing our relationships, let's return to one of the initial questions in the Focus Activity at the start of this chapter: "What are the problems, issues, and interests that those with whom I interact see or hold right now? How might these be different from the ones I see or hold?" Acknowledging the differences in your interests and those with whom you are working is a good place to start as you decolonize your inquiry practice and think about how to respectfully negotiate relationships.

BOX 4.3: CPI IN GUATEMALA

Through his inquiry project in Guatemala, Giovanni has worked alongside a nonprofit partner and a Kaqchikel Maya community. Although he had an existing relationship with nonprofit staff, he did not have one with the community. Nonprofit staff who are trusted partners with the Indigenous community were able to introduce him to community members; in other words, working with gatekeepers can facilitate dialogue and relationships where they do not currently exist. Before arriving on the community's land, however, Giovanni felt a sense of unease about proposing a project or starting preplanned data gathering or analysis activities. The last thing he wanted was to arrive and use community members as passive producers of data, as many had been involved in traditional research where their stories were used in publications with little benefit to them.

After reading more about traditional customs and consulting with nonprofit staff, it was clear that—to create a collective—they could establish mutual respect by gathering and starting with open dialogue. By coming to their land and accepting an invitation to hold a community consultation in their *nimajay,* or traditional community lodge, Giovanni and the nonprofit partner were showing that they were willing to make the effort to travel and meet with all interested members before proposing a project or setting research questions. Introductions were not a formal affair where a dry consent form was read aloud but mirrored a community gathering. The community leader started with an introduction, and Giovanni and his primary nonprofit partner then thanked the community for their invitation. Giovanni's introduction included personal notes about his background and family—as if he were meeting friends, not research subjects.

To understand how the community creates knowledge, Giovanni did his own homework, learning about the importance of oral history and storytelling among the Kaqchikel (more on this in Chapter 6). This was an important step in decolonizing his mind as a researcher to ensure he did not privilege particular methods or Eurocentric ways of validating knowledge. Rather than keeping his distance from community members, he took walks with them around the site, learning about symbols depicted in murals, local history, and the significance of the land. As the community would do after a traditional gathering, they all shared a meal together, speaking not only about their burgeoning inquiry project but exchanging stories about family and daily life. Several weeks later, the nonprofit partner arranged transportation and invited community co-researchers to visit their office. This was a way to open up their own space, conduct additional data analysis activities, and share another meal. The purpose of these activities was to establish reciprocity and respect so all could negotiate and nurture this relationship and ensure that the benefits outweighed the costs. Costs to the community, however, continue to be a point that Giovanni struggles with, but these reflexive questions should not be internalized; they can lead to further action. How much time is too much for community co-researchers to spend on this project, given that it could take time away from income-generating activities? How can community co-researchers be repaid or compensated for their time and knowledge? How would remuneration need to be justified for IRB purposes or to other researchers? Might others see compensation as unethical?

PRACTICAL CONSIDERATIONS

To this point in this chapter, we have focused on considering epistemology and ethics in the relationships we form or engage through and with CPI. It is important to understand these roots in order to put them into practice. This section will focus on practical considerations for building (on) relationships through and for critical participatory inquiry.

When you are building on existing relationships, you might make assumptions about who people are, their identities and positionalities, the experiences they have had, and the perspectives they hold. We often also make these assumptions when we do not know people or when we are forming new relationships. It is important to be intentional, to foreground dialogue, to be explicit about power dynamics, and to practice humility and care—no matter if the relationships are new or well established. We created Figure 4.2 to get you thinking about your own relationships and how or if you might engage in CPI through them.

We can walk through an example of how you might make such a decision. Perhaps you are a new program manager working for a jurisdiction or municipality that has recently created several goals related to increasing health equity for young adults who self-identify as LGBTQ+. You are a recent graduate of a top-rated graduate school, but your degree is in public affairs, not public health. You were introduced to CPI during your graduate studies, and you know you would like to propose a CPI project to make sure the jurisdiction's goals are aligned with the needs and assets of the community. You take a look at the decision tree above. You feel like you not have any close existing relationships in the communities that would easily facilitate beginning a CPI project. So, you examine your networks. You have met a few people within the local government and in your office, so you could probably talk to them. You also exercise every morning at the local community health club and are friendly with a few front desk staff members there—maybe someone there would be willing to think with you. You also volunteer monthly in your community's soup kitchen—maybe they would be interested. You decide to share brief thoughts on possibilities with two friends in your

FIGURE 4.2 ■ Inquiry Relationship Decision Tree

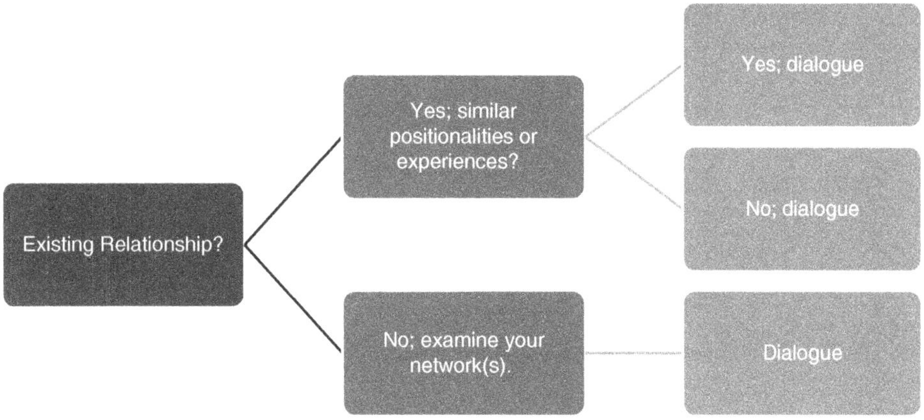

office. You ask the front desk staff members at your community health club if you can speak with someone in charge of programming or outreach. You float your ideas with her. You also mention CPI and your ideas the next time you are serving food at the community soup kitchen. It seems like your ideas really land with the outreach coordinator of your community health club. She says that she can advertise over the next few weeks and gather a group of community members for an introductory interest/brainstorming meeting in one of the rooms at the club. She suggests you identify three or four people from the local jurisdiction to join. You are on your way!

Notice how, in the above example, an everyday issue is at play: a jurisdiction's goals around health equity. The goals will most likely be addressed one way or another. It takes someone like you to simply bring up the possibility of CPI in your own networks. We have noticed in our own inquiry work that people are generally quite responsive to and excited about participatory approaches to research and evaluation—it just needs to be introduced. It is often easier than we may think—as simple as starting a conversation.

Of course, conversations can be difficult to start, depending on a variety of contextual factors. The next two sections walk through more details of what to consider when you do have a preexisting relationship that lends itself to CPI as well as what to do when, like the example above, you may not have an existing relationship. You will see we focus on questions of positionality, transparency, humility, and dialogue.

When There Is a Preexisting Relationship

Of course, Figure 4.2 does not cover every nuance of how or when or even whether to engage in CPI with existing or potential relationships; it is simply a starting point. If you decide that you have an existing relationship that may lend itself to engaging in critical participatory inquiry, you need to consider your own positionality in relation to theirs. From your perspective, will you be coming at the issue or concern in similar ways? Do you share similar experiences related to the issue? Do you share similar worldviews? If you think the answer to these questions is yes, test out your assumptions. You may ask someone out for coffee or tea or initiate an informal conversation that is transparent and honest: "Hey, I'm thinking about maybe doing a project that would help our jurisdiction better understand the needs and assets of our community related to health equity. I feel like you and I sort of share similar ideas on this, but I want to make sure my assumptions are right. When you think about future projects, what do you envision?" A question as open and honest as that can open doors to greater understanding.

You should also ask yourself if you have a trusting, authentic relationship with the person or group you hope to work with—or if there is potential to build that type of relationship. If you have concerns around positionality or power dynamics, you should consider whether the relationship is an appropriate one through which to engage in CPI. Perhaps it is not appropriate, and you reconsider other options. This would arise in our example about health equity if it appears community members may harbor significant mistrust of public officials, for example. In consultation with colleagues, you should discuss how you might seek to improve those relationships. Maybe something happened several years ago that led to this mistrust. Or perhaps mistrust has built up over time. It might be a symptom of deep-rooted structural or systemic inequity. Some of these could be addressed through dialogue, while others may take years to address in meaningful ways. Consider how much time you think your jurisdiction would give to a CPI approach. Also, think through to what extent attempts to build trust would be valued or taken seriously by community members. All of these questions and considerations must be weighed before jumping in the proverbial deep end.

As you consider possibilities for inquiry relationships, you must also consider how including differing experiences and positionalities would benefit the process. Earlier, we asked you to consider how you see the issue or concern compared to others you may work with. We do not want to suggest that you have to be in total agreement with the others you conduct CPI with. In fact, as is the case in everyday life, most often we have found that working with people who have different perspectives or experiences than our own only enhances the work done. We will discuss this later in this chapter as well as in Chapter 5. Suffice it to say here, be intentional about who you approach, when, and how. If you have existing relationships with people who have vastly different life experiences or perspectives than you do, think creatively and humbly about how each of you could add value to a joint inquiry effort. Do *not* rely on your own assumptions. Always. Rely. On. Dialogue. We cannot stress that enough. Clarify and then check your assumptions through open dialogue. If you feel uncomfortable approaching someone directly, seek advice and guidance from a trusted third party. In the example of the recently hired program manager, you could ask for advice from a trusted colleague (insider) or from one of your graduate studies advisors who is totally removed from the situation (outsider). It can often be helpful to ask for advice from both insiders and outsiders and then balance the guidance received.

Reflexive, dialogic praxis does not stop once you have decided whether or not to pursue CPI through an existing relationship. If you choose to pursue CPI through an existing relationship, you need to consider your obligation of care toward co-inquirers at every step along the way. Do not wait until something comes up to make decisions. Things might be too difficult then. You may make a decision in haste or without thinking through all the ramifications. As you have these introductory dialogues with yourself and your existing friends and colleagues, include questions about who benefits from the project. Will you consider publishing the work? If so, how will you make authorship decisions? How will you handle situations if things get hard, awkward, distressing, or overwhelming? When will you back off or call it quits? You should also clarify for yourself if you will try to separate the existing relationship (friend, coworker, partner) from the inquiry relationship. Will you do different things in different spaces? Will you discuss the CPI project at specific times, and it will be off-limits at other times? Or will these spaces and times be blended or blurred? Having these conversations and making these decisions ahead of time—and together—will help to set expectations and avoid difficulties later on. We will talk more about all of these issues in the next chapter, but it is important to clarify from the very beginning that all of these considerations are part of a critically reflexive process.

When There Is No Preexisting Relationship

While starting an inquiry project with existing friends, family members, coworkers, or community members has its challenges and opportunities, beginning a new research project at the same time you are building a new relationship can be difficult or uncomfortable but also highly rewarding. First, it is worth noting where you might look for potential inquiry relationships. We urge you to first examine the networks and connections you already have—you saw how the program manager did that in the example earlier in the chapter. You may not know the exact person or group you will eventually engage in inquiry with, but you may somehow already be plugged in. For example, imagine you are the head of a local government agency that is rolling out a program to help justice-involved women transition into civilian life after leaving prison. You would like to conduct a needs assessment and have heard about participatory inquiry but do not know anyone who specializes in it. Your funder seems to be supportive of a participatory approach. You could reach out to your funder, as they fund numerous programs across your country and may have a technical assistance provider or scholar within their network with whom they could connect you. You could also look to your local university for connections, calling a law school or research methodology program for help. You may also go to other local nonprofit organizations and ask if they have ever done participatory work or have any ideas of who might partner with you. By leveraging existing networks and connections, you have a good chance of finding someone you may be able to build a relationship and a project with.

Or perhaps you are a doctoral student. You took a research methods class that briefly mentioned participatory research. You feel drawn to that approach to inquiry but have no idea where to start and, as far as you can tell, no faculty members specialize in CPI or similar approaches. Also, you are really unsure about how to start forming ideas for a project. Luckily, you are early enough in your program that you have a few years before your dissertation. You decide to look up literature on CPI and contact three or four authors you see repeatedly. You mention your interest in CPI and you schedule informational interviews with each scholar. You realize one of them is at a university only 10 miles away. He has an ongoing CPI project happening through a local school district and says you are welcome to join the project. Over the next year, you participate with that group and get a feel for how CPI works. By the time you reach the dissertation proposal stage, you have developed some solid ideas and connections in your own community and are ready to move forward on your own!

These examples are meant to illustrate that in trying to start a new project through new relationships, you may look to the networks and connections you already have. Of course, just like in our everyday relationship-seeking moments, these may not work out. Another opportunity lies with **community gatekeepers**; that is, the people who are part of the community in which you are interested and who are recognized and trusted as leaders by that community. For example, look back to Box 4.3 and think about how Giovanni engaged with local nonprofit leaders who were already working alongside Kaqchikel Maya communities in Guatemala. In this case, members of the collective had similar priorities before they even became a collective. In the example about justice-involved women in transition, you may look to leaders of local nonprofit organizations that provide services to the same or similar populations. You may also look to religious leaders who serve these groups. If they do not work directly with the people you want to connect with, they may have other ideas for you. In the example of the doctoral student, you looked to leaders within academia, and they then connected you to other opportunities.

Clarifying and Balancing Interests

As you reach out to your networks, existing connections, or community gatekeepers, it is vital to make your agenda clear from the very beginning. We cannot overemphasize that you should never attempt to hide your interests, the purposes of your work, or any aspect of your goals. Just like in our everyday relationships, total honesty is required in order to build authentic relationships of trust. However, being honest and open does not mean you should ever put yourself at risk. If you are, for example, a teacher interested in exploring how school administrators can support more equitable classroom models, but you are concerned about the political implications for you in your place of employment, it may be better to partner with teachers or administrators outside of your own school so you can be open about your interests rather than put yourself at risk at your school. In addition, if CPI is risky in your context due to authoritarian governance or other power structures, you may choose to adapt CPI, as Melissa has in her dissertation research. Always protect yourself and the people with whom you may work.

In addition to being clear about your interests, it is important to balance your own agenda with the interests of your partners or inquiry collective. For example, in Giovanni's work in Guatemala, his nonprofit partner was interested in learning more about evaluation methods in order to evaluate a community memorial site, while Giovanni was interested in exploring whether inquiry could serve a restorative function for those who have experienced trauma. To balance these interests, Giovanni facilitated learning sessions where the nonprofit partner and Kaqchikel Maya community members could practice participatory methods so they could then start evaluating the relevance of their community memorial site and the Kaqchikel community's priorities going forward. On the other hand, Giovanni participated in a series of learning events held by the nonprofit and community, where he learned about their collective work and history. Through this act of reciprocity, the nonprofit partner has continued their participatory evaluation work with the community while all are now co-researchers in a project exploring Giovanni's initial line of inquiry.

As you try to balance the interests of everyone involved, it is important, first, to not make assumptions about your co-researchers' interests, and second, to constantly work to resist **transactional relationships**; that is, do not feel like everything has to be equal—I got one thing out of this, so you have to get one thing, too. This also can occur when people talk about a "give back" or even when paying community member researchers is considered. While we (the three authors of this book) all believe that paying all co-researchers working on a project is necessary when and where possible (if I claim to see co-researchers as my equals and I am being paid to be there, so should everyone else), it is not always preferable or possible. Imagine a doctoral student who is conducting an unfunded dissertation. She is not getting paid to do the project, so it would seem appropriate to not pay co-researchers. Or perhaps you are in a situation in which you are engaging in CPI with people who are not living in your community legally. Paying them may create a challenging or risky situation for them. There are as many possibilities as there are types of relationships and CPI projects, so the important thing is to never make assumptions about someone's interests. If you have funding for a project and are in a position to pay co-researchers, ask them if that would be helpful or meaningful to them, and then respect their wishes.

Keep in mind, though, that paying co-researchers can set up uncomfortable and unequal power dynamics that are not in keeping with the epistemology of CPI. There are other ways to balance interests while resisting transactional relationships. Many of these opportunities are rooted in care. Think about it—if you care for your co-researchers and they mention that they will be applying to university in the next year, you would naturally (as you would in everyday relationships) offer to write a letter of recommendation or support if that would be useful to them. You could find ways to co-author a paper or present at a scholarly or practitioner-oriented conference together. These opportunities may not always present themselves as someone (such as yourself) in a relatively greater position of power leveraging their positionality to provide things a co-researcher could not otherwise access, although that can often be the case. For example, you may have access to policy makers, resources, or professional or educational opportunities that co-researchers do not.

At the same time, someone may be participating as a CPI co-researcher because they are interested in making new friends or feeling a greater sense of connection within their community. In this case, balancing interests would look very different than the examples above. For example, if a co-researcher mentions they are having a hard time with one of their children, you might share how you have experienced similar challenges in your own family. Perhaps as you are analyzing data together, your co-researcher says they have nothing to do that night. You could invite everyone to a happy hour at a local pub or to a sunset walk. Being open, sincere, and caring in your inquiry relationship is one meaningful way to balance interests. We will continue this discussion in the next chapter, and you can see an example from the *Amigas de la Comunidad* case study in the Appendix.

Finally, it is important to never assume a "we" within the inquiry group. While working toward a feeling of cohesion, friendship, and equal partnership is necessary, in a participatory inquiry project we also need to be honest with ourselves and each other about how our different positionalities and life experiences create what is often referred to as a **contact zone** (Bettencourt, 2020; Patel, 2012; Pratt, 1991; Torre et al., 2008). While the concept of contact zones has been taken up for the past 10 years or so—particularly in the context of critical participatory inquiry and participatory action research—Mary Louise Pratt defined them in 1991 as

> . . . the social spaces where cultures meet, clash, and grapple with each other, often in contexts of highly asymmetrical relations of power, such as colonialism, slavery, or their aftermaths as they are lived out in many parts of the world today. (p. 34)

As Patel (2012) observes, the most important part of Pratt's (1991) introduction to the idea of contact zones is not that they exist in our everyday lives, but that "they all too often exist without ensuing engaged discourse that productively lifts up difference, discord, power differentials and conflicts" (p. 334). Participatory inquiry collectives will undoubtedly be contact zones because, whether you are working with existing or new relationships, any grouping of people will bring together different positionalities, perspectives, and life experiences—even in the most supposedly homogenous group. Engaging conflict, disagreement, and difference is an ongoing process of dialogue. The key is to fold this into the process, getting more and more comfortable with seeking to better understand and leverage difference and not avoiding it out of discomfort or because you think it will be easier. It might be easier, but it definitely will not be as productive, as you will miss out on the authentic relationships necessary to conduct valid (strong) inquiry.

CONCLUSION

In this chapter, we have discussed the very beginnings of critical participatory inquiry—the inquiry relationship. We have offered lots of suggestions and advice about where and how to build new inquiry relationships as well as how and when to build on existing relationships. We have given lots of examples for you to consider in relation to your own context, and we hope these have been helpful to you. As you conclude this chapter, take a look at the suggested activities. You might select one or two of them to solidify your understanding of the ethical, validity, and practical considerations of building (on) relationships for critical participatory inquiry. In addition, these activities can help you move your CPI project to the next phase—actually getting started in your inquiry. We will cover all the details of that in the next chapter. See you there!

RECOMMENDED PRACTICE 4.1: CONSIDER YOUR INSIDER-OUTSIDER STATUSES

Revisit Figure 4.1 earlier in this chapter. Consider your insider and outsider positions in relation to your future project or a community of interest to you. Try to map it out visually. As you engage in CPI as a researcher, practitioner, or both, consider (1) how you are an insider, and (2) how you are an outsider. How does engaging in a CPI project affect your existing relationships? How will it affect your new relationships? Does the continuum work well for you to visualize this? Is there some other way that is more helpful for you as you grapple with these dynamic and complex relationships?

SUMMARY OF KEY POINTS

- The relationships in a CPI project will seem different than those you may have studied in traditional research structures or protocols. Whereas traditional or positivist research approaches may call for a distanced observer, CPI requires the researcher to be a co-learner, as knowledge resides with all those who participate in an inquiry collective.
- Always rely on dialogue. CPI is a relational and dialogic approach—meaning that it requires us to nurture respectful relationships, which are rooted in open and honest dialogue. Communicating—by not only speaking but listening to others—allows you the opportunity to learn and create something greater than you would have on your own.
- CPI projects can start with preexisting relationships—with family or friends, at work—or you can nurture new relationships. In preexisting networks, you will need to examine

your positionality and agenda in comparison to those you know. If establishing new relationships, you will need to do the same after you get to know your new colleagues. In any case, these processes are all grounded in dialogue.

- The question of being an insider or outsider in any given situation is not all or nothing; there are gradients of belongingness. It is important to engage in reflexivity and question your position and assumptions. How do you consider yourself an insider or outsider? Would others define you as an insider or outsider? Are there particular positionalities that resource or constrain your inquiry?
- Authentic relationships are not always easy; they require effort to establish and maintain open communication and mutual understanding. Although participants will not always agree, conflict can yield new and interesting insights and strengthen relationships.

SUGGESTED ACTIVITIES

1. Journal about your positionality in relation to the community you intend to conduct participatory inquiry with. In what ways are you an insider? In what ways are you an outsider? What potential advantages or challenges could emerge as a result, and how might you plan differently in light of these insights?
2. Return to the opening focus questions and create a research relationship matrix based on your answers to these questions. Remember, those with whom you interact and build relationships will most likely identify problems and issues that are different than the ones you have identified. Refer to the Appendix for a sample research relationship matrix.
3. Go back to the Inquiry Relationship Decision Tree (Figure 4.2) and work through the reflexive process either individually or with a classmate to think about how you could build (on) relationships, brainstorm possibilities, and predict what kinds of dilemmas might emerge.
4. Choose a study cited in this chapter and examine how relationships with co-researchers are described. Were they preexisting or new? How did the outside researchers access the community, and to what extent did they acknowledge their positionality in the paper? Are decisions guided by apparent assumptions or by dialogue? How are co-researchers or participants compensated for their labor? What other details would you like to know about their interactions, and what might you do differently?

KEY TERMS

community gatekeepers
contact zones
insider–outsider
reciprocity
transactional relationships

5 GETTING STARTED

LEARNING OBJECTIVES

By the end of this chapter, you will be able to

- Reflect on power dynamics and their implications on a CPI project.
- Explain how critical consciousness and dialogue are vital in CPI.
- Understand how to utilize various approaches (e.g., community needs/assets mapping) to prioritize a CPI project.
- Co-create community consent forms/agreements and an inquiry plan.

FOCUS ACTIVITY 5.1: MEMORY SCAN

Think back to a time when, in your personal or professional life, you really cared about something—an issue, a policy, an injustice, a practice . . . anything. When have you wanted to make a change? Think about the following questions:

1. What was needed to make the change?
2. Did you have everything you needed?
3. Who supported you? Who stood in your way?
4. Were there forces at play that made it easier to make the change? Harder?

These are all questions you will need to discuss with your group of co-researchers before launching into a critical participatory inquiry (CPI) project.

Critical participatory inquiry is all about the power of people to create change. This requires trusting and open relationships between co-researchers, in most cases, building trust between groups with very different backgrounds and experiences of power dynamics. For example, in the photovoice project we mentioned in Chapter 2 (see Call-Cummings, Hauber-Özer, Byers et al., 2019), Meagan was a new university professor and Melissa was graduate student working with middle school English learners[1] under the leadership of a male senior faculty member

(Dr. Williams). Multiple and intersecting power dynamics complicated our interactions and relationships: age, gender, race, ethnicity, socioeconomic class, education level, professional experience, language proficiency, migration status, and so on. The classroom teacher, Dr. Radford, had invited Dr. Williams—her former PhD advisor and a literacy specialist who had done many similar projects with non-immigrant youth—to launch a photovoice project with her students and the other two English as a second language (ESL) classes in the middle school, which were separated by proficiency level. Dr. Williams had asked Meagan to co-facilitate, and both had invited several of their graduate students to join in. We planned to visit the school for about two hours each Wednesday for 10 weeks, creating small groups of three or four middle school students with each graduate student facilitator to work through the process of taking and selecting photographs and drafting and editing accompanying narratives. On the first day, the facilitators—professors and graduate students—met with Dr. Radford in an empty computer lab to decide on the project theme: problems in the community and possible solutions. Excluding student co-researchers from this decision was our first mistake and revealed that our (Meagan and Melissa) critical, democratic approach to photovoice was not shared by the other facilitators or that we had not developed the trusting relationships necessary for the open dialogue that might have allowed us to address these concerns.

After an introduction to the photovoice process, we led a collaborative brainstorming activity where students wrote problems and solutions on sticky notes and stuck them to a large piece of poster paper under the categories "school," "community," and "world." Then we broke up into small groups to brainstorm ideas for taking pictures, which the students would do before the following week's meeting. Melissa found, however, that it took several weeks to build trust with and between the two boys in her group—sixth graders from Ethiopia and Morocco in different levels of English—to the extent that they were willing to discuss problems, share their ideas about the pictures they had taken, and write the narratives. She also felt uncomfortable as a stranger prying into their lives and spent the following few sessions primarily building rapport—chatting about shared religious and cultural traditions. She felt that she needed to open up to the student co-researchers before expecting them to reciprocate.

Also, as an experienced English language teacher, Melissa felt uneasy about the approach taken during whole-group activities where instructions were given in English and then Spanish, the most common home language, leaving the students who spoke Arabic, Bengali, or other languages to interpret among themselves. This seemed to put an undue burden on non-Spanish speaking students and set up a language hierarchy in the group. Melissa brought up this issue in the pre-session facilitator meeting, but her concern was not addressed, perhaps because all the facilitators were simply unsure how to negotiate the complicated dynamics. Reflecting on the project later, we both felt lingering discomfort with how issues of power and trust had been addressed, prompting us to consider these aspects more deeply in our later work. For us, this mismatch highlighted the importance of addressing roles, dynamics, and dilemmas before and during the life of a project.

In this chapter, we move from the focus of Chapter 4 on creating or identifying potential inquiry relationships to gathering an **inquiry collective**, identifying an issue or area of concern, and creating an inquiry plan. As in previous chapters, we will first drill down on some key concepts and definitions before moving into a discussion of ethical considerations as well as practical considerations for these early steps in the CPI process.

CONCEPTS AND DEFINITIONAL ISSUES

Toward the end of Chapter 4, we introduced the concept of contact zones. Meagan and Melissa's photovoice project with middle school students, teachers, doctoral students, and university professors is a perfect example of what could have been a contact zone: It brought together people with varying life experiences and positionalities as well as highly diverse relationships to power in the context of a photovoice project. However, we believe it fell short of becoming a contact zone because we failed to grapple with power dynamics and build trust in a way that was meaningful for everyone involved. By maintaining the school's teacher–student hierarchy, we reproduced inequitable power structures, which, in turn, made the project into yet another opportunity for the students to feel marginalized and disempowered. In order for such spaces to be truly democratic and participatory, we need to explicitly address power dynamics and build trust across differences of age, language, gender, and so on (Dennis et al., 2019; Garnett et al., 2019). There are several approaches and strategies for explicitly addressing power dynamics within contact zones. In this section of the chapter, we highlight the concepts of humility, care, dialogue, critical consciousness, knowledge creation, and evidence as key to addressing power dynamics within contact zones and building trust among co-researchers.

REFLEXIVITY QUESTION

Consider the communities of which you are a part (educational, religious, familial, geographical, racial/ethnic, etc.). What is your role in each of these communities? Do you find yourself "stuck" in one role, or does your role sometimes shift? Would you consider any of these to be a contact zone? Why or why not?

Humility and Care

Caraballo and Soleimany (2019) describe creating "transformative third spaces in which traditional roles and hierarchies might be temporarily suspended" through an "ethic of care, grounded in affective relationships" (p. 84). These "third spaces" require explicit recognition and negotiation of roles in order to share power with those typically disenfranchised in institutional or structural dynamics (Caraballo & Soleimany, 2019). This must start by building relationships with co-researchers and valuing their multiple identities, experiences, and priorities (DeNicolo et al., 2017). DeNicolo et al. (2017) and Cahill et al. (2019) advocate for a *cariño conscientizado*, a culturally grounded praxis of care that displaces dominant cultural values and transactional research practices in favor of intentional engagement with difference. This also disrupts the "researcher as expert" façade and facilitates solidarity around community co-researchers' concerns and priorities (Cahill et al., 2019; Dennis et al., 2019; Garnett et al., 2019). We agree with these scholars that only by first building relationships of trust, mutual care, and radical solidarity can we work together toward personal and community transformation.

In our middle school photovoice project, if we outside facilitators (doctoral students and university faculty) had first worked to create this type of "third space" along with students and teachers, the experience could have been very different for all involved. We know Dr. Radford to be a caring and effective teacher—after all, she invited us into her school to facilitate an empowering learning experience for her students—yet she was constrained by institutional hierarchies, curricular standards, and district accountability measures. Because of our outsider status, we had the opportunity to set a different tone for the project. We should have focused first on building trust and mutual respect (Dennis et al., 2019) with students and teachers and working through power dynamics and language practices in order to create a contact zone in which typical school hierarchies were suspended. For example, instead of using Spanish as the default dominant language and letting minority language speakers fend for themselves, we should have worked to position all students' home languages as resources for making meaning together, co-creating a glossary of key terms or a set of instructions in all languages represented. Then, and only then, should we have decided on a topic *with* the students and moved into the "action" phase of the project. This very likely would have required a longer term engagement with the students; as we have mentioned, CPI takes time in large part because of the need for a relational foundation.

Dialogue and Critical Consciousness

Also, as we discussed in the first four chapters, the entire process of CPI is relational: It requires community engagement and dialogue. As Paulo Freire (1970) wrote, **dialogue** creates the foundation for *conscientização* (i.e., a process of critical consciousness borne out of mutual respect), which allows an individual to understand (1) their own history and place in society (i.e., self-actualization), (2) the role of power and the oppressor (i.e., mutual understanding), and (3) how to resolve systems of oppression (i.e., action, but more specifically, social transformation). As illustrated in Figure 5.1, the process of conscientizaçao is not a neat, linear process; it is a multidirectional system. While certain situations call for individuals to begin by understanding themselves (self-actualization), which helps them to understand others (mutual understanding); in other cases, an individual may hear an advocate speak and understand where they are coming from (mutual understanding), leading them toward action (social transformation) and to later understand their own place in the world (self-actualization).

When it comes to critically thinking about one's place in the world, though, it is necessary to consider the multiplicity behind one's identity. One individual may be affected by various forms of historical and societal oppression (e.g., coloniality, ageism, racism), but the same individual may also outwardly manifest these in their own negative ways. In other words, it is necessary to not only understand how the world affects you, but also how you affect the world by acknowledging your personal accountability and responsibility to others. It helps to think of *conscientizaçao* as a holistic system where each part cannot be isolated from the whole; it requires us to understand the

FIGURE 5.1 ■ Multidirectional Influences for *Conscientização*

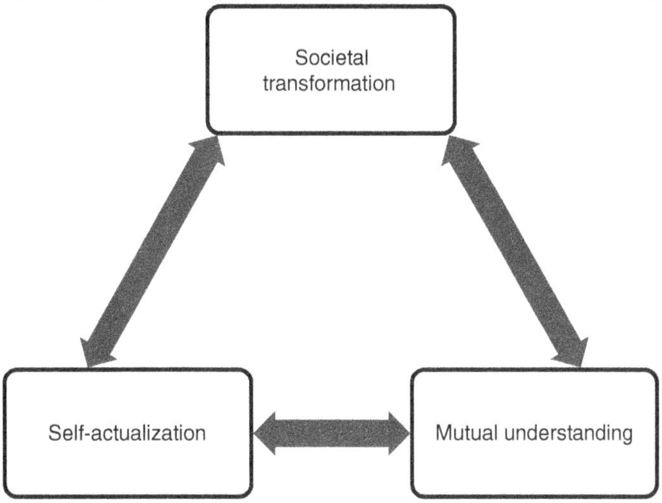

system rather than reducing it to its parts. You cannot start your CPI project without establishing relationships with community members and potential co-researchers. In the first three chapters of this book, we emphasized that our epistemological and ethical commitments to CPI require us to build trust and nurture relationships. Think about the relationships in your personal life: You can probably communicate openly and compromise as you trust the other individual(s). The same goes for CPI: Dialogue is the easiest way to build trust and relationships.

By nurturing relationships through dialogue, there is an opportunity to seek emancipatory goals. When we speak about a dialogic process, though, this process should not only be seen as spoken dialogue since that could be exclusionary. Conversations occur in many forms, from spoken to written word, but in the end, it is necessary to understand that through dialogue, we are creating an opportunity for exchange. Through participatory inquiry, we are able to facilitate opportunities for dialogue and critical consciousness through structured (e.g., card sorting) and semi- or unstructured (e.g., conversational interviews, written surveys) methods. We will talk more about exactly how to utilize these methods in Chapter 6, but for now we offer a brief example.

In his work in Guatemala, Giovanni and his co-researchers sought to include various methods as a way to open dialogue among three generations of Kaqchikel community members. This was done to understand and plot priorities for a community memorial site honoring those killed or still missing as a result of the country's armed conflict. Through community consultations where individuals were able to speak out and structured activities where co-researchers wrote or illustrated priorities, all of these methods were used to open up conversations. Community members spoke out, children and adults drew, several co-researchers listened and transcribed notes for nonliterate community members or those who felt uncomfortable illustrating their thoughts. As you can see, if we had prioritized or privileged one form of "dialogue" over another, we could have excluded community members based on their age, literacy skills, comfort level for speaking publicly. In the end, these activities facilitated dialogue and critical consciousness. We discussed Kaqchikel community members' priorities about the memorial site, the historical and structural issues affecting the community, what needed to change, who should be involved, and how it could all get done.

In this example, you can see a few of the basic techniques that Colombian scholar–practitioner Fals-Borda (Fals-Borda & Rahman, 1991) identified as important when starting participatory inquiry; or, as he termed it, the *people's science.* In Giovanni's work in Guatemala, these basics included a form of collective research that used dialogue and discussion as core values; the utilization of everyday forms of dialogue or folk culture familiar to the Kaqchikel (e.g., oral tradition, storytelling), which were used to document and recover their historical memory and possibly counter the accounts of others with more power or class interests; and co-production of new knowledge with Kaqchikel co-researchers that could be diffused through various media, including written reports, spoken word, and art. As you get started, remember that it is not all on you—as the "all-knowing" researcher—to tell community members and co-researchers how and why data will be gathered and analyzed. Through open dialogue, you will see that decisions can be discussed and made alongside co-researchers. The effects are manifold: In releasing power and control, the researcher shows co-researchers that they have agency over the CPI process as well; co-researchers can identify folk or everyday forms of dialogue and inquiry for the data gathering and analysis process; and co-researchers feel empowered to act, think critically, and continue discussing inquiry and action. Perhaps the loss of this control is what makes it so difficult to talk about getting started, but as you think about launching a project, remember that you do not need to plot everything out specifically. While it is necessary to be able to answer questions related to your purpose and principles (like those that we pose at the start of each chapter and in the reflexivity questions) and to incorporate some basic ingredients (as Fals-Borda and Rahman [1991] describe); the success of a CPI project is not based on your ability to foresee how the entire process unfolds but on your ability to hold true to its epistemological and ethical commitments.

Knowledge Production vs. Knowledge Creation

As we consider ways in which we can explicitly confront power dynamics and build trust within inquiry collectives, it is important to clarify how knowledge is created. Through CPI, unlike many other forms of research, we are not solely (or even primarily) interested in creating knowledge that is published within scholarly journals primarily read by academics. While this can be one objective, it is also necessary to think about how members of a research collective will collaboratively create (or co-create) knowledge by engaging in inquiry, reflection, and action.

Before we get to what knowledge creation may look like through CPI, consider what others might think when they hear the word *research.* If you have taken an introductory methodology or statistics course, you may have learned that a researcher is often seen as an expert who is capable of creating knowledge. They may gather data from other individuals (respondents) and then analyze it on their own or with other researchers. After this is all done, this individual may then write up an article and send it to an academic journal, where other academics or experts assess the quality of their work (peer review). These peer reviewers will assess quality by checking if the author(s) use(s) the correct terminology and draw(s) on the right academic theories. In this case, knowledge is created by academics and primarily presented for other academics. This, of course, is an oversimplification of the research process, but it does represent how some researchers see knowledge production.

When we think about this type of knowledge creation, however, it seems almost mechanical and devoid of relationships and dialogue, which are core to our epistemological commitments in CPI. This is not to say that this type of research is not valid or systematically conducted; rather, its framework for validity rests on the ideals that the researcher must keep relationships at a distance and that knowledge creation is neutral. Think back to Chapter 3, where we mentioned that validity simply means "strong," and this strength is based on the framework that is relevant to our form of inquiry. In CPI, our inquiry is *strong* when we are methodologically and epistemologically committed to democratizing knowledge creation (Call-Cummings, 2017). Now, think back to our hypothetical distanced researcher or expert: Although peer reviewers may see the quality of their work as relevant, what might respondents say when presented with an academic journal article that interprets and summarizes their data or stories without their input? These community members may not see it as valid or a strong interpretation. The academic theories used may not align with what they see in their everyday lives. This work may not be grounded in their realities, identities, and ways of knowing.

This is why it is necessary to reflect on how knowledge is created—which we can do through the reflexive exercises introduced in Chapter 4—to better understand if we are upholding our methodological and epistemological commitments. As we engage community members in CPI, in turn, democratizing the knowledge creation process, we need to see inquiry as both a social and educational process (Kemmis & McTaggart, 2005). This includes shared learning among co-researchers, where we do not privilege certain forms of learning or method over another. What would this look like in practice? While academic co-researchers may facilitate learning sessions on more traditional data collection practices (e.g., surveys), community co-researchers may teach academics how certain folk methods (e.g., storytelling) could be used. As co-researchers are involved in decision-making processes, they are able to demonstrate how knowledge is created, showing how we need to account for both the social and educational aspects of CPI. By continuing to reflect on how we engage in dialogue and build relationships for the purpose of animating critical consciousness, we can start to see how democratizing our inquiry processes and the methods we use can support our intention to unify theory and action (or *praxis*—a practical-critical activity).

Considering "Evidence"

Although **evidence** seems like an unassuming term, it is often used to make political arguments on what is considered valid or objective science. However, certain policies—for example, neoliberal policies on scientific evidence in education in the United States, Britain, and Canada (Shahjahan, 2011)—have illustrated how a simple term can be co-opted to promote particular values on what is considered valid evidence or an effective policy. In many cases, policies on scientific evidence encourage the use of randomized control trials (RCT), simplifying debates into a one-size-fits-all mentality where one method can solve everything rather than thinking about the most appropriate questions and processes that can solve a particular issue or advance an opportunity.

In this chapter, we have talked about the need for dialogue, critical consciousness, and the democratization of knowledge creation in CPI, but these ideas are not necessarily shared by all in the research community, nor will they be shared by all those you engage as co-researchers. As we have mentioned, even when we teach courses on participatory action research (PAR), doctoral students question whether certain aspects of PAR—such as the inclusion of community members as co-researchers—makes the evidence gathered and produced less objective or valid (Call-Cummings, Hauber-Özer, & Dazzo, 2019). As we learn from feminist scholar, Donna Haraway's (1988) work, knowledge (or evidence) is situated; It is not divorced from the hierarchies of class, gender, race, geography, or the many other societal structures we live within (Grosfoguel, 2007).

Evidence can be politicized to encourage particular social or economic policies or used to privilege certain ways of knowing over others. When used for these means, knowledge creation or evidence-based research can be seen as injustice, as noted by philosopher Miranda Fricker (2007). In her work, Fricker shows that when we limit epistemology to dominant paradigms, it can lead entire groups of people to feel wronged or excluded from scientific inquiry (and, in turn, have their thoughts and practices described as outside the realm of truth or knowledge).

Historically, this occurred systematically through colonial processes. For instance, across the Americas, Indigenous peoples were dispossessed from land and knowledge as universities – which they could not attend since enrollment was initially limited to men of European descent – were built (Hall & Tandon, 2017). Thus, as universities were built and Western and Global North knowledge systems proliferated through the exportation of written text, Indigenous and Global South systems were displaced and considered less-than. From Haraway's (1988) work, we can see that this occurs in the way that male thought processes were privileged over women's ways of knowing and being (Belenky et al., 1997). Considering the historical and social processes behind what constitutes evidence will help as you get started. By reflecting on these points, you will be able to reflect on how communities may see research, how they or their ancestors may have been involved in research (for better or worse), and whether their ways of knowing have been considered evidence or deprioritized through particular policy agendas. As you get started, think about the necessity to question what you think of as evidence. This is not only a personal endeavor but requires you to push against the hierarchical and colonial processes that have entrenched themselves in our systems for education and inquiry, socializing us to limit what we consider valid evidence.

RECOMMENDED PRACTICE 5.1: PLOTTING OUT POWER DYNAMICS

Think about the concepts we just covered: critical consciousness, humility, knowledge creation, evidence. In your existing or future CPI project, how will power dynamics and power differentials affect how these concepts are considered and enacted by you and your co-researchers? Create a list or visual map that shows how certain actors (e.g., you, co-researchers, community members, decision makers) and factors (e.g., policies, institutions, broader social and cultural norms) help or hinder critical consciousness, humility, for example. When thinking about power dynamics, move beyond the simply you (as researcher) versus them (as community members) perspective. Broaden your perspective and think about relationships and power dynamics among co-researchers in the CPI collective and the dynamics between the CPI collective and other institutions (e.g., schools, business, government agency). Plotting out these dynamics will help you to understand how power, control, and authority affect how a CPI project is conducted and how they affect your intended goals.

ETHICAL CONSIDERATIONS

Because the goal of CPI is the intentional creation of contact zones (Pratt, 1991; Torre, 2010), or groups of people with varying life experiences and perspectives working together in an equitable way toward a common goal, it is important to consider the ethical implications of how contact zones operate. In this section, we discuss three central ways in which the CPI contact zone can create possibilities for equitable, and potentially transformational, knowledge creation: resisting academia and accolades, navigating power, and disrupting assumed roles.

Resisting Academia and Accolades

While we have foregrounded the idea of power so far in this chapter, we thought it would be important to take a step back before directly addressing how to navigate power to discuss why power dynamics can be such a major hurdle or tension in CPI and other forms of social inquiry. First, it is crucial to acknowledge that power dynamics are not specific to CPI. Of course, there are power dynamics in other forms of social inquiry. The difference is that in CPI we seek to foreground, make explicit, and ultimately shift these power dynamics. In other forms of social inquiry, these structures are taken for granted, not acknowledged, or not considered important or salient to the research itself. We believe that inquiry is actually made stronger—more valid—by intentionally addressing power dynamics.

In terms of power dynamics, we know that positionality plays a huge part (and we have discussed that previously). There are also structures and systems at play that are often difficult to free ourselves from or operate outside of. Academia is one of those systems, and the desire for individual recognition is a normative structure that is deeply connected to—or a product of—academia. Here we discuss three aspects of academia that can be difficult to resist and will almost always affect how CPI plays out: the allure of funding, expectations of production, and the necessity of individual recognition.

The Allure of Funding

While we would all like to believe universities are benevolent spaces for academics to freely pursue the creation and sharing of new knowledge, we know that that is often not the case. Universities, especially public universities, are under a great deal of pressure to stay afloat financially, and this can lead to university administrators placing heavy expectations on faculty to seek external funding for their research. Some universities even require that faculty receive a certain amount of funding in order to receive tenure or be promoted. This may be an unwritten rule, or it can be spelled out in contracts or procedural handbooks.

While having funding can feel good to a researcher because it may act as recognition of the worth of their research, it can also be dangerous. As in other sectors, funding often leads to "mission drift." That is, we may have a particular research question or goal in mind, but then we find a funder who wants us to do something slightly different, so we may rewrite our goals or add more goals that take away from our original, singular focus. In addition, external funding often requires a significant administrative burden. If the university is not equipped to handle grant administration, much of the burden can fall on individual faculty members, reducing the amount of time and energy they can spend doing the research they had planned to do. Finally, most funders to do not understand CPI. They are used to funding research that follows a more traditional approach. This means a CPI researcher may need to "translate" their work into language and methods a funder can understand—and value—in order to receive the funding. This can again require time and energy that could be spent conducting the actual research.

We (Meagan, Melissa, and Giovanni) have been successful in receiving small amounts of funding here and there for our own work, but never large grants. In addition, we have conducted many CPI projects with minimal or no funding at all. We have found that the flexibility and freedom needed to conduct CPI that adheres to its underlying epistemological commitments is most often connected to not having external funding. That said, we know we live in the real world. As academics, we need jobs and tenure and promotion to provide for our families and reach our own professional and personal goals. We continue to seek external funding but are committed to only accepting grants that will allow us to maintain our epistemological commitments to equitable, dialogic inquiry.

Expectations of Production

In addition to external funding, there are also specific expectations around academic "production." Again, what is considered productive at one university may not transfer to another institution. Most often, though, university research faculty are expected to publish articles in scholarly, peer-reviewed journals—the more prestigious, the better. Some institutions and disciplines may prefer researchers to publish books. Overall, though, the mantra within academia is "publish or perish"—and publishing for and with community members often does not "count" or is not seen as rigorous or useful. When we tell you in later chapters that it is important to (1) consider co-authoring with your community-based co-researchers and (2) share findings in ways that are accessible and useful to your community, you may wonder how you can do that if all your institution cares about is top-tier journal articles. We understand: We have been there. In fact, we are there right now!

First of all, we want to be clear that some academic institutions have woken up to community-engaged research and have written into their own policies alternative ways in which CPI practitioners can be "productive"—like publishing in practitioner journals, being active (and recognized) on social media, giving interviews on podcasts, and more. However, these are the exceptions, not the rule. Most often, if you hold an academic position, you will need to figure out creative ways to both publish peer-reviewed journal articles *and* share findings in ways and through methods that are accessible to and useful for the community with which you are engaging. For Meagan, this meant that her CPI dissertation took the form of three scholarly journal articles along with a website co-created with her high school student co-researchers. For Melissa, her CPI dissertation took a more traditional form (five chapters), but instead of synthesizing themes across cases, her findings chapter featured each participant's individual story as a narrative portrait (Smyth & McInerney, 2013) constructed directly from their interview and photovoice products. She selected this less traditional approach to emphasize participants' unique identities, experiences, and strategies and to push back against common stereotypes of refugees. In response to participants' desire to share their creations more widely, she also created a web-based photovoice exhibition[2] (featured in the 2021 virtual conference of the Comparative and International Education Society).

The Necessity of Individual Recognition

In addition to the need to obtain external funding and the requirement to be productive by publishing journal articles, within academia there is an almost ubiquitous desire for individual recognition. Of course, this desire is something most people feel—you want to be recognized for your work. This is normal and natural. The concern here is that in academia, research is often more valued, seen as more important, when it is an individual endeavor—or when it is framed as individually accomplished. This may look like journal articles with only one author or external funding counting only if you are listed as the principal investigator (i.e., the boss). It may also mean individual awards given by a university, professional organization, or other group. Typically, these awards are given to a person, not to a group of twenty community members. Of course, all of these traditions and practices fly in the face of a participatory approach. Meagan has always tried to publish with her co-researchers, which has meant that she has very few single-authored papers to offer up as evidence of her individual achievements. She has explained this in her annual review narratives by making the connection to her participatory inquiry. For the most part, she has been successful in helping review committees understand the necessity of co-authorship with community members. If your department or discipline requires a predominance of single-authored papers or other examples of individual achievement, consider how you can fight that fight or whether you want to. Ask others more senior than you for advice. Build a team that can support you as you move forward. Meagan has found that her team of supporters, which includes practitioner—scholars from various disciplines and with experience pushing back against inequitable academic structures, has given her invaluable advice that has helped her be successful.

If you are not a scholar or do not hold an academic position, maybe you are a nurse thinking about CPI to improve health equity in your community. Perhaps you identify with that program manager we introduced in the last chapter. Or maybe you are a teacher who is trying to get your administrators' attention to do better by your immigrant students. Whatever your position, consider that at some point you may need or want to partner with a university researcher for your CPI project. You will need to understand that they have specific constraints. While we do not expect you to bow to these constraints, understanding them will help you know what to expect ahead of time as well as what to discuss with future academic partners as you decide how or whether to work together.

Overall, it can be really difficult to stick to our epistemological commitments while at the same time completing a degree, looking for a job, or working for tenure or promotion. The sets of values at play seem totally at odds. Nevertheless, we believe there is hope, and we believe there are opportunities for critical participatory inquiry in the context of academia. Indeed, we have seen significant changes at institutions across the globe that suggest community-engaged research and scholarship is valued now more than ever before. To be fair, we have seen some universities leading efforts to institutionalize opportunities for community-based and participatory inquiry. However, we would argue that no matter where you are, there is ample space for institutional change. If you see that your university is not particularly friendly to or understanding of CPI, you can be the one (perhaps with some allies) to work for change. There are countless universities that have published materials online on how they conduct community-engaged research—some even include templates and tools (see the University of Kansas's *Community Tool Box*, or the University of Illinois Chicago's *Community Engagement Toolbox*)—so you are not starting from zero. Reading through these types of materials can provide inspiration and you can build on these efforts with your own ideas for change. After all, change is at the heart of CPI.

Navigating Power

In any situation where relationships need to be negotiated and nurtured, there comes a need to balance agendas, control, and ownership. In CPI, this is no different. However, given that many community members will have experience with research—either direct (i.e., previous participation) or indirect (i.e., hearing about it from others or reading about it)—they may start with the assumption that you, as the researcher, wants to be in full control of the situation. This is an important factor to consider, though, because if you are interested in sharing power and control within an inquiry project, this is not always understood, believed, or thoroughly enacted. With all this in mind, it helps to practice some of the reflexive exercises we have included in each chapter to understand how power can be navigated and where you may need to do the most work in establishing roles and sharing control in your project. Another thing to remember as you begin CPI is that although researchers often talk about entering a research site, you are visiting someone's community or neighborhood where they live and work. Although you have needs as a researcher, it helps to put it all in perspective: Community members have their own priorities to attend to other than inquiry. Starting from this point helps to unpack how your project fits within someone else's life, not how they fit into your research.

RECOMMENDED PRACTICE 5.2: BALANCING NEEDS

As you get started with your CPI project, it is important to balance your needs with those of your community partners. How does your project fit within someone else's life? If you have not done so already, start engaging with and speaking to community members to create a list of their priorities. How do community members' priorities differ from your own? What will you need to do to balance your needs as a researcher or practitioner, and community members' priorities? Do any community members have priorities that vastly differ from others? How will this affect who is involved or included in the collective? How will it affect how you engage with existing or potential members of your CPI collective?

In their synthesis and review of educational action research projects that included students as co-researchers and partners, Susan Groundwater-Smith and Nicole Mockler (2016) show how the inclusion of community co-researchers can be tricky. They observed that researchers often grappled with one fundamental question in their projects: Were co-researchers—in this case, students—included as a way to share power or to maintain the status quo (by seeking buy-in through a veneer of tokenistic inclusion)? As you get started with your CPI project, reflect on this point. Are you including community members as co-researchers because you seek to engage them as true partners who share ownership and make decisions on the types of methods utilized and the way findings are presented? Or is their involvement superficial in that you are conducting research and simply validating what you wanted to do in the first place (what Lodge [2005] refers to as quality control)? Reflecting on these questions as you get started (and throughout your CPI project), will make you more alert to questions of power and authority. In the end, it will help in making the inquiry process more inclusive and democratic.

Reflecting on difficult questions like this should not stop us from including students, or those who may have less power and authority, in CPI projects; rather, the intention is to question whether we are engaging co-researchers in ways that encourage dialogue, critical consciousness, and positive change while respecting their agency. How are you defining key concepts such as power, authority, ownership, and participation (think back to the ladder of participation in Chapter 2) in your CPI project? A good place to start is to ask co-researchers how they would define these concepts—or how the concepts play out—in your collective. Several of the aspects that we have mentioned in this chapter—respect, communication, mutual understanding—can form a good foundation as you start. As education scholar Alison Cook-Sather (2011) notes, students and teachers mention the importance of respect and communication when sharing power in action research. Additionally, it requires us to actively listen to all in a collective rather than treating groups as having one voice (Cook-Sather, 2011). Through active listening, it becomes easier to navigate questions of power so co-researchers can begin to negotiate roles as you move through your CPI project.

Disrupting Assumed Roles

Unlike traditional research, in which roles are strictly defined and delineated, participatory inquiry requires collective members to negotiate roles throughout the process. Various members' levels or types of participation might fluctuate depending on the direction the project takes as well as external constraints or other obligations. This is often seen clearly in participatory inquiry conducted in schools. Youth who participate have many different commitments, including schoolwork, family demands, and social lives, which pull them in many other directions, so it can be hard to maintain a consistent schedule or workflow. In addition, schools are so hierarchical, with rigid power structures at play, that students and teachers are often only seen as their institutionally defined roles: students as learners, teachers as knowers, controllers, and keepers of knowledge. It can be difficult to disrupt our assumptions about who people are and what roles they can or should play in the context of school-based inquiry. We have experienced this in our own school-based CPI project, *Courageous Conversations* (see Introduction).

During the first year of our work together, a group of 10 high school students shared much of the leadership responsibility for data collection, analysis, and sharing findings. The youth created, administered, collected, and analyzed a survey that asked other students how and where they felt safe in school. Students then conducted interviews with their peers based on the survey and then led focus groups to further drill down on their interests. The adult co-researchers, which included Meagan, two doctoral students, and Mrs. Barnes, their teacher co-researcher and host, all took on organizational roles, setting times and dates for research meetings, communicating with the school principal, securing permissions for the work to be done, and even bringing treats on meeting days. When the school year ended, everything pretty much stopped until the next fall.

When the next school year started, some of those who had been leaders the previous year found themselves applying for college, stressing out about standardized tests, or feeling more complacent. Meagan and Mrs. Barnes felt like they had to take more of a leadership role to recruit other students into the group to keep it going, which took a few months. Once more students were involved, several took on leadership roles once again, and Meagan and Mrs. Barnes took more of a backseat. As time went by and everyone got more comfortable around one another, it became easier to recognize when a youth co-researcher was too burdened with other tasks to carry on as a leader or when Meagan's expertise called for her to lead in some aspect of the work.

We include this example to illustrate that the more a group works together, the more natural it will feel to navigate shifting roles. Meagan was not always the Knower ("expert" researcher). Mrs. Barnes was not always the Decider (the teacher "in control" because we met in her face-to-face or virtual classroom). Youth were not always the student leaders (in need of experience to bolster their resumes) or followers (learners because of their age). We switched roles constantly depending on our interests, abilities, and sets of expertise.

Melissa has also seen how fluid roles can be in her own dissertation work. As we mentioned in the Introduction and Chapter 4, she had carefully designed her dissertation research with Syrian refugee students in Turkey to be explicitly participatory. With the help of a key informant, a Syrian student who chose the pseudonym Samar, she planned to recruit a core group of participants—an advisory council—from one university where she had existing relationships with faculty and students. Through regular meetings, she would build relationships with these participants and incorporate their insights and priorities into each stage of the research, developing the interview protocol based on ideas shared at an initial meeting or focus group and through a written questionnaire. They would conduct data analysis together, and emerging findings would inform a series of photovoice workshops and, if there were interest, digital storytelling workshops. She wanted participation to be an enjoyable and worthwhile experience for the students, a chance to tell their stories and advocate for improvements.

However, just as Melissa was about to start recruitment in March 2020, the Turkish Higher Education Council announced that all universities would be closed for 3 weeks to prevent the spread of COVID-19. Students were sent home, and classes were then moved online for the remainder of the semester as well as, eventually, the following fall semester. Now that in-person meetings were impossible, she had to shift her entire research plan to remote recruitment and data collection, making it much more difficult to build relationships and incorporate participant feedback into each stage. Potential participants were scattered around Turkey, in many cases depending on limited and unreliable internet connections, so in consultation with Samar, she decided that it was too logistically difficult and too much to ask of participants to meet regularly as a group. As a result, participants completed the questionnaire online and were invited to complete an interview: With a few exceptions, the interview was the first time Melissa had met them. One advantage to this shift was that initial relationship and rapport building is captured in the interview transcriptions instead of lost in the memory of weekly meetings (as shown in Box 4.1 in Chapter 4). Reading through the transcriptions later, Melissa could identify specific choices that she made to create connections, such as sharing her own struggles with and strategies for learning Turkish or being a foreigner in Turkey. This seemed to help participants feel more at ease, to establish rapport, and to increase intersubjective understanding through shared experience. In a somewhat volatile sociopolitical context, dispersed, remote data collection also protected participants' privacy, preventing suspicious students or administrators from happening on research meetings or overhearing critical comments about the university or Turkish society, for example.

Instead of collaborative analysis with the whole group, which might have become complicated with personalities and power dynamics, Melissa worked closely with Samar to check her interpretations, which gave Samar the opportunity to learn more about research methods, something she had expressed interest in. Samar served as a community representative here, drawing on her lived experience, language skills (the data were in English, Turkish, and Arabic), and familiarity with the questionnaire, interview, and photovoice data to inform the analysis process. Melissa also shared the drafted narrative portraits with participants to ensure that she had accurately represented their experiences and incorporated corrections into her dissertation. Despite a sense of loss about the intended participatory design, Melissa felt that she had found ways to hold true to her ontoepistemological commitments and that protecting participants and ensuring their comfort with the process were more important in the end.

PRACTICAL CONSIDERATIONS

Once you have connected with a few people, shared what CPI is, and discussed your own interests as well as others', it is time to gather an inquiry collective and get to work. This section of the chapter will help you understand practical strategies for gathering your collective, identifying an area of concern, and creating an inquiry plan while staying true to CPI's epistemological commitments to equitable knowledge creation. In addition, we will offer ideas for ways in which you can anticipate and plan for sharing your group's findings and also how you can acknowledge the constraints within which your group will work.

Forming an Inquiry Collective

In the last chapter, we gave you practical advice for how to build—or build on—relationships in order to work toward starting a CPI project. This relationship-building phase may take a few weeks or a few years. However long it takes, once you and your co-inquirers have agreed to work together, you need to officially form an inquiry collective. This does not mean that all of a sudden everything becomes formal and your more informal relationship disappears. It just means that you need to set some expectations or guidelines so that you are all on the same page about how you will move forward. One of the ways in which this is done is through a process of obtaining consent.

When you hear about obtaining consent from research participants, you are probably thinking about a fairly short document that asks if the individual agrees to provide data to a researcher. These are important documents, but they are only templates that, in our view, need to be tailored to the project and participants. In one of his projects in Burma/Myanmar, Giovanni worked with community members—in this case, former political prisoners—to co-create consent forms before starting a 2-day community consultation. Although this process seems participatory and inclusive, it can sometimes confuse participants who have been involved in research, either as researcher or "researched." In this case, participants were a little perplexed at the thought of modifying a consent form, especially as many had experience as researchers. After introducing a template, Giovanni explained that he was interested in involving community members as co-researchers and having discussions on the ways they deemed appropriate for their data and any content produced (photos, video, stories) to be used. If you are interested in the process of co-creating consent forms, we offer step-by-step instructions for a structured activity in Chapter 6, as well as an example in this chapter, in Figure 5.2.

As you get started, though, think about this process as being more about steering your collective in the right direction (toward respectful engagement), rather than the usual concept of liability. When co-creating consent forms, we are still seeking to *do no harm*, but we are also seeking to *do good* by including co-researchers' voices in the process. If you are operating within a university, you will likely still need to use the general template provided by your institutional review board, and you may not be able to replace the university-approved form with a co-created agreement. Regardless, co-created consent forms can be seen as group agreements where the collective can negotiate relationships, power, authority, and control. This can be a place to explicitly document the collective's ground rules—how co-researchers will engage with one another, how concepts such as confidentiality are defined, and what data ownership and control look like. In Figure 5.2, we provide an example of what a group agreement could look like.

To spur conversation, it can help to ask community members if (1) they have ever signed a consent form but wished that they had not; (2) wanted to take back something they said during an interview; or (3) wondered how, and for how long, their stories were being used by researchers. By using these guiding questions, discussion often starts about the necessity of the consent form but also addresses how it inhibits good relationships and keeps power and authority in the hands of the researcher. During these discussions, changes can be made in front of the group—by projecting your screen or making edits on a flipchart or posterboard. The revised forms can then be printed and signed by all.

FIGURE 5.2 ■ Group Agreement/Co-created Consent Form

GROUP AGREEMENT
[PROJECT OR COLLECTIVE TITLE]

In this research collective, we, as co-researchers, are interested in [*include project topic, e.g., exploring possibilities to improve our schools*]. In this collective, we will co-design research procedures such as the development of research questions, data collection and analysis protocols, and processes for sharing findings.

PARTICIPATION

As part of our collective, we have also collaboratively developed this group agreement to make our expectations of one another explicit. As a co-researcher, if you agree to participate in this collective, you will be asked to follow these guidelines and ground rules:

- *Power.* Consider power dynamics/differentials when discussing and deliberating on topics. Be aware of your own and co-researchers' positionalities (step up, step back). Honor and respect that others are being brave when they share.
- *Active listening.* Listen to understand, not to provide answers. Do not force individuals to speak; let each person decide when to share. Understanding that being quiet and listening are forms of active participation.
- *Confidentiality and ownership.* Seek permission from an individual or group before you share their story outside the collective.
- *Humanization.* See everyone as an expert who contributes to knowledge and understanding. Challenge ideas, not the person (defer judgment, ask for clarification). As co-researchers, push one another to understand and participate.
- *Participation.* Consider multiple and varied opportunities for engagement, beyond large group discussions. Encourage participation, but do not push. Provide opportunities for everyone to lead in their own way.

CONSENT AND AGREEMENT

As a co-researcher, I have not only read this form but have been involved in discussing and deliberating on its contents with other co-researchers. My questions have been answered, and I agree to participate as a co-researcher in this collective. [*If a separate consent form is needed by your institution's Institutional Review Board, it is helpful to also include a note here, i.e., I have also received and reviewed the institutional consent form, which was reviewed according to [insert university or organization] procedures, under IRB#. I am aware of who I can contact at [insert university or organization] if I have any questions or concerns related to this research.*]

Co-researchers' signature: ______________________________

Date: ____________________

Keep in mind that this step of forming an inquiry collective is not really a distinct step but rather an ongoing process. Creating, agreeing on, and signing a consent form does not mean that everyone will be okay with everything all the way through a CPI process no matter what. Remember the goal of creating a contact zone: Surely there will be conflict, disagreement, or confusion at almost every step along the way. Another part of this initial collective formation is agreeing on processes for dealing with conflict and disagreement.

This is accomplished through open dialogue. Take a few hours during a meeting of the collective to simply ask, "Okay, we know we won't always agree on everything. What do we do when conflict arises?" Talk through ideas, consider a process, and work together to make sure you all know what to expect.

RECOMMENDED PRACTICE 5.3: CO-CREATING A GROUP AGREEMENT/CONSENT FORM

As you get started, outline a few areas that you would like to include within a group agreement. What principles are important to you? Follow or adapt the steps noted earlier in this section and in Figure 5.2 to form a group agreement or co-created consent form. Invite members of your CPI collective to respond and provide their feedback. Try to have a preliminary or draft agreement before you start moving to other parts of your project (e.g., identifying areas of concern, gathering data). As a step, it is important to explicitly outline your expectations as a group.

Finally, you will need to equalize power relationships up front. This can be really uncomfortable. You might be tempted to skip this part. Without addressing power dynamics early and often, your CPI project will not be able to fully realize its epistemological underpinnings. Leaving power unquestioned is just not an option. Like the ongoing consent process, the process of confronting and shifting relationships to power is continuous, but it needs to start somewhere. One way to begin this process may be through open dialogue. There are more structured ways to approach this as well, and you may have some great ideas for how to do this. We offer a few possibilities here. You can also refer to the Appendix cases or to articles we have referenced to see how others approach this.

One creative way to dig into power is by exploring the ways in which you feel constrained by expectations, norms, and your own positionality. Meagan tried this once with her *Courageous Conversations* group, and it was fun and lead to some useful conversations. Each co-inquirer has a piece of paper and pencil. Each person draws a box and some representation of themselves inside the box. Then they take a few minutes to label sides of the box with forces, expectations, identities, norms, or other things that keep them inside that box. Once everyone draws their own representations, they can exchange papers and review them silently or each person can take turns describing their pictures aloud, or some combination, depending on what the group decides.

The important part of this exercise is to dedicate time to dialogue. Perhaps you end by asking each person to suggest one way to open a person's box. Or maybe it would be interesting to think about ways to connect boxes or tear sides of boxes down. Whatever way your dialogue goes, make sure you are giving time and space for each person to participate, but also that you give each person the opportunity to pass or to listen instead of speak. In addition, make sure that each person who opens up is in charge of the time dedicated to talking about or questioning their own drawing. We do not want this exercise to trigger or traumatize anyone. The person who is sharing must be in a position of power to determine how the dialogue proceeds, what is shared, and what is left unsaid.

Identifying an Area of Concern

Once your inquiry collective has co-created consent forms or processes, grappled with positionality and power, and made plans for conflict and disagreement, it is time to identify the group's area of concern. You may already know what that is—often a CPI group comes together for a specific reason, at a particular time, for a unique reason. Other times the concern or issue may be more amorphous. It is important to make sure everyone agrees with what the group's goals are exactly so that miscommunication is avoided (although of course it is impossible to avoid all miscommunication as humans). The first task is to articulate individual and shared goals, which can be done in many ways. You could simply share goals verbally around a table. You could also make a list of goals on a chalkboard or poster paper. The most important part is to share openly and through dialogue, hopefully making connections between individual and shared goals and being honest about individual goals that may conflict with shared goals.

Another way to approach this articulation of goals is to step back and seek to understand a community's assets and needs. Often, we see researchers and evaluators focus exclusively on needs. You can see this in a plethora of publications and handbooks on conducting needs assessments. We believe that it is crucial to recognize, foreground, and celebrate a community's assets before seeking to address needs. Missing this step can lead you to take a deficit approach to the inquiry. If you immediately focus on needs you will most likely see the community as in need or "at risk," which is not in keeping with CPI's underlying epistemology. By taking a more appreciative approach, the process will be more equitable. Here we offer two methods to learn about a community's capacities: community needs and asset assessments and community mapping.

Community Needs and Asset Assessments

In introductory research methods courses, you may have noticed that the research process often starts by identifying a problem or need. To understand needs, we can think of it as a gap between what is and what should be (Altschuld & Kumar, 2010). While a similar approach can be followed by working with co-researchers in a CPI project, it is also necessary to assess community assets so you have the full picture. By understanding what a community needs as well as its strengths, you can then recognize whether gaps exist. This allows the inquiry collective to not only outline priorities but also uncover what capacities or resources are available so the collective can build on those rather than assuming everything needs to be done by university researchers or others outside the community. As a reflexive exercise, think about this: Imagine if an outside researcher visited your neighborhood and only asked you what was wrong and what you needed. Of course, there are things that could be improved in every neighborhood, but if you are only asked about what is wrong, you may start to think that your community is somehow deficient, simply through the language and methods that this researcher is using. As a critical inquirer, though, it is vital that you facilitate projects that provide space for co-researchers and community members to identify their strengths and contribute their own knowledge.

So, how do we go about conducting a needs and asset assessment? First—depending on the community you are working alongside—you should learn whether it is a good idea to call it an assessment (some individuals associate assessments with tests, and people really hate tests) or if you need an alternative name. As Giovanni usually facilitates needs or assets assessments through open dialogue or interactive methods (e.g., storyboards; see Chapter 7 for an example), he usually uses the term *community consultation* since the group discusses priorities and strengths during these sessions. You can also learn about needs and assets during community mapping and just refer to the method you are using rather than calling it an assessment.

When you are working with co-researchers, it is ideal to expand how you think about needs or assets, as many people get stuck thinking about inanimate objects (e.g., books, funds). As illustrated in Figure 5.3, which can be used as a planning matrix during a community consultation, needs or assets can be people, places, or processes.

Considering these three "Ps"—people, places, and processes—helps to answer the questions that we posed at the beginning of the chapter in the memory scan focus activity. Consider *people* first: Think about the community members or groups of people (organizations, nonprofits) that can offer their expertise or skills (*assets*), or those we *need* to speak to or influence. Think back to Question 3 in our memory scan: Who supported you? Who stood in your way? Are there *places* (e.g., community centers, library meeting rooms) that community members can identify for meetings? Or, are there *processes*—anything from community members feeling that they are listened to and acknowledged to the library offering printing services—that can facilitate your inquiry?

FIGURE 5.3 ■ Planning Matrix for Community Needs and Assets Assessment

	People	Places	Processes
Needs: What do we need to complete our project or achieve our goals?			
Assets: What strengths and capacities can support our project or goals?			

In working with community co-researchers, the planning matrix can be used as a way to prompt discussion. Through discussion, your collective can start listing the people, places, and processes that are needed and to those which the community already has access. One area that you will need to look out for during discussions, however, is the close connection between *needs* and *solutions* (Altschuld & Kumar, 2010). When asked about needs, many people will go straight to solutions. Take for example this statement: The community needs training. Training, however, is something that can be done—a solution. Training is usually the solution for a lack of knowledge, but this gap could be due to a lack of translated materials or the local government not posting information about services. For this reason, it is helpful to question the reason behind the gap and what can be addressed, especially if your mind goes straight to solutions.

It is also a good idea to reassess needs and assets as your CPI project moves forward. By periodically reassessing needs and assets, the collective can start to reprioritize needs, assess whether certain people can now be considered supporters (*assets*), and understand which gaps or needs have been addressed and which are important to move forward. While the assessment provides useful information to start your project, it can also be a useful check-in activity to document achievements and motivate co-researchers.

RECOMMENDED PRACTICE 5.4: ASSESSING NEEDS AND CAPACITY

As mentioned, the planning matrix in Figure 5.3 can be used as an easy way to start a community needs and assets assessment, but this is not the only method. The assessment can take the form of a survey, mapping exercise, interview, focus group, or community meeting (Altschuld & Kumar, 2010; Rotary, n.d.). As you are getting started, think of the assessment as a mini research project. In this process, there are a few tips to think through—as outlined in the previous four chapters—to plot out your plan. These steps can include organizing and recruiting a core group to co-lead the assessment (people), defining areas of interest and what your collective needs to learn (questions), how you will learn about needs and assets (data, existing and new), and outlining who is responsible and how data will be collected and analyzed (methods). In your initial discussions with your collective, use the planning matrix in Figure 5.3 to plot out these needs and assets. This can be done in one afternoon or spread across several meetings. As you navigate your CPI project, remember to revisit the matrix to consider if needs or assets have changed.

Community Mapping

The planning matrix (see Figure 5.3) that we just discussed may be helpful in conducting a community needs and assets assessment, but this can be done in a number of ways. In some cases, if the purpose of your inquiry project is related to the geography of the community where you are living or working, it may make sense to co-create a map of community needs and assets. For example, think back to the hypothetical situation from Chapter 4: You are a new program manager working for a jurisdiction that has recently created several goals related to increasing health equity for young adults who identify as LGBTQ+. In this instance, you may want to work with co-researchers to map out health-related needs and assets. In terms of health equity assets, co-researchers could identify the community health club on a map. Local parks and playgrounds may be highlighted as assets. As you begin to talk more about what is on the map, you may naturally gravitate to what is missing (needs or gaps). Are these assets accessible to everyone? Does the community health club advertise to a broad swathe of residents, appealing to the diversity of the neighborhood or to just one group (e.g., English speakers)? Are supermarkets geographically dispersed so the majority of residents have access?

How you conduct the mapping process will depend on the resources that you have at your disposal and what makes most sense for your collective. In the example in the last paragraph, we seem to be working in a neighborhood that is established on a city plan or grid. In that case, we could probably print out a map from a search engine and then ask co-researchers to make notes on the map based on our discussion. In cases where a detailed map may not be available, it is possible to gather and design the map together by drawing landmarks and road markings. As you gather co-researchers for this activity, there are a few important considerations: Do you have good community representation among co-researchers? The map can look quite different based on who is present for the community mapping activity. If elderly community members are missing from the group, certain needs and resources may not be mapped. Mapping and dialogue can be useful ways to think about power dynamics and how they affect an individual's perceptions of resources. As you work on your CPI project, you can also revisit the map as a way to document changes. Box 5.1 offers a step-by-step guide for how to approach this type of exercise.

BOX 5.1: STEP-BY-STEP: COMMUNITY MAPPING

Step 1. Gather community members around a map of their environment (or draw a map if one is not available).

Step 2. Ask co-researchers to share information about access to resources. What assets or resources exist?

Step 3. Ask co-researchers if there are particular gaps when it comes to resources or if particular issues exist in geographic areas. What needs do community members have? What types of issues exist and where do they happen?

Step 4. Use the map as a tool for discussion. Through dialogue, map assets (and possible individuals or groups who can support your project), outline needs, and document community priorities.

As you think more about this method, consider how your CPI collective could utilize community mapping as a way to open up dialogue about issues or priorities that you would like to focus on for your project.

Creating an Inquiry Plan

As the collective assesses needs and assets, co-researchers may start to identify evidence gaps (*needs*) or data that they have or can easily obtain (*assets*). When the topic of evidence comes up though, it is important to define what type of data are valid. As we have mentioned in previous chapters, the decision on what counts as evidence and whose evidence counts is not neutral (Fine, 2012). Based on previous experiences with research, however, many individuals may only think that quantitative findings (or anything that mentions statistical significance) are valid. If you are facilitating a session on creating an inquiry plan, this is why it is important to communicate that co-researchers should be able to identify what counts as evidence. This does not mean that you are not rigorously thinking about, collecting, and analyzing data; you still need to be systematic. As we mentioned in Chapter 3, this simply means that you can still aim for rigor while taking an approach that democratizes knowledge (Hall & Tandon, 2017).

To structure conversations around the creation of an inquiry plan, it may help to focus on the following questions:

1. What counts as evidence?
2. What evidence do we need?
3. What evidence do people (inside and outside our collective) value?

As the collective discusses and answers these questions, you may start to see that the responses across these questions do not sync. For instance, community co-researchers may want to prioritize their own stories, choosing to speak to their direct experiences around a certain issue. However, members of the collective may find that their city councilmembers only respond to statistics. For this reason, it then helps to plot out the types of data that already exist (e.g., administrative data and statistics collected by a city office) versus the data that co-researchers will need to collect (e.g., collecting community members' stories through interviews). This creates a clearer picture of whether the collective will need to focus their efforts on using qualitative techniques such as interviews or focus groups, quantitative techniques like surveys, or taking a mixed-method approach that combines qualitative and quantitative collection and analysis (Mertens, 2009). Before the collective goes out and starts designing survey tools and collecting data though, it is necessary to prioritize what is necessary—what you *need to know*—versus what would be *nice to know*. With any inquiry project, there are limitations on funding and time, so co-researchers will need to outline which pieces of evidence are most important to collect, which types the collective has expertise collecting, and where you may need some support (i.e., you may need someone experienced in survey design).

As the collective discusses and prioritizes the types of evidence that could be collected, some co-researchers may grow disillusioned and state that they do not have experience with research methods. This is likely untrue, though, as research is based on curiosity, and curiosity is a human trait. If discussions begin to go awry (or even before they move in that direction), you can introduce the concept that all communities have their own forms of data collection and analysis methods; they just may not be seen in that way because they are not conducted by university-based researchers. In his work, Giovanni begins his inquiry projects from a place he refers to as **known methods**—those that community members already use in their daily lives. When we talk about knowledge democratization (Hall & Tandon, 2017) and questioning what counts as evidence, we can think back to the work of Ignacio Martín-Baró (1994), a Salvadoran social psychologist and priest, who spoke of the need for researchers and community activists to *de-ideologize* everyday experience. From the perspective of research methods, this means that we can work with communities to co-construct data through routine practice. For instance, community members may meet each evening and discuss their days, rehashing their experiences and asking one another specific questions. While this may not be initially identified as an unstructured focus group discussion, that is essentially what they are doing. While you, as a researcher, may have methods that are familiar to you, including those that we talk about in this textbook (e.g., ripples of change, storyboards), community members may have their own knowledge systems and cultural traditions. By recognizing that all co-researchers have their own methods, you begin to decenter your own experience by acknowledging that community members hold knowledge that resides in their own expertise.

RECOMMENDED PRACTICE 5.5: CREATING AN INQUIRY PLAN

Invite your co-researchers to a meeting and write out the following questions on a white-board or flipchart paper: (1) What counts as evidence? (2) What evidence do we need? (3) What evidence do people (inside and outside our collective) value? Consider the power dynamics and differentials in your group: Will everyone feel comfortable speaking out and providing responses? If not, hand out index cards or sticky notes to everyone. Ask everyone to write out their ideas on the cards or notes (one idea per card or note). Collect the cards and notes and place them near the corresponding question. Use these ideas to facilitate dialogue toward the creation of an inquiry plan.

Anticipating Sharing Findings

It will come as no surprise when we say that decisions about sharing research findings should also be made by the collective and that all co-researchers' contributions should be recognized to the extent possible. In many cases, this will require creativity, considering multiple options and avenues for sharing what you have learned and advocating for change. It will also require careful thought and discussion about whether and how to include community co-researchers, especially those from marginalized or vulnerable groups, as authors or presenters. For example, a collaborative autoethnography about one refugee student's experiences in U.K. universities published in the prestigious *Journal of Refugee Studies* lists "R. Student" as the first author, a creative way to give the student credit for his intellectual property without jeopardizing his immigration status (Student et al., 2017). Similarly, an article describing a photovoice project with ex-prisoners lists 'Deer' as the second author, a pseudonym chosen by the participant co-author to protect her identity (Jarldorn & 'Deer,' 2017). University ethics boards will typically require the use of pseudonyms to protect participants who may, in fact, wish to use their real names in research reports. Balancing these institutional requirements and participant wishes can produce tricky dilemmas for the CPI collective.

Melissa has attempted to balance these considerations by including her research assistant Samar as a co-author and presenter (under her real name) in virtual conferences based outside of Turkey (one benefit of COVID-19 restrictions was the plethora of online conferences), where her involvement should not pose a risk. This is a valuable learning and CV-building experience for Samar, as she is interested in pursuing a PhD abroad in the future. For presentations and publications within Turkey or in Turkish that took a critical stance toward national policies or practices, Melissa served as sole author to protect her refugee participants, Samar included. As a Turkish citizen and academic with U.S. credentials, Melissa has both more influence and more legal stability on which to push for needed changes, which she seeks to leverage strategically. She also draws on her personal and professional connections to get this knowledge into the hands of those who can do something with it; for example, she shared initial findings about crucial shortcomings in the available Turkish language courses and her participants' strategies for supplementing formal learning opportunities in a webinar hosted by an association of Turkish language educators (YADOT).[3] In addition to the online photovoice exhibition mentioned earlier, Melissa presented findings regarding the role of NGOs and oversights in services intended to support refugee students at the 2021 virtual CIES conference, which draws a large segment of its an audience from nonprofit organizations and agencies. She plans to develop other practical outputs, including a white paper for policymakers and a workshop for faculty members interested in better supporting their refugee students, along with scholarly publications co-authored with interested participants. Finally, she sees this project as just the start of her work with Syrian young adults making their way in Turkey and other asylum and resettlement contexts and is pursuing external funding to expand the study into a long-term participatory advocacy effort.

CONCLUSION

In this chapter, we reinforced the relational nature of critical participatory inquiry. We offered our own experiences in the context of various CPI projects to underscore the necessity of equitable engagement rooted in dialogue and the importance of nurturing our inquiry relationships in order to provide opportunities to seek emancipatory goals together. We described several ethical considerations of working in contact zones, including thoughts on how to navigate power dynamics and when and how to disrupt assumed roles. Finally, we walked through the steps of forming and inquiry collective, identifying a focus area, and creating an inquiry plan.

SUMMARY OF KEY POINTS

- Creating positive contact zones, especially in hierarchical institutions like schools, requires intentional relationship building and negotiation of power relations among co-researchers.
- The process is characterized by open dialogue and *conscientizaçao* (critical consciousness).
- In traditional research, knowledge is controlled by and produced for academics, while in CPI, knowledge is created through a relational, dialogic process that accounts for individual and communal experience.
- CPI is, in many ways, incompatible with traditional expectations of academia, funding, and publishing. Those who commit to this approach need to identify parallel ways to meet these expectations (e.g., through publications co-authored with co-researchers) and share findings in more publicly accessible ways (such as a web-based exhibit).
- Researchers should deeply consider potential issues of power related to procedures and roles that could emerge and evolve during CPI and address these with community co-researchers.
- Consent forms can (and should) be tailored to the community's literacy practices, age, preferred language, for example. They can be co-constructed along with community members.
- Community assets and needs to be addressed through inquiry can be mapped using a variety of participatory approaches.

SUGGESTED ACTIVITIES

1. Journal about the community you are considering starting inquiry with. What types of interpersonal, institutional, or structural power dynamics, cultural differences, and language barriers might you encounter? How could you build a mutually respectful contact zone or "third space" with co-researchers and navigate roles? How can you prepare now (e.g., learning greetings in the community languages)?
2. Create a basic budget for a CPI project you have in mind. What realistic expenses do you anticipate? Could the project be done on a shoestring budget or without funding? What are some potential external sources of funding, and what are the application procedures?
3. Represent the forces that constrain you in a drawing or other visual. Label the identities, expectations, or forces that keep you acting inside that "box." What can free you? If you feel comfortable, share this with a friend or colleague and ask them for ideas.
4. Take a walk in your own community. Bring along a notepad or voice recorder. Walk slowly. Notice all the good things about your community. Write those assets down or record them.

5. Brainstorm possibilities to share project findings that are relevant to your discipline and professional setting: academic or practitioner-focused conferences, scholarly journals, reports, webinars, blogs, social media platforms—the sky is the limit! What do you need professionally, and what outlets might lead to positive change in the issue you are investigating? Also, consider how you could meaningfully and ethically include co-researchers in this stage.

KEY TERMS

dialogue
evidence
inquiry collective
known methods

ENDNOTES

1. There are multiple terms used for this population and the programs in which they are enrolled, and some are considered controversial; here, we use the terms employed by the school in which the project occurred.
2. https://melbeth27.wixsite.com/melissahauber/gallery
3. A recording of the webinar (in Turkish with auto-translated subtitles) is available at: https://www.youtube.com/watch?v=lZ2VewRh1Q8

6 GATHERING DATA AND MAKING MEANING: MAKING TRADITIONAL APPROACHES MORE PARTICIPATORY

LEARNING OBJECTIVES

By the end of this chapter, you will be able to

- Articulate the main goals of critical participatory inquiry.
- Reframe traditional data collection and analysis methods to be more participatory.
- Facilitate semi- and unstructured conversational methods, structured methods, and 'Pon the Corner methods of participatory data collection and analysis.

FOCUS ACTIVITY 6.1: EVERYDAY LIFE APPROACHES TO INQUIRY

Think of a problem you have encountered recently in your everyday, personal life. How did you go about trying to find a solution?

1. How did you "gather data"?
2. How did you analyze that data?
3. How did you arrive at findings?
4. Consider mapping out the process you went through visually. Is it clean and tidy? Or do phases of solution finding overlap?

At this point you have built (or built on) a relationship toward trust and openness through dialogue and have gathered an inquiry collective. You have come together around a common goal and have begun the ongoing process of creating knowledge equitably. The next three chapters are meant to offer practical suggestions and options for gathering data (or evidence) and making meaning of that data. We have intentionally blurred the lines between what are traditionally known as the data collection and analysis phases because in reality these are almost always blurred—conducted simultaneously or iteratively rather than in distinct and separate phases. Also, most, if not all, of the methods and techniques we suggest can be used for both data collection and analysis.[1] In addition to these blurred collection-analysis approaches, we have also interspersed purely analytic approaches (e.g., thematic analysis, narrative and visual inquiry) across each chapter. These examples are meant to show how inquirers can analyze data together with co-researchers, ensure evidence remains with and is relevant to communities, and, possibly, share findings with those outside the CPI project, including the general public, the institutional review board (IRB), academic journals, news outlets, and funders.

As always, we will start by providing some thoughts on concepts and definitions of key terms or ideas before diving into step-by-step guidance on approaches. This chapter centers on making traditional approaches to gathering data and making meaning participatory. Chapter 7 will emphasize arts-based approaches, and Chapter 8 will cover digital and multimedia approaches. While we have separated these into three categories for the purposes of communicating them through this book, in reality all of them can be combined or adapted depending on your circumstances, contexts, and local needs and practices.

CONCEPTS AND DEFINITIONAL ISSUES

Many of the methods used in a CPI project will be similar to those you may have studied in other research methods courses, like interviews, focus groups, and surveys. Similar to any research project, the overall objective is to gather data. However, the underlying rationale in using these methods may differ as we are also seeking to honor respectful relationships and improve mutual understanding and dialogue among individuals. Additionally, depending on the level of participation, participants not only provide data (e.g., narratives, art, survey responses) as they would in a traditional research project, but, as co-researchers, they can also be involved in the creation of data gathering tools (e.g., interview questions, survey forms) and analyzing data. Taking all of this into account, we need to ensure that we are gathering and analyzing data in ways that engage co-researchers respectfully so they are not left feeling as if they are simply passive producers of data. Rather, co-researchers should feel a sense of ownership and control over the protocols and processes developed. No matter what, the underlying rationale of any method used in CPI should be intersubjective understanding, which we discuss in the following section.

Intersubjective Understanding

Meagan conducted a participatory evaluation project for an Afrocentric transitional housing program for justice-involved women of Color who also have a history of addiction. After she submitted her initial report to the evaluation collective, she received feedback from one member of the team that the report seemed one-sided and included things that were patently untrue. It took Meagan a day or two to grapple with these comments from someone she considered an ally and friend—someone who understood Meagan's desire to be humble, caring, and also accurate in her inquiry. During those few days, Meagan began to realize that she had not been clear about the goal of the evaluation report. It was not to provide one truth or to draw a line between fact and fiction. Instead, it was to offer up the many varied experiences related to the transitional housing program, to center the experiences of women who had resided in the home, and to help outsiders better understand those experiences.

In our research methods classes, we refer to this understanding as **intersubjectivity, or intersubjective understanding**. In Chapter 3, we discussed the concepts of objectivity and subjectivity. Instead of equating objectivity with truth or validity and subjectivity with bias or lack of validity and truth, we introduced these concepts differently. Objectivity, we said, operates according to a principle of multiple access. That is, many individuals have access to the knowledge, culture, and language needed to understand a concept. Subjectivity, on the other hand, operates according to the principle of privileged access—unique access to knowledge that is internal to me or my world. Extending this, *inter*subjectivity relates to the idea of reaching toward greater or better understanding of another person through dialogue. Full and complete knowledge of another person or a person's position, experiences, or identity can never happen. Reaching toward understanding—that is the key.

The goal of CPI is not to establish truth; rather, it is to build or reach toward greater intersubjective understanding. This is not to say that we will not arrive at verifiable facts through our inquiry—quite the contrary. However, the primary goal of all the methods and techniques we offer in this and subsequent chapters is intersubjective understanding.

REFLEXIVITY QUESTION

How are you feeling about not pursuing "truth" as a main goal of CPI? Does this resonate with you? How does this fit into your own previous training, your disciplinary perspective, or your personal inquiry goals? Do you have concerns? Consider journaling about your goals, thoughts, and concerns, or discussing them with a trusted colleague.

Blurred Data Collection and Analysis

As you orient your inquiry toward intersubjective understanding, it is also important to debunk the myth (often anchored in scientism and positivism) that data collection and data analysis must always be separate and distinct processes. This reinforces an epistemology (how we know or come to know) that frames a university-based researcher as the expert and Knower and others as mere participants in a researcher's study. According to this view, data collection and analysis are separated from their everydayness and have become technical, dependent on an elite, "researchy" language. Think about it: Have you ever been sitting in a conference or meeting with a researcher who is reviewing evidence or findings and thought, "I'm completely lost." or "They're speaking another language!" This is not an accident! In order to maintain our status as Knowers, university-based researchers often buy into the idea that research (and all aspects of it) must be technical, set apart from the everyday, and reserved for only a select few. Hence, we use language that makes inquiry seem complex and beyond the reach of others. This practice of excluding non-researchers from inquiry processes is deeply rooted in academic circles. Think back to this chapter's opening focus activity: When you walked through a recent problem you encountered in your everyday life, the collection of data (information or evidence) and analysis of that data were not distinct phases but blurred together, right? That is often what happens in social science inquiry—particularly in participatory inquiry. We collect some data and, almost simultaneously, make meaning of or with it. As we make meaning, we may realize we need to collect more or different data, so we may change the questions we ask, approach different people, or seek other forms of data. As we do that, we interpret those data, and so forth.

As you move forward in learning techniques and approaches, remember that almost all of the methods we offer in this and the next few chapters can be used as both data collection and analysis. And they are not very fancy or technical. Recently, we presented a few of these techniques to some of our colleagues and one friend remarked, "I thought to myself, 'Oh! I can do this!'" These approaches are not reserved for those of us with the letters "PhD" after our names. They do not require extensive training or expensive equipment. They are anchored in dialogue and intended to promote equitable participation.

ETHICAL CONSIDERATIONS

Before diving into methods and techniques, let's briefly discuss how you will eventually make decisions about which methods to use, when, with whom, and why. As we make these decisions, we will center our conceptualization of ethics and urge you to always fall back on our touchstone—dialogue. Always engage in dialogue with your collective when making these decisions or when weighing options and possibilities. As you do this, it can be useful to focus on three components of the inquiry: the collective, the moment, and the audience (Figure 6.1).

FIGURE 6.1 ■ Three Components of Inquiry

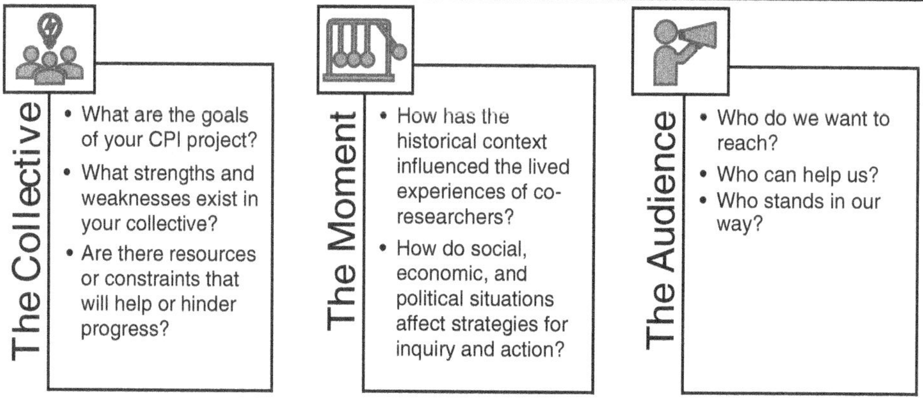

RECOMMENDED PRACTICE 6.1: APPROPRIATE, NECESSARY, HELPFUL

As you consider each of these (collective, moment, audience), ponder these three questions:

1. What is appropriate?
2. What is necessary?
3. What is helpful?

We have found that asking—and answering—these questions at the beginning of the inquiry process and then consistently as you move forward will help to keep you and the collective tethered to your ontological and epistemological commitments. Consider these questions and write them down. Make sure to include a date so you can note changes when you revisit these in the future.

Let's walk through how you might take stock of what is appropriate, necessary, and helpful for the collective, in the moment, and for your intended audience. Then, we can move into possibilities for making traditional inquiry methods more participatory. First, the collective. As you consider the many options for methods of data collection and analysis, it can be useful to remind yourselves of your goals as a collective. If you have not done so to this point, write these down somewhere you can see them. You might review them at the beginning of each meeting or put them in a place where you can see and reference them. It is also important to take stock of your collective's strengths, weaknesses, resources, and constraints. We urge you to write these down and reference them as you make decisions and engage in the inquiry process. For example, you would not want to plan to create a community survey if no one in your collective had ever done that before. Similarly, you would want to know if a member of your collective had a background in graphic design, as this would be helpful in sharing findings. You would also want to know if people have limits on their time or schedules so you can plan to hold meetings that are accessible for everyone. What if you have monetary constraints or resources? All this is crucial to know before making concrete plans. As you continuously review all these considerations, you will be in a strong position to make plans that build on your strengths, take advantage of your resources, stay true to your goals, and acknowledge your constraints.

Once you have explored everything your collective brings to the table, it can be useful to consider the moment in which your collective is conducting the inquiry. In 2020 (when we started writing this book), you would have wanted to be clear about the sociopolitical context, including the Black Lives Matter movement, the COVID-19 pandemic, various political regimes, and so on. Your collective needs to be aware of what is important to others, such as what social forces are stronger and weaker, who holds power, and what people are paying attention to. All of these contextual forces would impact how or even *if* you approach others. Remembering the historical and contemporary context of your inquiry is key.

Finally, your inquiry collective needs to consider your intended audience. Reminding yourselves of who you eventually want to reach with your inquiry will determine many of the steps you take. Are you interested in reaching academic audiences? The local community?

Community leaders? Practitioners? National policymakers? Perhaps a combination of these? Thinking strategically about who you want to influence—and why—will put you in a good position to make decisions about what you need in order to do that.

As you focus on these three points, remember to ask yourselves the following: "What is appropriate? What is necessary? What is helpful?" By asking—and answering—these questions collaboratively, you will be practicing critical, dialogic reflexivity, centering questions of ethics; and balancing your own interests with the interests, needs, and assets of the community in which you are working. As you reflect on these questions, take a look at the case studies in the Appendix, where the authors provide practical examples of how this can be done.

METHODS: SEMI- AND UNSTRUCTURED CONVERSATIONS

The good news is that if you have already taken a research methods course or two, you probably have a lot of tools in your methodological toolbelt that can be useful for CPI! If you have taken a qualitative methods course, you have learned about interviewing, and if you have taken a quantitative methods course, you have learned about surveys. Often, CPI takes some of these more "traditional" methods and reworks them a bit to make sure they are in line with the overarching goal of intersubjective understanding. This section will delve into how we can make interviews, focus groups, and surveys more participatory, democratic, and dialogic so that we can increase our mutual understanding of and with co-researchers and participants. As we offer suggestions, we will provide examples from our own and others' CPI work. Following these narrative descriptions, we will provide short, step-by-step guides for your quick reference. At the end of the chapter, we provide suggestions for further reading, including resources that may remind you of the basics of some of these methods.

Interviews as Storytelling

When we learn about developing interview protocols in introductory methods courses, we are taught to tie our interview questions to our overarching research questions and our purpose. We are also taught to stay away from leading questions (i.e., those that will steer a respondent toward what you would like to hear) and to find subtle ways to inquire about additional information (i.e., using probing or follow-up questions, nonverbal affirmations like head nodding, and verbal affirmations like "uh-huh"). These are all good tips, but some of what we are taught—such as coming up with a list of questions to be asked in the same order to all individuals (*structured interviews*)—can sometimes make an interview feel like a dry affair, divorcing it from communication and dialogue. When overly structured, the interview becomes a one-sided event where the interviewer gets what they want while the respondent may not be able to develop their own narrative. Have you ever been interviewed and thought, "When is this person going to stop asking me questions so I can finally speak?" or "I wonder why they don't ask me about this. I could tell a more interesting story if they did." Through structured interviews, although the researcher learns what they intended to learn about, it stays there—boxed in by the expertise and interest of the individual asking the questions. When we do not meaningfully involve co-researchers or simply position them as data providers, we can lose sight of the questions that are important to them and information that may lead to action.

On the other hand, if we see interviews as a form of storytelling and less as a way to simply collect responses, natural conversations can flow. This is not to say that you do not need a plan: It is still good practice to tie your interview back to the collective's research questions and purpose. When we say that it helps to see interviews as storytelling, we mean that respondents–co-researchers should have the space and control to develop their own narratives, to tell you if you are asking the wrong questions as the collective develops interview protocols or even during the interview, and to tell their stories as they please, rather than being inhibited by the interviewer's rigidity.

One example of informal conversational interviews (Patton, 2014), which include open-ended questions (i.e., those that allow for broad interpretation and let conversation flow), comes from Blodgett et al. (2010). In this example, university co-researchers and Aboriginal co-researchers in Canada worked together—refining a research agenda, developing interview guides, and analyzing data (i.e., identifying themes from interviews)—to explore community-based recommendations on how researchers could work with Aboriginal communities to design sports and exercise programs. To gather data, the collective sought to develop an interview protocol around general guiding topics and included examples of open-ended questions rather than a long list of rigid prompts. This provided space for respondents to speak about their experiences without being barraged by interviewers. Depending on the direction of the response, the interviewer could then use the general guiding topics to follow the interviewer's lead.

Responding to the open-ended nature of the questions, Aboriginal community members told stories of mainstream researchers coming in and making them feel dysfunctional because of the culturally inappropriate or insensitive questions they asked. They brought up examples of researchers collecting data and then disappearing, never to hear from the researcher again or learn how the data were being used. After gathering data, they collaboratively analyzed the interview data, showing how Aboriginal communities often felt overresearched yet misunderstood due to ineffective research strategies and the inability of mainstream researchers to develop community relationships. Based on the exploration of these themes, the collective then explored how researchers might be able to better develop relationships and take a more community-driven approach when working with Aboriginal people. In Table 6.1, we have adapted the interview guide developed by Blodgett et al. (2010) to show how this can be done (we encourage you to go straight to the source and read this article for more information). From this example, we can see how the use of informal conversational interviews was helpful because the purpose of

TABLE 6.1 ■ Informal Interview Guide (Adapted from Blodgett et al., 2010)

Interview Guide Topic	Possible Questions
Past research experience in the community	Can you describe any past research experiences you have had with outside researchers in the community?
	Could you tell me about why this research experience worked well? What could have worked better?

inquiry was exploratory (e.g., setting agendas, improving understanding around a topic, plotting feasibility for other studies or projects).

To help conversations flow during an interview, you can choose to use a *semistructured* or *unstructured* approach. With semistructured interviews, the researcher develops a few predetermined questions but then asks follow-up questions based on the participants' response. This allows the researcher to set a direction—as would be done in a structured interview where all questions are predetermined and asked in the same order—with the flexibility of the unstructured interview, where questions are not planned in advance. The collective can determine which approach would be best depending on whether it is appropriate and necessary for all individuals to answer a set of similar questions (semistructured) or whether it would be more beneficial to ask different questions as they arise (unstructured). Box 6.1 is a step-by-step guide to help you design your interview.

BOX 6.1: STEP-BY-STEP: DESIGNING INTERVIEWS

In this example, we outline how an interview could be developed. The steps here are outlined for explanatory purposes. These steps do not need to be followed precisely but offer some insight into how you could go about collaboratively developing an interview protocol that is grounded in methodological thinking and epistemologically consistent with CPI.

Step 1. Hold unstructured conversations with co-researchers to explore topics of interest. This step can often flow naturally when you speak with acquaintances or those in your networks. In reality, you may not even know you are conducting this step, as inquiry can often arise when we least expect it (e.g., having coffee with a friend, venting about community issues with a neighbor, speaking to a student about school expectations).

Step 2. Invite co-researchers to a brainstorming session to workshop questions. Brainstorming sessions can be unstructured, or you can follow one of the structured activities in the next section of this chapter (e.g., ripples of change, card priority sorting).

Step 3. After identifying concepts—these can be problems or issues to solve, strengths to amplify, strategies to define and refine, or co-researchers' hopes and expectations—develop questions. Question development can be a daunting task, especially if it is your first CPI project or you are not familiar with methodology. To formulate questions in a systematic way but still allow for the flexibility needed to let conversations flow, we often use Carspecken's (1996) critical ethnographic approach to interviewing. Here are a few tips on question development:

a. *Identify topic domain.* As you have identified important concepts, this will allow you to identify a *topic domain.* Topic domains are broad categories of interest (e.g., students' classroom experiences, neighbors' perceptions of police violence). Your interview questions should be broadly applicable to your topic domain, which is like a signpost to keep you on track.

b. *Develop a lead-off question.* A lead-off question is often called a "grand tour" question. It is open-ended and allows respondents to develop their own narrative. It often starts like this: "Could you tell me about your experience?" or "Can you recall a time when . . . ?". Remember that it is important to offer respondents space to develop their own story.

c. *List covert categories. Covert categories* are one more way to keep us on track. These are topics that the co-researchers would like interviewees to speak about but that will not be asked explicitly, as it may lead the discussion toward the interviewer's preconceived notions. The covert categories include participants' views of participatory research; participants' views of performance as a liberating, empowering, or transformative experience; and participants' implicit theories of power and privilege.

Co-constructing questions can be approached in a number of ways. Here are two examples that can be followed as is or mixed and matched:

a. *Free form*: Ask co-researchers to each develop a few interview questions. This can be done on their own time or when you meet as a group. Collect the questions and vote on the most relevant and appropriate ones for the collective. Refine the questions as a group—this is where bits and pieces of one individual's question can help to refine the question posed by another.
b. *Refinement and validation*: The lead researcher or a group of co-researchers can develop interview questions and then pose them to the larger collective. Collective members then select those that are most relevant and appropriate and continue to refine them as a group.

Focus Groups as Conversations and Community Consultation

In addition to interviews, we often learn about focus group discussions or group dialogue as a primary data collection method. Focus groups can be structured similarly to interviews, in that you can take a more or less structured approach, but as the name suggests, these conversations happen in a group setting (usually between six and 12 participants). Also, focus groups are helpful for talking about topics that individuals are familiar with but that are not particularly sensitive (Merriam & Tisdell, 2015): You would not want to cause harm or discomfort to participants by asking them about things that they would not want others to know about. Although interviews can be intimidating in that you are face-to-face with just one person, focus groups require additional skills for effective facilitation and moderation. It is important to ensure that all individuals feel comfortable speaking (e.g., think about power dynamics if elected officials and constituents are in the same group) or that you frame questions in culturally appropriate and respectful ways. Much of this can be mitigated with proper planning—asking co-researchers or community members about how questions should be worded or who can be in a group together so conversation is not stymied. Lastly, prior to holding a focus group, it is always a good idea to pilot your question guide with co-researchers or individuals who are familiar with the topic and community where you are conducting inquiry.

As an example of how a focus group discussion can be used for community consultation, in one project, Giovanni invited former political prisoners in Burma/Myanmar to discuss strategies for societal reintegration after prison release. In this case, the focus group format was helpful because community members shared similar experiences (i.e., imprisonment for political demonstrations and human rights work), were fairly homogenous (i.e., shared similar political motivations and socioeconomic status), and were comfortable speaking about the topic of reintegration in front of one another. The community consultation format was mentioned to community gatekeepers—staff from an organization assisting former political prisoners (staff were also former political prisoners themselves)—and they discussed its utility. Rather than dictating the direction of inquiry and action, it was decided that the community consultation would be used to outline priority areas and types of assistance that the affected group would consider relevant for their own societal reintegration.

Community consultations can be utilized for a number of collaborative purposes, from co-creating consent forms (see Box 6.2) to setting the agenda for your CPI project to gathering and analyzing data. Additionally, community consultations do not need to follow a particular format; rather, you can integrate traditional practices to maintain cultural relevance for those involved. In his work in Guatemala, Giovanni learned that Kaqchikel community members use oral traditions, such as *story/sharing circles*, and their collective used this as a way for community members to tell their stories about their lost loved ones and outline priorities for their community memorial site. In a way, story circles can be likened to focus groups, but there are several important differences (Kovach, 2009). As Margaret Kovach (2009), an academic of Plains Cree and Saulteaux ancestry, notes, many communities consider the story circle to be a sacred ritual or ceremony; thus, it is important that you consider whether those you are working alongside already use this method in their daily lives. If so, it is important to respect the process and how this is conducted (e.g., does it begin with prayer or an offering before individuals speak?). If not, it is important to consider whether it is appropriate to export it to another cultural setting. If you do, it is necessary to detail the history of the method you use and to give credit where it is due.

BOX 6.2: STEP-BY-STEP: CO-CREATING CONSENT FORMS

Prior to gathering any data, you can co-create consent forms with a group during a community consultation. By co-creating consent forms during the community consultation, you can concretely ground your CPI project in the principle of *reciprocity* (Mertens, 2009)—balancing researcher and community needs. Rather than handing participants–co-researchers a consent form and asking them to sign it, the co-creation of consent forms embeds community ownership and control into the inquiry design process.

Step 1. After introducing the purpose of the community consultation, ask participants if they are familiar with consent forms (remember, consent forms are used in academic settings, so participants might not be familiar with their purpose). If not, explain that consent forms describe how information will be protected (confidentiality and/or anonymity) and how data are stored and used.

Step 2. Explain to co-researchers that you would like to co-create consent forms to ensure that they are able to dictate how their data (e.g., stories, photos, art, videos) are used for this project and beyond.

Step 3. After opening this is up discussion or a question-and-answer session, begin co-creating the form. This can be done in a number of ways:

a. *Full co-creation.* Ask participants for what they would like to see in the consent form. If participants are unfamiliar, outline several areas that are needed—e.g., confidentiality and privacy, how data are used, and how long data will be used. Write out ideas and phrases on a flipchart. Write out or type the entire consent form so the group can then view it and refine wording if needed.

b. *Refinement and additions.* If participants are more comfortable refining a consent form, you can also start with a template. This helps if you have certain requirements from your IRB or organization. In this case, you can go through each section of the form and discuss revisions and additions. Use a projector or large screen to display the consent form to the group, and then make changes on your computer so the entire group can see what is being done.

Step 4. Print and invite all co-researchers to sign their own copy of the consent form. This can be easily done by holding a coffee or tea break after ***Step 3***. During the break, participants can sign their forms and request a copy. Reconvene and continue using the community consultation for collaborative data gathering and analysis.

Second, unlike focus groups, the moderator or leader does not interrupt or steer the conversation. Instead, the group sharing circle is an open conversational method. The moderator can simply ask one open-ended question at the start of the circle, and each individual then tells their story without interruption. Whoever is speaking has the time and space to develop their own narrative, without prompts. This is quite difficult if you have been trained to conduct interviews or focus groups because it requires you to listen to what individuals would like to tell you rather than press for what you would like to hear. Even if the individual seems like they are starting to deviate from your question, it is important to give each person their space because you never know what they would like to tell you or how they tell stories (i.e., some people are straightforward, while others follow a more circuitous process). After an individual is done, they can then pass to the next person. See Box 6.3 for a step-by-step guide to using storytelling in your CPI work.

BOX 6.3: STEP-BY-STEP: STORYTELLING AS DATA

Storytelling presents co-researchers with the space to develop their own narrative. Rather than the usual format—the interviewer or moderator asks a question, waits for a response, asks others if they agree or disagree, follows up with another question, calls on an individual to speak, then repeats the process—storytelling (e.g., oral traditions, story/sharing circles, spoken word) places more control in the hands of the speaker. Remember, some communities may consider a storytelling practice, such as a story circle, to be sacred (Kovach, 2009). Prior to utilizing any method, it is important to understand if and how it is or is not a part of a group's cultural practices. Recall that the methods we use in CPI can draw from everyday ways of knowing and creating knowledge. Before using any method, though, it is important to grapple with whether your use of a method could be seen as appropriation or co-optation.

Step 1. Acknowledge the history and tradition of the storytelling practice. Explain how the process will work to participants (prior to this, the collective can decide the best method for facilitation). It is important to note that sharing is voluntary: Participants should not be pushed to share if they are not comfortable. Ask all participants to confirm that they will listen when others speak and not to interrupt. From your consent form, it should be clear if video or audio recording or note-taking are appropriate.

Step 2. Pose an open-ended question to the group. In Giovanni's work in Guatemala, the following co-created question was posed: What was the significance of having a family member identified during the forensic process? (How) has it changed your life?

Step 3. Invite the first individual to speak. Remember that cultural traditions should be followed. In some cultures, elders or those with a particular title are invited to speak first (prior to the session, this is a helpful point to discuss with co-researchers). Actively listen as the individual tells their story. Give them space to pause and reflect.

Step 4. As the first individual ends, invite the next speaker, or invite the first speaker to choose the next. Repeat ***Step 3*** until all have had a chance to speak or pass.

Step 5. Depending on the amount of time or the structure of your session, you can facilitate a collaborative data analysis or reflection session with the group. If conducted immediately after, details from stories will still be fresh in participants' minds. Conducting this immediately after is also helpful in that participants can ask questions to others, if clarification is needed for interpretation and understanding (remember, you are trying to improve intersubjective understanding). Here are a few questions to prompt discussion and reflection:

- **a.** Did you notice any similarities (i.e., what researchers often refer to as themes) across the stories that were told?
- **b.** Were they any surprises?
- **c.** Did a particular individual's story call out to you?
- **d.** Are there any points where you would like additional clarification, or would you like to ask anyone a specific question?

Step 6. Compile data and share back with the group, immediately after or on another day. Continue to refine and use stories as data.

METHODS: STRUCTURED ACTIVITIES

In addition to adapting these traditional approaches to data collection for participatory use, there are several collaborative data collection and analysis methods that we have found useful in our inquiry work. These approaches are designed to enable university-based and community co-researchers to gather data in a structured way. These can be used to generate project ideas, assess needs and assets, determine questions and priorities, and serve as alternatives to standard data gathering approaches such as interviews.

Brainstorming Through Ripples of Change

Ripples of change (Action Aid, n.d.) is a helpful, structured way to define and differentiate concepts. In this activity, the facilitator prepares three concentric circles (or more, depending on the levels of change to be discussed). This can be done using tape on a floor or drawing circles on a flipchart or poster board (see Figure 6.2). Participants are then asked to write or draw concepts and place them in the circles, depending on the level of change. To make this method more participatory, group members can be invited to define each level of change. For instance, if you are evaluating the outcomes of a project, co-researchers may want to understand micro/personal, meso/community, or macro/policy level changes. If you are trying to understand co-researchers' expected priorities for change, there may be an interest in understanding how change would take place within various institutions or among certain people (micro/by students, meso/by school administrators, macro/by school board officials).

In Giovanni's work in Guatemala, co-researchers used the ripples of change method to explore priorities for their community memorial site. The following question was co-created during a community consultation and then explored during a collaborative data gathering and analysis session: "What are your hopes for your memorial over the next five years?" Co-researchers then defined two levels of change: (1) personal or individual-level hope or outcome (inside the circle) or (2) larger scale or community-based or external to the memorial (outside the circle). Co-researchers were then asked to write or illustrate these changes on cards (one concept per card). If a co-researcher was not print literate

FIGURE 6.2 ■ Cards Detailing "What Needs to Change" Across Three Different Levels

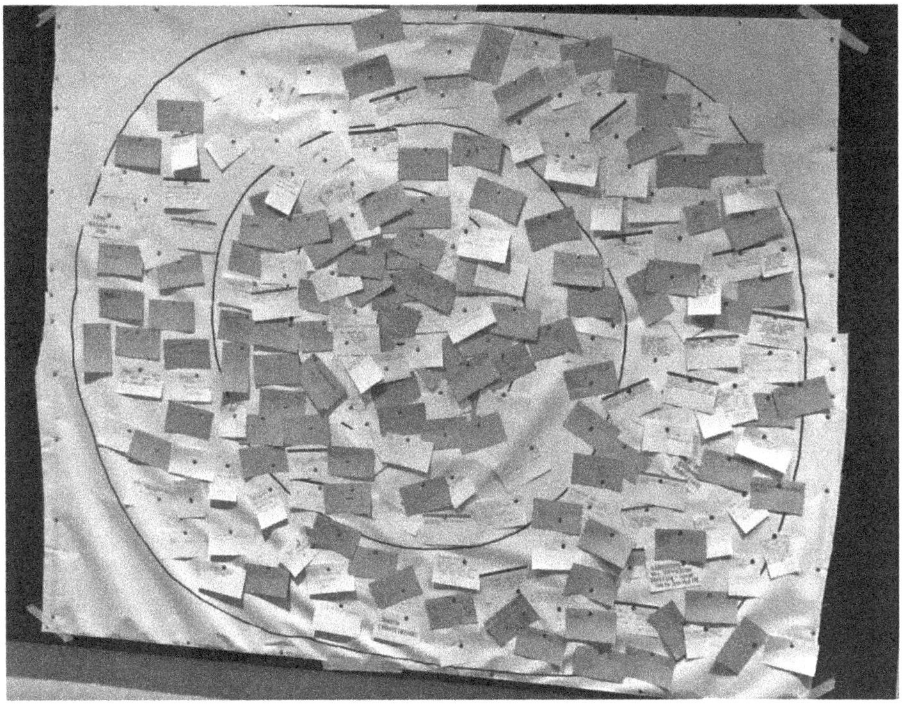

or did not feel comfortable drawing on a card, other co-researchers were ready to assist. Co-researchers then placed their cards in the ripple where they felt it belonged. We then used the cards to facilitate a discussion on these expectations. To facilitate discussion, several exploratory questions were used: "Why did you place this card in this circle?" "Are there any other cards with similar ideas?" "What types of priorities seem significant to you?" "Is anything missing?" During this collective analysis session, several co-researchers listened and took notes. These notes, along with the actual index cards, were then used to co-construct themes (see Box 6.4). With this method, co-researchers reinforced their expectations for the memorial going forward, and through reflection and analysis, they had data to (1) form an action plan, (2) determine the actions or roles that nonprofit staff and community members should take, and (3) explore what types of outcomes may be sustainable given available resources.

Many of the interactive, structured activities in this section (e.g., ripples of change, card sorting) will produce a significant amount of data (see Figure 6.2, which displays the hundreds of cards written by high school students during a *Courageous Conversations* event). When moving into meaning making, it is important to consider how your collective will demonstrate these points, depending on the audience you seek to inform or influence. For instance, policymakers or funders may not have time to come to your office and view all cards from a ripples of change activity. Or you may be responding to a call for proposals where a funder would like you to synthesize your preliminary data, so they can decide whether your initiative aligns to their goals. In these cases, thematic analysis (Braun & Clarke, 2006) is one way to organize and visualize data. Just as we have done with other methods, we do caution you to consider whether this analytic method is culturally appropriate, as some communities may not believe that data should be reduced to categories.

BOX 6.4: STEP-BY-STEP: COLLABORATIVE THEMATIC ANALYSIS

The steps below summarize the helpful steps outlined by Braun and Clarke (2006), adapted as a collaborative thematic analysis activity.

Step 1. Organize data in a way that allows co-researchers to view and familiarize themselves with it. This can be done in several ways, depending on the size and orientation of the group: taking photos of each card and uploading the digital files to a shared folder; typing up notes from each card in various colored cells in a spreadsheet (helpful if different colors were used to differentiate co-researcher identities, e.g., students/teachers/administrators, elders/youth); posting the flipchart in a room and having space for co-researchers to view it and take notes. During this step, you can ask co-researchers to make initial notes based on their observations of the cards. This is like the process of generating initial codes. Later in this chapter, you will see a photo of an index card that reads: "Adults need to learn that just because I'm young doesn't mean what I think isn't important" (see Figure 6.5). Co-researchers may construct a number of initial codes from this piece of data and similar cards: for example, adults do not listen to youth,; youth do not feel listened to, youth have important things to say, power dynamics between adults and youth. As you can see, these initial codes pull out semantic features within this piece of data.

Step 2a. Facilitate a discussion to learn what co-researchers see. It is often helpful to have a series of questions to facilitate dialogue among the group. This can be done collaboratively by asking the group to communicate their exploratory questions. Examples include the following: "Do you see similar ideas expressed across cards (i.e., convergent themes)?" "Are there any ideas that only show up once or a few times, but seem significant (i.e., outliers)?" "Are any ideas counter to one another (i.e., divergent issues)?" "Does anything seem surprising?" "Are any topics missing?" During this step, it is important to have a few co-researchers acting as notetakers. One individual can write themes or important ideas on a flipchart or whiteboard so the entire group can see, while other notetakers write in notebooks. This will deepen opportunities for collective meaning making while also facilitating the report writing or data sharing process.

Step 2b. After it seems like the collective has exhausted dialogue around initial coding, ideas can be systematically organized in groups, often called themes. This is the next step after initial coding and discussion. As a unit of analysis, themes provide a broader interpretation of the data. As mentioned by Braun and Clarke (2006), it is important to work through the entire data set (e.g., all interviews, all index cards). When searching for themes, it is often helpful to visualize it through mapping. This can be done by connecting main themes to smaller subthemes or units that make it up. Let's take for example the case of the card in Figure 6.5 ("adults need to learn"): If there are quite a few cards expressing a similar sentiment, it is possible that the idea, "adults need to learn from youth" could be a unifying theme for a number of subthemes (e.g., power differentials between adults and youth, youth do not feel listened to, adults do not listen to youth, youth feel disenfranchised, youth have ideas for outlets to voice their opinions to adults).

Step 4. After generating themes and a conceptual map, it is necessary to review these themes with the group. The exploratory questions in ***Step 2a*** can be revisited here to ensure the group's thematic map represents the data.

Step 5. Once themes have been constructed, it is often helpful to define and name themes. This is an important step before sharing your data with an outside audience.

Step 6. Reporting can be done in a number of ways, including policy briefs, infographics, data postcards (i.e., small cards with a printout of important themes and representative quotes). Recall that it is important to consider who your collective is interested in reaching.

Brainwriting Through Card (Priority) Sorting

Card sorting activities (Chambers, 2002) can be used to prioritize various data pieces—from themes (as identified during community consultations or interviews), community needs and assets (when discussing these topics with co-researchers or in surveys) or ranking the most pressing problems to address through inquiry and action. Prioritizing concepts can be achieved through dialogue, but at times a structured activity may help. For instance, imagine you have students who feel uneasy about speaking out in front of classmates or you are discussing sensitive topics and community members do not want to draw attention to themselves while identifying a particular problem. With card sorting, these concerns can be mitigated through a structured activity that calls for **brainwriting**. Much like a brainstorming session, which provides an opportunity for group members to build off the thoughts of others, brainwriting provides quiet time so individuals have time to compose their thoughts on cards and then discuss these with others. This is an excellent alternative to focus groups or brainstorming if you want each co-researcher to have a chance to contribute to the conversation without individuals feeling pressured to speak out.

To prioritize inquiry for the *Courageous Conversations* collective, we had university-based co-researchers work with high school co-researchers to prioritize topics of inquiry. During these sessions, university co-researchers mentioned various aspects of a participatory event, from the transformative nature of spoken word poetry to the actions that students might take as a result of inquiry. After each university co-researcher mentioned their idea, all co-researchers – university and high school based—were asked to write their thoughts on cards without speaking to other members of the group (i.e., brainwriting) for about seven minutes. To ensure university co-researchers' topics were appropriate, necessary, and helpful for the collective, we asked high school co-researchers to then prioritize the ideas and questions on cards as high, medium, or low priority. By using card sorting, all co-researchers contributed to the discussion without exposing their initial thoughts. Additionally, as a way to prioritize ideas for inquiry, this served as member checking (Stake, 1995). By having high school co-researchers prioritize data without interruption from university co-researchers, we were also intentionally redistributing power and control of the inquiry process. Once cards were prioritized, this approach provided a natural space to launch into dialogue as a group and to discuss where views converged or diverged. Box 6.5 offers a step-by-step guide for this activity.

BOX 6.5: STEP-BY-STEP: CARD (PRIORITY) SORTING

Card sorting provides a quick and easy way to prioritize concepts with co-researchers and community members. This structured and timed brainwriting activity can be used to prompt individuals' thoughts and ideas, without the pressure to speak out in a larger group.

Step 1. Explain the method of card (priority) sorting to participants. Topics to prioritize can range from (but are not limited to) needs, problems, assets, expected outcomes, and hopes.

Step 2. Provide participants with index cards or Post-it Notes. Ask participants to write or draw their thoughts, questions, and ideas about the topic being discussed on the cards or notes. To facilitate prioritization, it helps if participants include only one concept per card or note (if multiple ideas are included on one card or note, it becomes difficult to prioritize). Provide a set time for participants to compose their thoughts—5 to 7 minutes often works well (*tip*: provide 7 minutes to start and reduce time as participants get used to the method).

Step 3. Ask participants to throw their cards in a pile and shuffle the cards. After shuffling the cards, evenly distribute cards to participants. Then, ask participants to prioritize cards in order of importance.

Step 4. After cards have been prioritized, use this as an opportunity to verify or spot-check priorities through group discussion. Continue discussions until all cards have been compared and prioritized.

Troubling Theories of Change

If you have had to manage or evaluate a program (Weiss, 1995) or have worked in a nonprofit or philanthropic setting, the term "theory of change" may be familiar to you. When creating a theory of change, we are often tasked with envisioning the outcomes we would like to see across a period of time—from the short to medium and long term. After thinking about and writing down what we would like to see happen (outcomes), we can then reflect on what needs to occur for these outcomes to actually come about (preconditions). By noting these preconditions and how they relate to each outcome, we can start to theorize a pathway toward change. This is a helpful strategy when we know what we would like to see happen but we are not quite sure how to get there.

During their work on *Courageous Conversations*, Giovanni and Meagan worked with high school co-researchers to envision how schools in the United States could be more empowering places for students. As we sat in a classroom after the school day ended, we discussed what high school students would like to see happen. We asked, "What do you want to see happen at your school?" As you can see in Figure 6.3, we noted tangible outcomes like an open-door policy

FIGURE 6.3 ■ Courageous Conversations Researchers Create Their Theory of Change for Empowering Schools in the United States

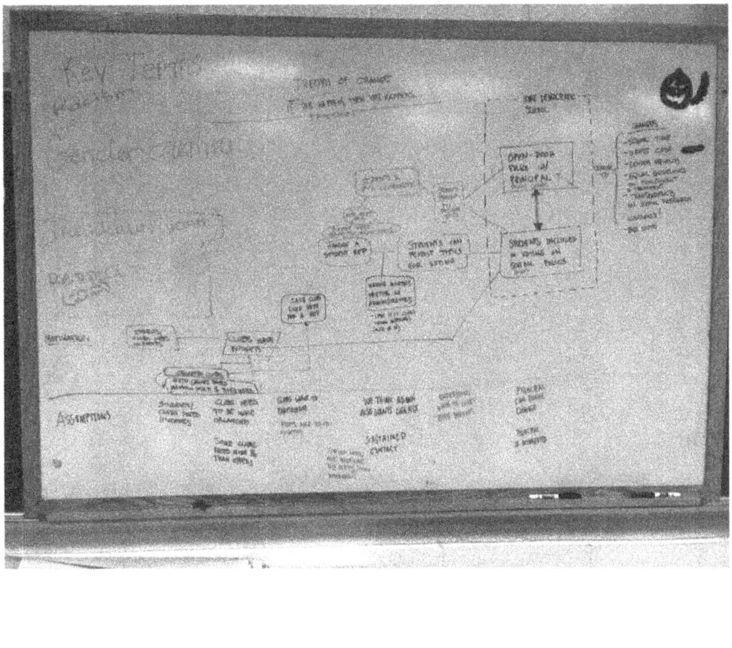

with administrators or including students when the school board votes on school policies. From there, we worked backward. We asked, "What needs to happen for this outcome to occur?" "Who do we need to work with?" "Who has power to change this?" "What do we need to do this work and succeed?" As we wrote down these preconditions and intermediate outcomes, our collective also started noting themes that came up in our discussion (e.g., gender equality, racism, respect, individual growth) and the assumptions behind our theory (i.e., how we think preconditions, outcomes, and goals are linked to one another). Through dialogue and mapping out our theory on a whiteboard, it helped the collective to document possible priorities, strategies, and needs.

METHODS: 'PON THE CORNER RESEARCH

Some of the most useful data collection and analysis can happen quickly and "on the fly." In our own inquiry, we have struggled to balance more structured methods with those that are flexible and can reach large groups of people quickly. One of the ways we have done this is through what we can 'Pon the Corner Research—that is, research that can literally be done on street corners!

In order to use these methods, it is important to make sure you have the right people on your team. You want buy-in from people whose corners you will be occupying. Whether they are full-fledged members of your collective or friends, key informants, or allies, you will need them on your side to help you gain access to communities in appropriate and ethical ways. You would never want to perpetuate a colonizing or extractive (or just plain weird) approach to inquiry by showing up in a community to which you have no connection or to which no one in a position of authority has given you access. This would be uncomfortable at best and unethical, damaging, or even unsafe at worst.

In the following sections, we describe several possibilities for methods that we have tried out in our own inquiry or that we have seen done well by people and groups we trust and respect. You will see that all of these are derived from some version of the traditional survey yet are markedly different in that they are created by and for the community members whom we (in CPI) see as experts and knowers. Also, these methods take an appreciative approach to inquiry, which is a hallmark of CPI. They are not asking what a community does *not* have. Rather, they focus on the assets of a community and elicit the thoughts, ideas, perspectives, and voices of those who are closest to an issue, problem, or phenomenon. As you consider these as options for your own participatory inquiry, we urge you to make them your own—adapt them to your own contexts, circumstances, and goals.

Mini Community Surveys

Earlier in this chapter, we discussed the use of surveys to gather information from community members. Unlike longer surveys, shorter, "mini" community surveys can be a great way to garner a lot of information in a short amount of time (see Box 6.6 for a step-by-step guide to mini surveys). First, we have to be very clear that these surveys are not meant to be the kind of validated instrument that some of our colleagues would argue are most appropriate for social inquiry. Instead, these are meant to gather targeted information from a wide swath of people in a short amount of time. There are, however, examples of larger scale surveys conducted by collectives (Fine et al., 2021; Stoudt, 2014, 2016). As Fine et al. (2021) note, survey methods require the inquirer to grapple with questions related to statistical (re)presentation (e.g., appropriateness of categorizing demographic data, pushing against the minimization or erasure of statistical outliers).

BOX 6.6: STEP-BY-STEP: MINI COMMUNITY SURVEYS

Mini community surveys are a great way to gather a lot of information in a short amount of time, usually around a targeted or narrow focus or topic. These can help you gather valuable information from a wide variety of people or from a targeted population.

Step 1: Once your collective has decided to do a mini community survey, discuss who you need to collect data from—who you need to reach.

Step 2: Write the survey. Brainstorm questions and different ways of asking the questions.

Step 3: Finalize the questions you will ask, the order in which you will ask them, and the ways you will use to ask them. Will you use a Likert-type scale? Open-ended questions? Other ways?

Step 4: Back track: Go back to your finalized survey. Make sure the questions you ask all contribute to your interests. Are there any that are not really necessary? If so, strike those. Is there anything missing? Make sure your final survey fits on one sheet of paper so they are quick for people to fill out.

Consider Meagan's work on her *Courageous Conversations* YPAR project. During the third year of the project, the collective found themselves at a crossroads. Up to that point they had been operating according to an understanding that students at the school did not feel like they were being heard by teachers. Much of the work they did revolved around this understanding, yet they wondered if they were missing anything. They did not want to move in a direction that was not in keeping with what the student body at their high school would deem appropriate or useful, so they decided to write a quick, one-page survey that would help them better understand where to go next. Because one of the members of their collective was a teacher at the school, she had the access needed to distribute the surveys to each student in the school through their English classrooms. In less than one week, each of the over 2,500 students in the school had the opportunity to fill out the survey. The collective also asked a friend who was a teacher at another school to pass out the survey to her students. In this way, they could compare responses to see what was specific to their school versus what might be a more widespread issue of concern.

Figure 6.4 is one of the more than 370 completed surveys the *Courageous Conversations* collective received back from students at their school. In about one week, the inquiry collective gathered a ton of information about how students feel heard and by whom. They were able to see trends related to gender identity, grade, and racial/ethnic identity, and they received some interesting insights about what students would say if they felt like they were heard through the last, open-ended question, "If you could say one thing and the whole world would listen, what would you say?"

Overall, the collective reached two conclusions that were new to the group. First, they noticed through their analysis of the survey results that students were more inclined to feel heard by their classroom teachers but less sure of being heard by administrators. This led the collective to focus their efforts on engaging administrators in future work. Second, the collective noticed

FIGURE 6.4 ■ Youth Respond to a Schoolwide Survey

Circle either Yes or No based on your GENERAL experience at your current school:

Do you feel like your **teachers** want to hear your opinions?	(Yes)	No
Do you feel like your **administrators** want to hear your opinions?	Yes	(No)
Do you feel like your **teachers** value your voice?	(Yes)	No
Do you feel like your **administrators** value your voice?	Yes	(No)
Would your **teachers** support you if you wanted to protest or make your voice heard through a public display (public protest or gathering, school walkout, etc.)?	Yes	(No)
Would your **administrators** support you if you wanted to protest or make your voice heard through a public display (public protest or gathering, school walkout, etc.)?	Yes	(No)
Have you ever felt silenced at school?	(Yes)	No
Have you ever NOT said something or expressed yourself at School because you thought you would not be heard?	(Yes)	No
Have you ever NOT done or said something related to your identity (race, gender identity, ethnicity, immigration status, religious affiliation, political affiliation, etc.) because you thought you would be silenced?	Yes	(No)

Where do you go to school? [redacted]

What grade are you in? 10

What's your gender identity? Female

What's your racial and/or ethnic identity? White

What other identities are important for us to know about you? ______

If you could say one thing and the whole world would listen, what would you say?

School, Should not be a place where Kids are Scared.

that over 60% of the students that filled out surveys answered the last question, "If you could say one thing and the whole world would listen, what would you say?" with some version of "I don't know" or "I don't have anything to say." At first, members of the collective thought students just did not want to answer the question or did not want to take the time to think deeply. The more they reviewed the surveys, however, the more strongly they felt that perhaps students are so used to not being asked their opinions or being put into a position of *learner* rather than *knower* that they stopped valuing their own voices, thoughts, and opinions. The collective wondered: If students felt their voices were not valued by others, did they stop valuing their own voices? This led the collective to place greater emphasis in their inquiry work on helping students articulate their own thoughts and see the value in their own experiences and perspectives.

Analyzing survey data is one area where the blurriness between data collection and meaning making tends to fade but not entirely disappear (see Box 6.7). As researchers, we generally hold a survey open for a particular amount of time (e.g., 3 weeks), and then wait for responses to come in before analyzing data. However, as CPI is grounded in multiple perspectives, analysis should be conducted by members of the collective. This means that collective meaning making generates additional data as group members question variables, constructs, and categories.

BOX 6.7: STEP-BY-STEP: ANALYZING COMMUNITY SURVEYS

In this box, we note several steps you can take to facilitate participatory survey analysis. For a more nuanced view, we encourage you to read Brett Stoudt's (2014, 2016) work on *stats-n-action.*

Step 1: Determine how data will be input. With the evolution of online survey tools, the need for data input has been minimized. However, if survey data must be collected through paper surveys, it is important to determine who will receive guidance and payment for data input. As Stoudt (2016), data input can actually be a generative meaning making activity as members of the collective are able "to read and respective individual surveys as whole people" (p. 192).

Step 2: Before beginning the analysis process, it is helpful to reorient the group with the type of data that were collected. It is helpful to go over the survey questions and the types of potential responses (e.g., open-ended, checkboxes, scales).

Step 3: After revisiting the data, the lead facilitator(s) can project the dataset to the group. In our experience working with youth, it is often helpful to have several sessions to demonstrate how survey data can be analyzed through various tools (e.g., Microsoft Excel, Google Sheets, SPSS). If a smaller group within the collective is interested, they can take on the role of analysts, utilizing software to compute descriptive and inferential statistics. Examples of analyses can include

- Tables showing descriptive statistics based on respondents' self-identifying demographic categories (e.g., gender identity, race/ethnicity). Consider whether you include checkboxes or open-ended responses.
- Computing correlations to show how marginalized and minoritized groups may be subjected to higher levels of discrimination than dominant groups. When composing charts, it may be necessary to show each demographic group on a separate visual.

Comparing different minoritized groups on one graphic may cause your audience to diminish the effects that discrimination may have for one group over another.

Step 4: Once the group has conducted their preliminary analysis, data outputs (e.g., tables, cross-tabulations) should be brought back to the group for interpretation and meaning making. This is an important step—analysis should not end with the output generated by the chosen software; it should generate dialogue among the group.

Step 5: Back track: Go back to the data outputs. As you facilitate a discussion on these outputs, it is important to ensure that the collective questions data that may normally be disregarded during typical quantitative analysis (e.g., outliers). As Fine et al. (2021), it is important that contradictions are not flattened. Rather than always seeking consensus, dialogue provides a space to "unearth and work through a wide range of perspectives; *a mosaic of counter-stories and outliers*" (p. 354). This can be helpful in questioning constructs such as gender to seeing pushing beyond binary interpretations often constructed through numerical data.

Whiteboard or Notecard Statements

Similar to mini community surveys, whiteboard or notecard statements can be a powerful method for gathering a lot of information in a short period of time (see Box 6.8). More than mini surveys, though, these statements are really targeted to answering just one question. These can help at any stage of the inquiry process, especially when your collective might be stuck on how to start, where to focus your energies or resources, what to do next, or how to share findings. In addition, this method can be a quick way to conduct an assessment of needs and assets.

BOX 6.8: STEP-BY-STEP: WHITEBOARD OR NOTECARD STATEMENTS

These statements can be useful, informal ways to get a lot of people involved in offering their experience (expertise), opinions, and thoughts on a given topic or area of interest. They are easy to use in a community, where real people with real lived experience are.

Step 1: Once your collective has decided to do this, discuss from whom you need to collect data—whom you need to reach.

Step 2: Brainstorm on the one question you will ask people to respond to on whiteboards or notecards. Narrow it down to just *one* question.

Step 3: Decide where you will go in the community and when to maximize the reach of this method. Vary days, times, and locations. Aim for at least three different data collection opportunities.

Perhaps your collective knows a lot about the needs of a particular population or community of interest. Needs are often well known and well documented by governmental organizations and groups because they typically take a deficit perspective of minoritized and historically disenfranchised populations: Where do they fall short? What do they not have? What do we need to give them? and so on. In order to focus more on assets and take an appreciative perspective, consider having a table at a Saturday farmers market or getting permission to set up an informal block party in the neighborhood you are interested in—even in the lobby of a hospital or before or after religious services. You may even do two or three of these on different days and at different times over the course of 1 or 2 weeks to catch as many people and perspectives as you can. Once you have decided where and when, the rest is easy. Get your hands on several whiteboards and markers, sheets of paper, or notecards. Find a way to display those that have been submitted—this could be on a corkboard—simply pin papers to it as they are completed. Or take pictures of statements on whiteboards and then erase them as use them again. Pictures can be uploaded onto a public website or blog and shared widely with community members as well as policymakers and other leaders.

The big decision is what to ask people to answer or reflect on. For the *Courageous Conversations* project, we asked students what they would say to administrators or other adults if they felt like they would listen and take action.

Within less than 30 minutes we collected hundreds of notecards, each with a statement directed at adults. Figure 6.5 says, "Adults need to learn that just because I'm young doesn't mean what I think isn't important." By gathering these perspectives and voices, we were able not only to better understand what students thought and how they felt, but also what they wanted our collective to communicate to the adults in their lives. We clarified who our audience was—or who it should be—based on what our community told us.

Banner Statements

Similar to whiteboard and notecard statements, banner statements allow inquiry collectives to take an appreciative approach (nondeficit oriented) to data collection and analysis (see Box 6.9). The goal of this method is to put the power into the hands of those responding to a question or prompt. The prompt should be really open-ended to see where respondents place focus. For *Courageous Conversations*, students were again asked the question, "If you could say anything and the whole world would listen, what would you say?" We put out all sorts of markers, papers,

FIGURE 6.5 ■ "Adults Need to Learn"

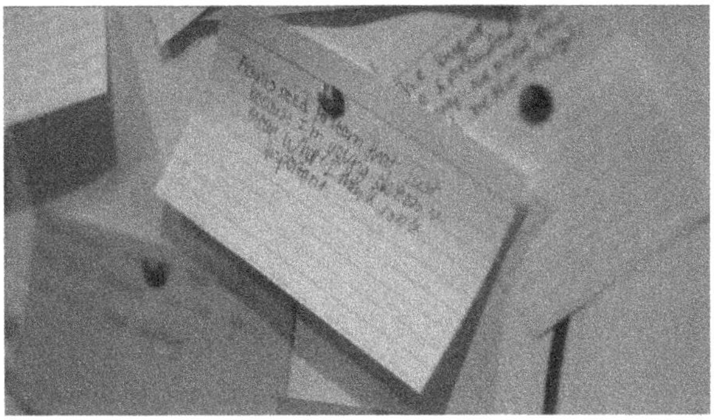

and art supplies in a hallway during one of our day-long arts-based inquiry workshops. When students were not busy doing something else, they could stop there and create a banner. Some worked on banners alone, while others worked in groups. They sat or lay on the floor working. Some took just a few minutes and others spent an hour crafting their messages. They all were clear, though, in what they were communicating. The students who created the banners in Figures 6.6 and 6.7, for example, were speaking directly to policymakers about the treatment of Hispanic and Latinx community members.

The banners created helped our collective understand that we needed to make sure to focus on issues of stereotyping and race and ethnicity-based bullying in our future work. They also became tools to help us share our findings. Although we did not have the opportunity because of the COVID-19 pandemic that broke out in 2020 shortly after these were created, we could have presented these banners at school board or immigration policy meetings as a way to advocate for student-centered policy recommendations at the local, state, and federal policy levels. However, because the pandemic forced the majority of our *Courageous Conversations* work to go virtual, we posted much of the data that we collected online, which helped us share our findings to wider audiences.

FIGURE 6.6 ■ "Just BC I'm Hispanic"

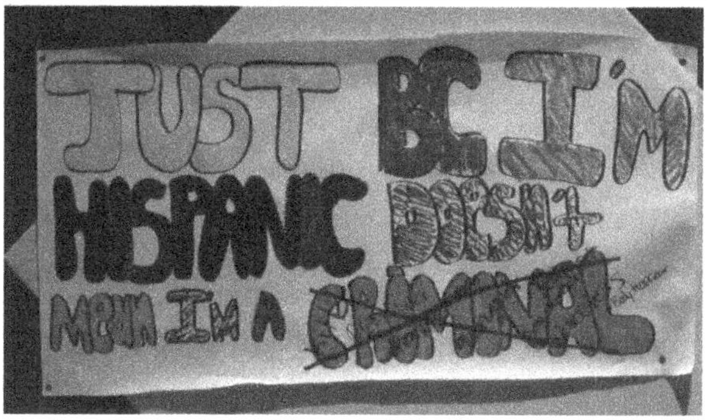

FIGURE 6.7 ■ *"Si Tú Puedes"*

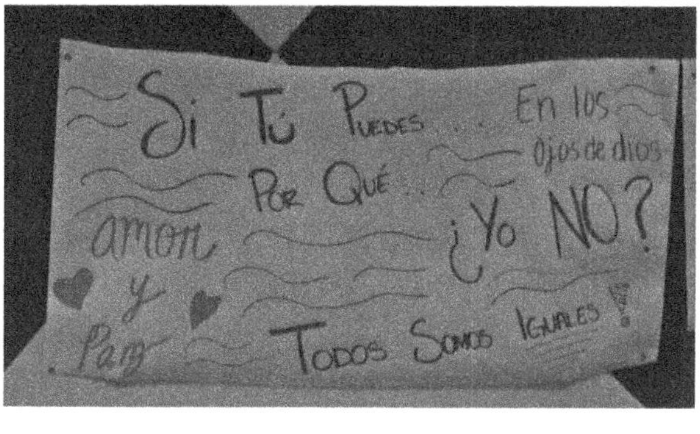

BOX 6.9: STEP-BY-STEP: BANNER STATEMENTS

Banner statements are a useful tool if you want to gather information in a creative, empowering way that simultaneously displays (shares) the information you are collecting. They can be a great means to call public attention to your inquiry project.

Step 1: Decide whom you want to engage in this approach and whom you need to reach.

Step 2: Choose one, broad question or prompt you will ask participants to respond or react to. It might be a question, but it could also be a picture, news article, or statement that you ask them to respond to.

Step 3: Decide where you will go in the community and when to maximize the reach of this method. Vary days, times, and locations. Depending on who you want to reach, you might be able to do this in just one opportunity or you may need to do it in more than one place, at more than one time.

CONCLUSION

In this chapter, we reinforced the idea that intersubjective understanding is the goal of critical participatory inquiry. We also introduced the often "blurred" nature of data collection and analysis in social science inquiry and especially in CPI because of its flexible, iterative, democratized nature. We have suggested that before you make decisions in your collective about which methods to use, you should remember the collective, the moment, and the audience of your inquiry, and consider what is appropriate, what is necessary, and what is useful for and in each of those. Finally, we offered several ideas for ways to turn traditional data collection approaches into more participatory methods of inquiry, including semi- and unstructured conversational approaches, structured activities, and 'Pon the Corner methods. Note that all of the methods we have provided are anchored in dialogue.

RECOMMENDED PRACTICE 6.3: HOW WILL YOU COLLECT AND MAKE MEANING?

As you meet with the co-researchers in your collective, start talking about how you will collect data and make meaning of these data. Go back to the inquiry plan where you talked about what counts as evidence and what type of evidence matters, as well as the areas of concern that you decided to explore. Consider the structured, semistructured, and unstructured methods from this chapter. Write out one area of concern on a piece of flipchart paper. Discuss which methods would create the type of evidence that matters most to the community and decision makers. Repeat this process until method(s) are selected for each area of concern. If the methods in this chapter will not produce the evidence you need, consider those in the following chapters (e.g., arts-based, digital and multimedia approaches).

SUMMARY OF KEY POINTS

- Unlike traditional, positivist research, the goal of CPI is not determining "truth" but establishing intersubjective (mutual) understanding of others' experiences. This requires ongoing dialogue and reflexivity in determining the goal(s) of inquiry and procedures to be followed.
- In CPI, data collection, analysis, and sharing findings are often blurred, iterative, and overlapping rather than distinct phases, and community co-researchers ideally participate in creating tools and collecting and analyzing data to ensure ownership and control over the process.
- Many traditional data collection methods (e.g., interviews, focus groups, and surveys) can be adapted to become more participatory, democratic, and dialogic.
- Other approaches (including ripples of change and card sorting) are designed to be collaborative and are useful for brainstorming and brainwriting, categorizing and analyzing, and prioritizing topics for inquiry.
- Still other approaches, which we call 'Pon the Corner methods, are useful for impromptu or efficient data gathering and sharing; these include mini surveys and whiteboard, notecard, and banner statements.

SUGGESTED ACTIVITIES

1. Look back at the reflexivity question about truth in this chapter. Consider journaling about your goals, thoughts, and concerns about pursuing intersubjective understanding through your inquiry. You may also choose to discuss your thoughts with a trusted colleague.
2. Conduct a ripples of change activity by yourself. Consider what types and levels of change you want to effect through your inquiry. You may draw it on a whiteboard, use an empty wall space in your home, or just note ideas down on a scratch piece of paper. This can help you focus as you engage with communities, as you discuss plans with committee members, or as you practice critical reflexivity on your own.
3. Make your own banner statement: If you could say anything in the world and everyone would listen, what would you say? Then journal about how it felt to make the banner, and how it feels to think everyone would listen to you. Consider putting the banner up in your home, facing outward in a window, on your office door, or somewhere else to let your voice be heard!
4. Interview a family member. Write three questions that would elicit stories about a phenomenon you are interested in. Interview the person and then debrief with them about how it felt to be interviewed in that way. Journal how it felt to you to ask for stories

instead of trying to extract data. Then switch roles to see how it feels to be interviewed and whether the questions feel too personal or lead you to a particular type of answer.

KEY TERMS

brainwriting
card (priority) sorting
intersubjectivity/intersubjective understanding
ripples of change

SUGGESTIONS FOR ADDITIONAL READING

ActionAid. (n.d.). *Tools and methods*. Reflection Action. https://www.reflectionaction.org/tools_and_methods/

Chambers, R. (2002). *Participatory workshops: A sourcebook of 21 sets of ideas and activities*. Earthscan.

Merriam, S. B., & Tisdell, E. J. (2015). *Qualitative research: A guide to design and implementation*. Jossey-Bass.

Patton, M. Q. (2014). *Qualitative evaluation and research methods*. SAGE.

ENDNOTE

1. There are many excellent resources on data analysis methods, so we have focused our discussion here on those that are distinctly participatory.

7 GATHERING DATA AND MAKING MEANING: ARTS-BASED APPROACHES

LEARNING OBJECTIVES

By the end of this chapter you will be able to

- Describe how arts-based data collection and analysis techniques may have a positive impact on individuals, communities, and academia.
- Identify and describe arts-based methods of data collection and analysis that are in line with a commitment to critical participatory inquiry.
- Explain ethical concerns of using arts-based methods of data collection and analysis.
- Describe how to mitigate any negative impacts of using arts-based methods of data collection and analysis.

FOCUS ACTIVITY 7.1: ART AS EVIDENCE

1. Examine what is foregrounded in this mural (Figure 7.1): What do you first notice?

FIGURE 7.1 ■ Exploring Murals with Community Co-Researchers during Mobile Interviews in Guatemala (2019)

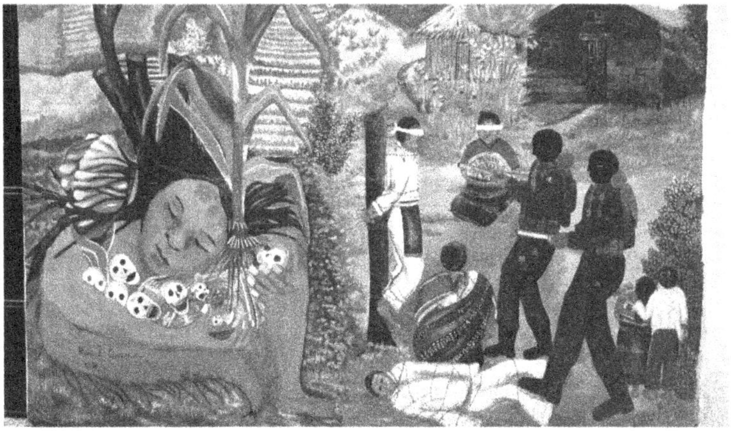

2. Examine what is in the midground in this mural: What do you notice that may not at first be most obvious?
3. Examine what is backgrounded in this mural: What do you notice that makes up the background of this image?
4. How does this mural provide evidence of both the human rights violations that occurred in Guatemala and what happened afterward among the people there?
5. Examine the left portion of the mural: What does the illustration say about the types of change or action that co-researchers have experienced or would like to see?
6. Can you identify potential forces at play that would make it easier or harder to make these changes?

As you examine the mural, outline ways that you could use art to gather and analyze data. How does your process engage co-researchers?

In English, there is a saying *a picture is worth a thousand words*. In Spanish, *una imagen vale más que mil palabras*. In Turkish, *Bir fotoğraf bin sözcüğe bedeldir*. Italian, *un'immagine vale più di mille parole*. No matter the language or culture, there seems to be an almost universal belief in the power of art to communicate what sometimes the tongue cannot. Art engages that affective part of understanding that is often so difficult to reach in other ways, as Giovanni experienced in his work with the Kaqchikel community members in Guatemala.

The mural depicted in this chapter's focus activity provides an example of how art—created by community members—can be analyzed with co-researchers. This art may already be in their neighborhoods, or it may be something that could be created as part of your own critical participatory inquiry (CPI) project. In this example, by walking around the community memorial site and using an existing mural as a point of dialogue, Giovanni and community co-researchers examined the difficult process of justice and reconciliation after the country's 36-year armed conflict. For some of us, our eyes may first gravitate to the right: In the foreground, we see a violent past where community members are being executed and their village burned. This scene signifies the genocidal past witnessed by community members during the country's internal armed conflict. Others may focus on the left: Here, we see a symbolic figure nurturing the bodies of the dead, from which corn now grows.

As we examine the backgrounded meaning within this mural, we see two disparate scenes: violence and pain on the right; peace and calm on the left. While the mural represents two different scenes, they share a common geographic site—the Kaqchikel community's land. The juxtaposition of violence and peace depicts the collective memory and history that the Kaqchikel would like to present. As Giovanni and community co-researchers spoke about the mural, he learned that the community chose to depict peace and reconciliation through a traditional symbolic figure. As co-researchers mentioned during group storytelling sessions, the pain of losing loved ones will never fade (see Chapter 6). From storytelling and art, our research collective learned about how important it is for the Kaqchikel to document these atrocities so that others may learn. However, community members also explained that the earth has nurtured those who were executed, and, in turn, the soil continues to regenerate and care for the current generation through the production of corn. By examining this mural with community co-researchers,

Giovanni learned about the community's priorities for their memorial site. For instance, when speaking about the necessity to tell difficult stories, Kaqchikel co-researchers explained that this was the rationale for leaving several of the empty mass graves open. By inserting a single pane of glass to preserve the hole in the ground, visitors to the site are able to witness loss. They can see the grave from which the remains of the disappeared were exhumed—empty holes that will never be filled, but that should be left uncovered so that we do not forget those who lost their lives.

REFLEXIVITY QUESTION

How has art deepened or challenged your everyday understandings and experiences? How has art helped you better understand *the Other*? How has art inspired you or someone else you know to change?

Remember in previous chapters we noted that whenever there is an opportunity to make decisions about data collection and analysis, you must consider the *collective* (What is important, useful, and valuable to the collective as a whole?), the *moment* (What is important, useful, and valuable in this historical moment?), and the *audience* (What is important, useful, and valuable to your intended audience?). In order words, ask yourselves as a collective and as individuals while you are making data collection and analysis decisions, "What is appropriate? What is necessary? What is helpful?"

As you ask yourselves these questions and engage in dialogue to clarify any assumptions or biases you may be bringing to this process, you will be better positioned to make ethical decisions and build the validity of the inquiry process. In this chapter, we ask that you continue to ponder these questions as we further discuss art as a multifaceted opportunity to reach toward intersubjective understanding through the inquiry process.

CONCEPTS AND DEFINITIONAL ISSUES

One of the most common assertions related to critical participatory inquiry is that this approach to research does not have broad impact. Many people will not see it as scalable. This idea of research not holding value because it may not reach broad audiences buys into postpositivist notions of **rigor**, which base goodness on external validity, reliability, and objectivity (Lincoln et al., 2011). As we have said throughout this book to this point, it is helpful in seeking to understand, or reframe, impact to remember and anchor ourselves in our epistemological commitments. CPI is committed to centering the experiences and expertise of those who are typically silenced or harmed by traditional research processes. This is the standard by which we should demand to be judged. If our inquiry is able to recenter or recover expertise that has been deemed not useful or invalid, knowledge that has been stolen, claimed as White or western, and repackaged or resold to its original owners, it has had an impact.

We believe that the impact of CPI can, and should, be seen and felt on multiple levels, in many ways. Of course, we know that not everyone will agree with our stance. As you read this chapter, think beyond the positive or negative binary of impact. Consider the complexity of how one action could potentially have both positive and negative effects on one individual, on and in the community, beyond the community, and within academia. For instance, while our inquiry may benefit one individual or group, it could also harm others. Or, while it may benefit us in some ways (e.g., publishable papers, funding), it could also harm us (e.g., politically motivated scrutiny, lack of promotion). Therefore, in this section we briefly cover some of the ways in which CPI can have impacts on the individual, on and in the community, beyond the community, and within academia. We hope that offering these examples and delineating the ways in which staying true to CPI's core epistemological commitments moves us toward impact will equip CPI practitioners with the ability to demand recognition for the impact of their work. As Julio Cammarota and Michelle Fine (2008) have said, participatory inquiry is a "radical epistemological challenge to the traditions of social science, most critically on the topic of where knowledge resides" (p. 215). While they were referring to youth participatory action research, the sentiment is the same. CPI is a radical challenge to the status quo of the research enterprise. As practitioners of CPI, we will find ourselves in a position of articulating, clarifying, and advocating for the impact of our work.

Impact on the Individual

Often we hear the word *empowerment* in the context of CPI's impact on the individual (Call-Cummings, 2015). This word, though, can assume a power dynamic that puts a person who holds power in a position to somehow give or bestow power on another. This, of course, is the opposite of what we are after. CPI aims for a more critical approach to empowerment, one through which practitioners of CPI create space and dedicate time to amplifying the voices and honoring the experiences of others. As people engage in CPI, they are better able to see, hear, and feel their own experiences as expertise and their knowledge as valuable and legitimate. They are able to claim power for themselves. *This* is what we mean by a more critical approach to empowerment.

Emily, a member of the *Courageous Conversations* research collective Meagan has worked with for several years, eloquently described an experience she had when she performed spoken word poetry at an arts-based inquiry retreat in front of her peers, parents, teachers, and community members. In this moment, she realized people wanted to hear what she had to say:

> It definitely took some pushing; I remember my friends were like, "Get up there, get up there. Here's the microphone." And we were like, "Okay." I think at the end you kind of have this high, this euphoric, "Oh my god, I just did that," and it kind of leaves you with this feeling like, "I could do that again. I could go back up on stage again." It was an amazing experience, and without that I definitely did not see myself ever doing something like that, getting up on stage and talking in front of all those people. But I think that I understood a little bit more that what I had to say, it was important, and people wanted to hear what I had to say. People, they agreed with what I said.

This realization that what she had to say was important is the epitome of critical empowerment—or what we have also discussed as transformation (Call-Cummings et al., 2021). This transformation is available to community-based and university-based researchers alike and should not be assumed to be reserved for community members. If we are to truly be a collective, all members must be open to experiencing the impact of their inquiry.

Freire (1970) discussed individual impact as emancipation. By engaging in praxis—which involves critical inquiry, reflection, and action—the process behind a CPI project may lead co-researchers to a better self-understanding. Freire (1970) referred to this as a "constant unveiling of reality" (p. 81), showing how someone can gradually begin to see their "reality in process, in transformation" (p. 83). Through this understanding of self and one's place in the world, including intersecting privileges and oppressions, the co-researcher has the opportunity to better understand others and then possibly move toward actions that remedy problems. When thinking about transformation, however, we should not think that co-researchers will achieve some type of resilience that will lead them to solve problems completely on their own. This would place the burden of their problems squarely on their shoulders and ignore the structural inequities and systematic barriers that exist. Rather, as CPI is collaborative in nature, we should understand transformation as a process that not only impacts how the individual co-researcher sees themselves, but also the ways that they relate to, understand, and work with others to critically question (reflect), examine (inquire), and remedy (action) issues, or more succinctly, engage in praxis. In the next paragraphs, we describe CPI's potential to go beyond individual impact and to create positive change on, in, and beyond communities.

Impact on, in, and Beyond the Community

As university-based researchers, we often carry with us assumptions of grand changes that will be seen at the community level and beyond. At a recent interview, Meagan was asked what changes she saw after she completed her dissertation work in rural Idaho (U.S.), which was focused on exposing White supremacist and racist attitudes, behaviors, and practices among teachers at a high school with a large population of Latinx students. The person asked what concrete changes were realized. Meagan answered that the impact she saw, beyond what she witnessed among the individual members of the *Why are our teachers racist?* collective, was an overall increased awareness that these Latinx students were paying attention. After student presentations at the local school board meeting and at service organizations traditionally led by White men, the research collective knew that these White adults better understood and saw for themselves the power these Latinx students had and their willingness to stand up and speak out against and name racism and White supremacy. These White adults could no longer act without consequence. They were seen. In fact, this increased awareness is a common marker of community impact in CPI work.

We also see concrete impacts in communities. The Public Science Project led a CPI effort in New York City to document the effects and then publicly challenge the constitutionality of the New York Police Department's Stop and Frisk policy, which, as the *Morris Justice Project* showed, unjustifiably targeted young men of color. By collecting data in various ways, the collective was able to provide evidence that the policy was not only unfair because it led to racial profiling and harassment but also ineffective in achieving its goals of reducing crime. In August 2012, U.S. District Court Judge Shira Scheindlin ruled that the policy violated the U.S. Constitution (Thompson, 2013). This is a clear example of concrete impact in and beyond one community.

Impact Within Institutions

As we have discussed in previous chapters, having impact within institutions, including academia, can be challenging because impact is often seen as meaning numbers of publications and citations and recognition as an expert among peers. We have found in our work that one way to have an impact within institutional settings, from academia to governmental agencies, is to challenge the status quo in various ways. We have offered workshops in participatory and anti-racist research, for example, that directly challenge the ways research is typically done, the ways institutions measure impact, and even the ways tenure reviews are completed in academia. Meagan convened a faculty learning community to organize for changes in promotion and tenure procedures. Melissa and Giovanni designed their dissertations to push against traditional norms of "good" or "rigorous" research, which future students can use as examples and to justify their own desires to follow their commitments to justice-oriented participatory inquiry. In his previous work in a government agency, Giovanni conducted and commissioned research projects that explored communities' interpretations of "validity" and "impact" and pushed for more participatory inquiry.

While there are many ways to have these kinds of impact within institutions, it can feel—and be—risky. You may risk various job prospects or grant funding. You may risk receiving promotion or tenure. You may risk the respect of certain faculty advisors, peers, colleagues, or senior scholars. You must decide what is worth the risk.

REFLEXIVITY QUESTION

Consider your level of comfort and ability to take risks to have a positive impact through your inquiry. What are you willing to risk? Where will you draw the line? What do you need to feel more comfortable?

As you think more about the burden of risk, it is necessary to reflect on the institutions where you operate. Your risk levels may be constrained by what your faculty advisors or supervisors allow. In this case, it helps to ask, "Are there individuals or institutions who can share the burden of risk and provide support so I can continue my work?" One way to feel more comfortable putting yourself, your career, or your reputation at risk is to find a mentor or advisor that will be in your corner supporting you, standing up for you, and fighting with you. All of us have found these types of mentors. Meagan's mentor, Barbara Dennis, told her at her dissertation defense that she is getting in good trouble through her dissertation. Melissa and Giovanni have had Meagan—and others—in their corners.

Understanding and Mitigating Negative Impacts

Within institutions, the notion of impact is often seen as solely a positive thing. While assembling her documents to submit for tenure in 2021, Meagan was required to show evidence of the "impact" of her research and scholarship. There was never a delineation between positive and negative impact. It was simply assumed that any impact or recognition would be positive. Of course, we know that this is not always the case. Even if our journal articles have hundreds or thousands of citations or our research findings are retweeted, this does mean our research has had a positive impact on the world or in the communities with whom we engage. To be sure, arts-based data collection and analysis hold great potential for positive impact; however, they can also lead to negative outcomes. Within each subsection of this chapter, we will emphasize the possibilities for positive as well as negative impact so that you and your research collective will be equipped to mitigate those potential negative impacts of your research choices. One area of particular concern to us is cultural appropriation of methods. Because Giovanni, Melissa, and Meagan have all worked and lived in various countries, cultures, and contexts across the world, we will bring in examples from our varied experiences, but we will be careful to warn against cultural appropriation, which relates to the use of culturally specific or culturally bound methods, practices, or rituals without appropriate permission, consent, or understanding. Cultural appropriation is closely connected to colonialism, and as we advocate for explicitly decolonial research practices, we are deeply concerned about any research that steals methods or ways of knowing or being from cultures, peoples, or contexts of which those researchers are not a part.

ARTS-BASED APPROACHES TO GATHERING DATA AND MAKING MEANING

Think back to this chapter's opening focus activity. When have you used art as evidence in your everyday life? Perhaps you illustrated a point through art during a professional presentation. Maybe you took a child to a theatrical performance and then engaged them in conversation about some of the themes that were brought out. Or maybe you have chatted with neighbors or colleagues about a political meme or cartoon that seemed to prove a point or that connected with your experiences or views. The point is, we use art as evidence to document, reflect, or communicate every day. In this section, we will offer several examples of ways that art can be used in critical participatory inquiry. Remember, though, that all of these methods can be used in nonparticipatory and noncritical ways, so as you read, continue to reflect back on our CPI touchstones: dialogue, relationships, shared ownership, humility in practice, and reflexivity. Many questions about process ("What do I do if . . . ?") can be answered by reflecting on and anchoring your practice in these epistemologically oriented values.

Visual Arts-Based Inquiry

Visual arts-based inquiry offers infinite possibilities for generating knowledge and returning findings to co-researchers and community members, practitioners, policymakers, and other stakeholders in accessible and effective ways (Boydell, 2019). In this section, we provide several examples of how visual media—from murals to paintings to storyboards—can be used to gather data and make meaning. It is important to note that art does not need to be created for the purpose of a CPI project. Just as you saw in the opening focus activity, Giovanni and co-researchers used existing art, including murals already on Kaqchikel land, to facilitate discussions. On the other hand, youth co-researchers in Meagan's *Courageous Conversations* project created paintings as a way to respond to research questions and then displayed them in an exhibit to which they invited peers, parents, educators, policymakers, and community members (Figure 7.2).

Through these examples, we can see how existing and new art can be used as a tool to elicit and create knowledge with co-researchers and can be shared with various audiences.

Murals

In Guatemala, Giovanni used murals as a way to encourage dialogue and elicit stories from co-researchers. After several hours of participatory data gathering and analysis sessions, members of the research collective took a break for lunch and Giovanni walked around the grounds of

FIGURE 7.2 ■ *Courageous Conversations* Art Exhibit, 2019

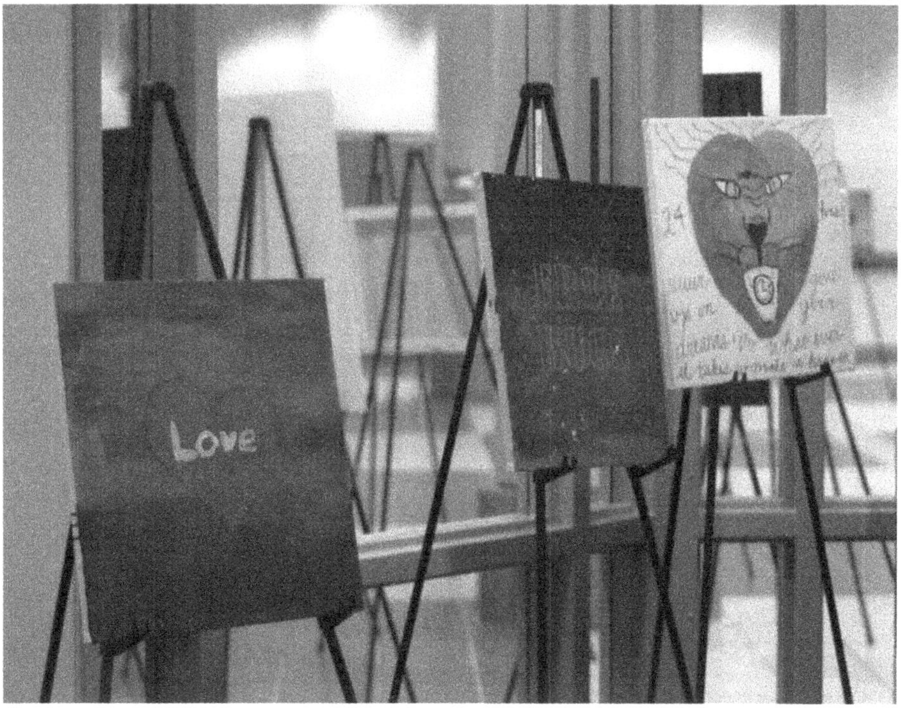

the community memorial site with co-researchers from the Kaqchikel community and a local nonprofit partner. While this group was walking, they stopped at the *nimajay* (community hall) and began discussing the murals painted on its walls. During this impromptu walk, Giovanni and nonprofit staff learned from Kaqchikel co-researchers as they spoke of the meaning behind the illustrations and symbols on these murals. During this discussion, it was interesting to hear Kaqchikel co-researchers speak about these visual depictions because similar themes had arisen during previous data gathering sessions, especially around what the community valued and how they interpreted topics of peace, conflict, justice, and reconciliation. This dialogue, which drew on questions from the focus group and storytelling protocols, soon became an opportunity for joint meaning making as Kaqchikel co-researchers related their intrinsic values, as illustrated in the murals, and how these should be prioritized in the design and development of the community memorial site. In this instance, it was possible to utilize the community's existing knowledge and cultural artifacts to elicit topics of discussion and relevant themes for inquiry and action.

Alternatively, murals can also be a product of a CPI project, especially when there are opportunities to utilize the medium to inform others in the larger community about co-researchers' priorities for action. For instance, Katherine Fobear (2017) reflects on her work supporting the organization of a community mural project with lesbian, gay, bisexual, and trans (LGBT) refugees in Canada. Through this project, called *Painted Stories*, a collective of 15 LGBT refugees worked with a local artist to co-create a large public mural showcasing their experiences at the Queer Arts Festival in Vancouver. Fobear (2017) observes how discussions and planning sessions with LGBT refugee community members provided an opportunity to critically reflect on the purpose behind the mural and whether this art project could create a space for understanding, mobilization, and solidarity. Initially in this project, organizers of the arts festival asked LGBT refugees to paint stories of the violence and trauma they experienced to their gender identity and sexual orientation, for the purpose of advocating for greater protection. Through dialogue and training sessions on anti-oppressive education, however, members of the collective pushed against depicting what they felt is often seen as the single story that LGBT refugees have to tell, that is, one revolving around their trauma. Rather, they chose to depict their experiences of violence, detention, and asylum alongside messages of hope, strength, and their personal insights on LGBT refugees' experiences and the policies that affect them. In this case, the mural served as a counternarrative against singular stories of victimhood, while also depicting LGBT refugees' agency and capacity.

In another example, Jesica Siham Fernández, a social-community psychologist working with Latinx youth in an after-school program, has used murals to document the community action projects initiated by youth co-researchers (Fernández, 2018). To design their mural, youth co-researchers conducted focus groups to explore problems, priorities, and solutions, and then conducted analysis to group these into themes. They then worked together during arts-based workshops to construct symbols to include in their mural. From these participatory data gathering and meaning making sessions, youth co-researchers came up with themes related to structures of power, such as protest, solidarity, and social justice, as well as the importance of education, diversity, and history. Since this mural was designed within a school, however, it required a final sign-off from school administrators, which presents an important lesson for those interested in conducting CPI: You must always consider power structures that may inhibit your ability to conduct the project in the ways you deem important or necessary.

In this case, when youth co-researchers presented their mural design, several administrators asked that one of the symbols (a sign of protest) be removed. Thus, while we may facilitate a space for knowledge generation and empowerment while gathering data and making meaning, we need to remember that our CPI projects always operate within larger structures of power and hierarchy. As we mentioned in previous chapters, it is necessary to reflect on the groups and forces that may inhibit your inquiry collective from achieving the types of action and change you feel are important. It is also worthwhile to consider how to strategize to engage those forces early on so that they will not be caught off guard by actions your collective takes. As they learn about your goals and ideas, they may even become unexpected partners! At the very least, they may pose less of a threat. If it does not seem appropriate to bring these forces or groups in, it may also be useful to discuss early on how to act outside of their sphere of control or in anonymous ways.

Street Art

Another form of visual arts-based inquiry involves the use of community street art projects as a participatory method and as a tool for neighborhood regeneration. An example of this includes a street mosaic project in Vilnius, Lithuania, developed by the neighborhood residents of Šnipiškės and an art collective, Laimikis.lt (Lavrinec, 2014). In this project, residents donated ceramic tiles, which were then used to beautify communal spaces around the area. After documenting the negative image of the neighborhood as portrayed by local media and the growing pressure to redevelop the area with high-rise buildings, residents and members of the art collective sought to disrupt this narrative through the use of history and art. During the 17th and 18th centuries, the neighborhood of Šnipiškės had been known for its ceramic tiles. Drawing on this piece of culture, the street mosaics evoked sensory metaphor and critical spatial research, calling on residents and passersby to question their view of the neighborhood.

In this case, we can see that the primary audience of this project was not necessarily academics but those living in and visiting the neighborhood. Additionally, if we think back to the touchstones of CPI, we can see how this project meets several criteria, including dialogue, relationships, and shared ownership. The process of creating the street mosaics led to dialogue, data gathering, and shared meaning making among residents and co-researchers, where they were able to come together and share stories about the neighborhood. Additionally, the final products (i.e., street mosaics throughout the neighborhood) likely provided a space for reflection or dialogue for anyone passing by. As we look at the possibility of forming street art, it is important to explore the history of this visual medium within the community where you are working. For instance, if an inquiry collective were to conduct a similar project in Portugal, they would be able to draw on the country's rich history of ceramic tilework (*azulejo*) that adorns its cities (Laimikis, 2021).

Smaller Pieces of Art

In our previous examples, the visual forms included murals and street art projects; however, visual arts-based inquiry does not need to take up much space to make an impact. For instance, in Meagan's *Courageous Conversations* project, youth co-researchers created their own paintings, with symbols and messages showing the types of change they would like to see in their schools and communities. As previously mentioned, visual arts-based inquiry can also rely on existing media, such as photographs from family scrapbooks and photo albums. Through their work with the Centre for Visual Methodologies and Social Change at the University of KwaZulu-Natal and the International Visual Methodology Project at McGill University, Mitchel and Allnutt (2008) describe a process where participants were asked to find, rather than take, several photos and then associate them with a narrative. In this case, this process could be made participatory by bringing participants together to discuss themes, generating knowledge and shared meaning making in the process. Much like photovoice (see Chapters 4 and 5), which requires co-researchers to take photos, this process of finding existing photographs could be engaged as a useful and meaningful method to involve co-researchers in historical inquiry. Imagine conducting a CPI project similar to the street mosaic workshops facilitated in Lithuania, but rather than using ceramic tiles, neighborhood residents could ask relatives and friends for photographs of their community. These photographs could then be used to create exhibits and advocacy campaigns, displaying residents' history and priorities.

Another small form of art is storyboards, which co-researchers can use to document problems and solutions (see Box 7.1). Giovanni drew on a process conceptualized by Pittaway et al. (2010) during the project in Myanmar where former political prisoners met to talk about the issues they experienced after being released from prison (see Chapter 6). Based on the core problems identified during a participatory root cause analysis, co-researchers were then asked to plot out their recommendations and solutions through storyboards (Dazzo, 2016). Using this technique, co-researchers prepared six panels in each storyboard, using any method (e.g., drawing, writing), with the purpose of moving from identifying problems to recommending solutions to policymakers. In the example in Figure 7.3, you can see how co-researchers used questions to gather data and make meaning of their experiences, priorities, and recommended actions. This storyboard illustrates how former political prisoners continue to face discrimination when searching for employment. Although these individuals were freely exercising their right to peacefully assemble and demonstrate, they now carry criminal records which limit their opportunities for employment. In the latter panels of the storyboard, they provide recommendations on skill-building sessions as well as the types of organizations that could help.

After identifying core issues in a previous session (participatory root cause analysis), co-researchers were asked to form small groups based on the problem they considered to be most prevalent in their lives. This was done to organize individuals in like-minded groups as a way to form relationships and provide a space to converse and strategize with others experiencing the same issues. After discussing their plans, participants plotted out the six panels, from problem to solution. As a way to facilitate dialogue and meaning making, each small group then presented their storyboards to the larger group.

FIGURE 7.3 ■ Storyboard Moving From Community-Identified Problem to Solution

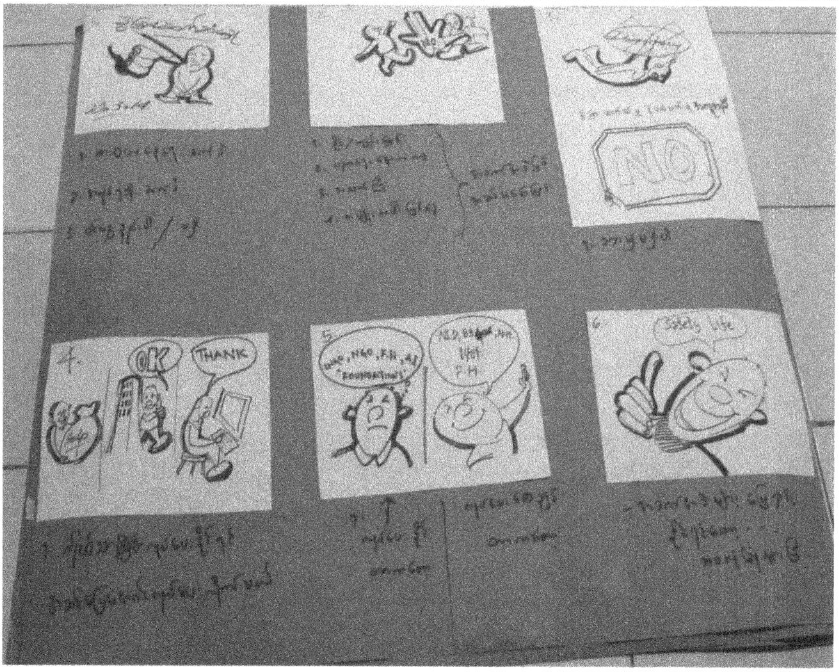

BOX 7.1: STEP-BY-STEP: STORYBOARDS

Using the method proposed by Pittaway et al. (2010), organize six panels on a large piece of paper or whiteboard. This can be done by pasting six pieces of paper on a larger poster-board, as shows in Figure 7.3. The six panels can be organized in this order:

1. Depict a problem or concern that you have experienced.
2. Identify the impact of this problem on you and your community.
3. Identify the type of assistance available and its effectiveness.
4. If you were in charge, what solutions would you provide?
5. Identify the institutions that could provide services.
6. Identify the best outcome for the community if this solution is implemented.

Along with co-researchers, answer these questions. This can be done as a large group or by organizing into smaller groups, based on co-researchers' interests or areas of concern. Use the storyboard to discuss issue areas and potential solutions, and how your collective can move toward these goals through research and action.

There are many art forms that may not at first seem (or be structured as) participatory in nature but lend themselves to a CPI approach. We encourage you to think broadly and creatively about opportunities to use the arts for inquiry aims. When Meagan was thinking with members of the *Courageous Conversations* collective about what other art forms they might use to help students' voices be heard, one of the co-researchers mentioned she really enjoyed doing henna art. This caught Meagan by surprise at first, not because she did not think henna art is beautiful, but because to her it did not seem at all research oriented. Of course, she realized that what was most important was relying on her co-researchers' knowledge, expertise, and interests. Your co-researchers may enjoy creating collages (Butler-Kisber, 2008), textual sculpture (de Cosson, 2008), or even upcycling (Coemans & Hannes, 2016) as a pastime. Of course, as a pastime the methods may not at first seem research oriented or "participatory enough." All it takes is a little creativity and recalling the CPI touchstones (dialogue, relationships, shared ownership, humility in practice, and reflexivity) to fold these methods into an innovative and affective inquiry experience. We urge you to remain open to your co-researchers' ways of knowing and being and to engage those through and in your critical participatory inquiry.

Understanding and Mitigating Negative Impacts

It is important to remember that art can always be interpreted in many ways, sometimes in ways the artist did not intend. This is a potential risk in using art for inquiry purposes. A student in one of Meagan's research methods classes did a practice ethnographic observation at a street art installation in Georgetown, Washington D.C. To Meagan, it sounded like a beautiful installation using different colored lights to depict the beauty of diversity. According to Meagan's student, the aim of the artwork was to begin conversations about LGBTQ rights, but this goal was never explicitly stated. As the student conducted her observation, she overhead many visitors wondering what the lights were about or not understanding the goals of the project. This was a shame, as the student described her experience, because she thought the installation could have had a much bigger impact than she thought it did.

In your own CPI work, it is important to strike a balance between using art for affective purposes and giving appropriate and necessary information so that audience members will understand the message you are trying to send. While each audience member may have a slightly different experience, your goal should be to try to help them understand the collective's experiences and perspectives. Without that guidance, you run the risk of people not understanding or misunderstanding your message.

Poetry, Memoir, Narrative

Amanda Gorman's stirring poem, "The Hill We Climb," which the 22-year-old U.S. youth poet laureate recited at President Joe Biden and Vice President Kamala Harris's January 2021 inauguration, calls for reconciliation amidst racial and political unrest in a country she declared is "not broken but simply unfinished" (Gorman, 2021). Just two weeks after the deadly insurrection at the U.S. Capitol, Gorman vividly denounced both violence and silence while expressing hope for healing and a call to work toward change:

> *being American is more than a pride we inherit,*
>
> *it's the past we step into*
>
> *and how we repair it.* (Gorman, 2021)

Gorman describes her poetry as activism, pointing out that "everything is political, especially art" (WBUR, 2021).

Poetry offers an alternative "way to know the world . . . to be and become in the world" (Leggo, 2008, para. 1), in other words, to understand and express our onto-epistemology both critically and creatively. It can communicate experience and provoke emotional responses in ways that prose cannot (Leggo, 2008), and has been used in and as inquiry in various forms and numerous disciplines (see Galvin & Prendergast, 2016; Lahman et al., 2010; Prendergast, 2015; Wang et al., 2017). For example, Tucker-Raymond et al. (2011) demonstrate how poetry can provide youth, in this case members of the Puerto Rican diaspora in the Midwestern United States, with an opportunity "to explore cultural, historical, and political dimensions of change, struggle, and persistence" (p. 271). Bishop and Willis (2014) use poetry writing as a way to investigate Australian youth's perspectives on hope, capturing evocative conceptual data of their subjective experiences. Traditional data, such as interview transcripts, can be crafted into and presented as poetry (Lahman et al., 2010), and poetic inquiry (Prendergast, 2009) can be used as a form of data analysis (Stapleton, 2021). For instance, Stapleton (2021) describes the use of poetic transcription (Glesne, 1997) in a participatory action research (PAR) project with experienced teachers in a low-income, urban district of the Midwestern United States, systematically crafting free-verse poems from transcripts and field notes to capture and clarify emergent themes.

Spoken Word Poetry

Spoken word poetry, a form with deep roots in African American culture, can be a powerful way to denounce systemic oppression (Johnson, 2017) and "disrupt hegemonic, middle-class norms" (Alim, 2011, p. 124). The writing and performance process is a type of critical literacy praxis—reflection, dialogue, and action—of creating and sharing knowledge (Endsley, 2014; Fisher, 2003, 2005, 2007; Jocson, 2006, 2008). It is increasingly used as a form of culturally relevant literacy instruction with "urban" youth that employs out-of-school literacies as a bridge to the "dominant" (White) language arts curriculum (e.g., Fisher, 2003; Jocson, 2005, 2006; Morrell, 2002, Morrell & Duncan-Andrade, 2004). However, this runs the risk of appropriating a cultural form for hegemonic purposes (Endsley, 2014), in fact, we urge researchers who are not members of Black communities to carefully consider whether it is appropriate to engage in this form at all.

During the second annual arts-based research event in Meagan's ongoing *Courageous Conversations* project, the group invited a local African American spoken word poet to facilitate a 3-hour workshop for youth participants, many of whom identified as Black, Latinx, or first- or second-generation immigrants (see Call-Cummings et al., 2020). The facilitator started the workshop with an introduction of spoken word poetry's development and cultural significance and performed one of his poems as an example; he then led participants in crafting collaborative spoken word poems on the theme the collective had selected, "my voice." Participants wrote a few lines of poetry while music (chosen by participants) played in the background. After a few minutes passed, the facilitator indicated participants should pass their papers to the left for another participant to add to the poetry, thus nurturing an exciting and fun collaboration (Figure 7.4).

FIGURE 7.4 ■ My Voice Is . . .

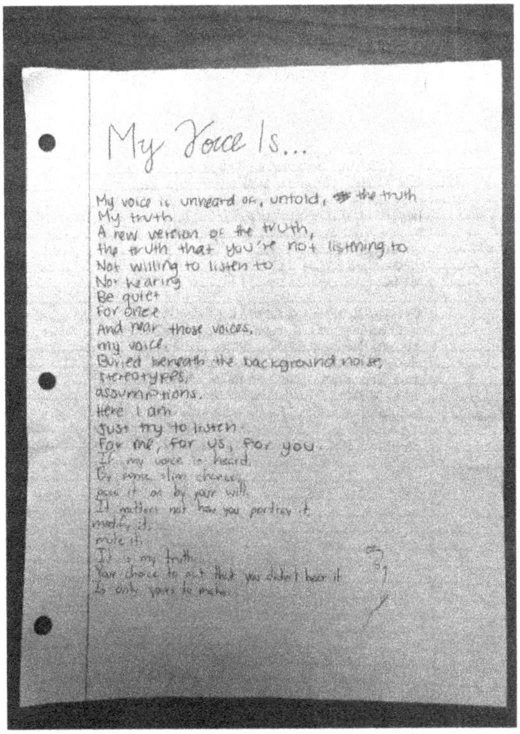

Participants were given more time to hone the poetry they started and were encouraged to share their work aloud at the end of the workshop as well as during an evening exhibition of the day's arts-based data collection activities. Participants grappled with school stress and self-doubt and spoke back to experiences of being silenced by teachers and parents. By creating the poetry collaboratively, they found safety and confidence in speaking as a "we." As one group wrote,

And we are powerful because we have a voice

And even if that voice is small, the words it speaks are powerful.

Participatory Narrative Approaches

Personal memoirs or autobiographies provide a forum for constructing and representing experience and identity for a real or imagined audience (Atkinson & Silverman, 1997; Bruner, 2001; Ellis & Berger, 2002). These can also be written collaboratively to recall, analyze, and communicate memory (Haug, 1987; Lapadat, 2009). For example, Lapadat (2009) describes engaging in collaborative autobiography with graduate students in her qualitative methods course: first, individually writing out a memory of a life challenge, discussing each with the class and looking for connections and differences across stories, and then reflectively rewriting individually and as a group, incorporating the class analyses and interpretations. This process demonstrates the blending of individual and collective knowledge as well as data collection and analysis and could be adapted to an infinite number of topics, contexts, and purposes.

Autobiographical timelines can also help co-researchers to document, reflect on, and make sense of their experiences (Leung, 2010). These artifacts can then become data in and of themselves or can be the basis for conversations, in-depth interviews, or personal narrative writing (Guenette & Marshall, 2009). If co-researchers are finding it difficult to start a timeline – perhaps they are not sure where to begin or may feel like the task is daunting—it can be useful to start small. You may suggest that those who are participating use small notecards to brainstorm ideas or to tell a story within a few sentences, such as is shown in Figure 7.5. This can feel less intimidating than giving them a large, blank sheet of paper they are supposed to fill.

Folk Storytelling

In Chapter 6, we talked about the use of story/sharing circles and showed how this everyday narrative form could be used to gather data and make meaning of co-researchers' experiences, priorities for action, and policy recommendations. In this chapter, we explore the use of oral histories and folk stories in the form of sound recordings. John Gaventa (1991), an early participatory inquirer who worked closely with communities from the Appalachian Mountain area in the United States, saw that folk storytelling, a traditional narrative form for this group, could be used as a way to document their expertise to counter dominant narratives. Much like the Lithuanian neighborhood of Šnipiškės, the expansive Appalachian cultural area in the United States has been portrayed negatively in media accounts, which has led to numerous stereotypes. To dispel these accounts, researchers like Gaventa worked with Appalachian communities to document folk stories, which question dominant forms of knowledge, expertise, and decision making that affect the daily lives of these individuals.

The documentation and recording of folk stories have been used outside the practice of participatory inquiry. The author, anthropologist, and folklorist, Zora Neale Hurston (1927),

FIGURE 7.5 ■ The time when . . . no one wanted to listen to me.

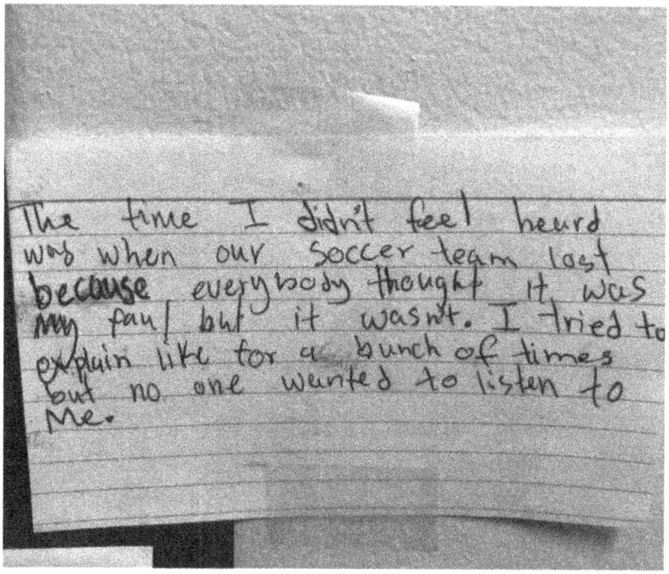

created sound recordings of former slaves across the Southern region of the United States. Hurston drew on this popular form of data gathering and meaning making to ensure these stories would not be lost. These sound and film recordings counter dominant historical accounts and provide a view into the lived experiences of people who were enslaved in their own words. Although these recordings were created in the 1920s and 1930s, they have been archived so we can all continue to listen and learn. This example shows how, in our own CPI projects, we can create visual and recorded artifacts from everyday narrative forms. Box 7.2 offers a step-by-step guide for conducting collaborative narrative and visual analysis.

BOX 7.2: STEP-BY-STEP: COLLABORATIVE NARRATIVE AND VISUAL ANALYSIS

In the previous chapter, we mentioned the use of thematic analysis to synthesize and make meaning. In this example, we will cover how narrative and visual forms of inquiry could be used. Drawing from the Focus Activity at the beginning of this chapter, we outline a few steps you can use to collaboratively explore the explicit and implicit narratives in arts-based inquiry.

Step 1. Organize co-researchers around a piece of art. This can be one that already exists, such as a mural in the community, or one that the group has developed as part of the CPI project. Depending on your purpose for analysis, make sure that co-researchers agree on what the output will be from your collaborative analysis sessions. If you are interested in organizing co-researchers' thoughts around several concepts, you can use thematic analysis (see Chapter 6, Box 6.4). If you are interested in presenting all ideas or constructing a narrative as part of your arts-based analysis activities, we recommend the following. This can be conducted as an organized activity, like a community consultation, or informally as part of your conversations with co-researchers.

Step 2a. Ask a series of open-ended questions to explore what co-researchers see and interpret from the piece(s) of art. Here are a few examples:

- When you look at this [image, poem, etc.], what do you first notice?
- Take some time to look at this [image, poem, etc.] a bit more. Is there anything you notice now that was not obvious at first?
- What about the background of this image? What do you notice?
- Are there any abstract or hidden messages that come to mind?
- As a [community member, co-researcher, project participant], what type of change or action does this [image, poem, etc.] inspire?
- What forms of power, oppression, or action exist and intersect throughout this [image, poem, etc.]?

Step 2b. During the discussion, make sure several co-researchers are taking notes. As mentioned in Chapter 6, this can be done in several ways: on a flipchart for the entire group to see, in individual notebooks, or a combination of the two.

Step 3. Work with co-researchers to construct write-ups around what was interpreted. It is possible to organize co-researchers into small groups and to ask them to write captions, stories, memos, memes, or poems that incorporate the ideas and concepts discussed during your collaborative analysis session(s). You can see here how a collaborative analysis session could generate more arts-based data and interpretation—an example of blurred data gathering and meaning making. When using narrative and visual approaches to analysis, it is important to note the purpose is not to reduce data to themes, but to construct a story around the whole.

Remember the type of analyses you use should relate back to your research questions or purpose, as well as considerations around the *collective* (What is important, useful, and valid to the collective as a whole?), the *moment* (What is important, useful, and valid in this historical moment?), and the *audience* (What is important, useful, and valid to your intended audience?). While arts-based approaches may be appealing to some groups, they may not produce the type of evidence that others regard as valid or rigorous. This is not to say that narrative and visual forms of analysis should not be used; rather, it is important to discuss what the collective values and how they want and need to portray messages to various audiences.

Understanding and Mitigating Negative Impacts

While we believe in and have witnessed the power of art to document and communicate the experiences and knowledges of marginalized groups, we also want to include a note of caution. As we have indicated at various points of this chapter, art also has the potential to be misinterpreted, misused, and appropriated. Great care should be taken in deciding—with co-researchers and participants—on which art forms are appropriate to use for the issue at hand and for the intended audience. With culturally rooted forms such as folk storytelling, rhetorical devices, vocabulary, and references might not be comprehensible to outsiders, and the experiences described in memoirs can be deeply personal and even traumatic or risky to recount. For example, during her dissertation research with Syrian refugees, Melissa carefully avoided asking about their experiences of civil war and their journeys to Turkey, which quite likely involved violence, loss of or separation from loved ones, unauthorized border crossings, and other potentially emotionally or politically treacherous admissions. In short, research collectives need to consider together what is appropriate and beneficial for the community when selecting and carrying out arts-based knowledge creation activities.

Theatre of the Oppressed

"And so, you can see, it is the re-enacting of these seemingly small moments that can lead to big change," Meagan pronounced as the *Courageous Conversations* Theatre of the Oppressed performance came to an end. Many in the auditorium, including teachers, parents of participating youth, and community members emphatically nodded in agreement. Perhaps Mrwa, one of the *Courageous Conversations* youth co-researchers, described the process best when she said, ". . . It's like a before and after picture, like before, that's not what should have happened and then after, that should have happened instead of what did happen."

Theatre of the Oppressed (Boal, 1979) was created by Augusto Boal, a theater director and friend of Paulo Freire, whose *Pedagogy of the Oppressed* (1970) argued that oppression is a relationship between oppressor and the oppressed and that neither on their own could free themselves or the other from that relationship. Boal, in his Theatre of the Oppressed, argued that when we become aware of how we act within moments of oppression—either as oppressor or oppressed—we can transform our ways of knowing and being in this world. We can release the oppressive relationship. Thus, the process in Theatre of the Oppressed is designed to first recognize and then change small, everyday moments of oppression through acting them out and then re-enacting them with compassion (Boal, 2002).

Theatre of the Oppressed is actually not one approach but a group of performance-oriented practices that address the oppressive relationship. Here, we cover four of Boal's most well-known methods: Image Theatre, Forum Theatre, and Cops in the Head. We have used all of these in our own CPI projects at various times and find that they are particularly useful to engage people who may have a hard time articulating their ideas or feelings. Of course, participation is never required or forced, and the decision to do any of these should come from the CPI collective.

Image Theatre

Image Theatre is one of the many tools developed by Augusto Boal under the umbrella of Theatre of the Oppressed. In Image Theatre, participants create still images with their bodies as a way of exploring and literally embodying abstract concepts that can be difficult to understand or even speak about. In this approach, participants quickly sculpt their bodies to express concepts like relationships or emotions and then bring them to life in various ways. This is one way to grapple with concepts like oppression. Image Theatre can be a useful entree into the world of Theatre of the Oppressed because participants do not have to have any background or formal training in drama or theatre to feel confident in participating. It often feels less intimidating than Boal's other approaches that are more in line with improvisational techniques.

Several of our colleagues once used Image Theatre at an academic conference to start dialogue about relationships between researchers and participants (Dennis et al., 2017). They began with a few easy exercises to get participants' bodies moving and warmed up and to get group members to know each other just a little. They then asked volunteers first to sculpt images using just their own bodies, not working together. Ultimately, after several iterations, participants were asked to work together to sculpt images, first as still images, but they ended up having these images come to life. Each stage of the process yielded dialogue that added to the group's nuanced understanding of what research relationships could look like.

Forum Theatre

Forum Theatre is another approach to Theatre of the Oppressed. In this case, participants act out a play or scene that usually connects to some experience of oppression. The participants can act out the scene numerous times. During the replay, any member of the audience—or what Boal called "spect-actors"—can yell "Stop!" or "Pause!" and can take the place of one of the actor–participants to try out a different way of acting the scene out. The goal is to show that the scene could have been acted out differently to reduce the oppression experienced.

Another version of Forum Theatre is called Cops in the Head, which adds a component of "cops" that live inside our minds, our subconscious, and often rehearse to us various oppressive concepts or ideas. Someone's cop may be the internalized voice of their mother, saying, "Real women don't ask a man to marry them. That's the man's job." Another cop could be a former teacher who says "Black girls should take classes more appropriate for their future job prospects—like cooking." These cops are like our internalized, oppressive voices. As we act out scenes of oppression, spect-actors can pause the scene and articulate what our cops in our heads might be saying. By so doing, we are better able to understand others' actions within oppressive situations.

Understanding and Mitigating Negative Impacts

One lesson we have learned as we have engaged in several iterations of Theatre of the Oppressed and drama-based inquiry is that there is great danger (ethical, validity, and moral) in not ensuring enough time for processing—before, during, and after participation. Because Theatre of the Oppressed is almost exclusively focused on teasing out, understanding, and grappling with oppression, it can trigger deep scars and raw emotion. Researchers are not (usually) trained mental health professionals and so will not be available to provide the level of care some might need. It is important to help people understand what they may experience before starting the process, to always give opportunity to volunteer and to not actively participate, and to process in ways that are useful to each participant. You should also always have a list of trained mental health professionals available in the local area. It is also helpful to have one of your team if that is possible (Box 7.3).

BOX 7.3: USING COLLABORATIVE PLAY BUILDING TO EXPLORE WHITENESS

Tanner (2014, 2016, 2018) engaged the Midwest Critical Whiteness Collective, incorporating play building and drama pedagogy to facilitate conversations about Whiteness, foster awareness of White supremacy, and encourage anti-racist action during an extracurricular theater program with mostly White-identifying high school students. Through a series of workshops, youth co-researchers collaboratively wrote and performed a play, *Blanchekreist: A Collaborative Play About Whiteness*, which addressed their experiences of Whiteness and how it operates in school and society. Tanner (2014) notes in his dissertation that "multiple perspectives should be allowed to challenge each other in order for something complicated and messy to emerge" (p. 5). Engaging many of the commitments and goals of Theatre of the Oppressed, Tanner's critical, theatrical approach to participatory inquiry helped "make room for the messiness that comes in allowing tensions to be made visible" (p. 5). Anchoring his choice of methods in Patti Lather's (2007) treatise, *Getting Lost*, Tanner describes his commitment to carefully packaging the messiness of multiple voices, competing ideologies, and deep tensions in ways that would both make sense to a reader or audience member and challenge them to think, and perhaps act, anew.

Other Forms of Art

We want to be clear that there are so many forms of art out there that it can be hard to cover them all in one chapter—or even a whole book. We often make decisions about arts-based forms of data collection and analysis as we learn about the methods members of our CPI collectives know and use in their own lives. Using these *known methods* can help to democratize the inquiry process as we learn together, with some as experts at some points of the process and others at other points. In this section, we offer arts-based approaches that do not fit neatly into a particular category.

Body Mapping

Body mapping—tracing an individual's body and filling the outline in with representations of their identities and lived experiences—has been employed for a variety of purposes, including education, advocacy, therapy, and research (Boydell, 2019; de Jager et al., 2016). Although practitioners adapt the process in varying ways, Solomon's (2002) guidelines describe producing a visual body map, accompanying ***testimonios*** or first-person narratives, and a key to symbols and text used on the map over the course of several participatory workshops. With strong ties to social justice and political activism (de Jager et al., 2016), this collaborative approach to gathering and sharing embodied knowledge has been particularly widely used in the domain of health, for example, to document young women's reproductive experiences in Jamaica (MacCormack & Draper, 1987), to reduce HIV/AIDS stigma and advocate for improved access to treatment in South Africa (MacGregor & Mills, 2011), to understand young people's experiences in drug and alcohol treatment (Macken et al., 2021) and to treat trauma (Crawford, 2010; Santen, 2014, 2015). The process is described as accessible for children and nonliterate adults and therapeutic or "empowering" for vulnerable and marginalized groups, and the completed body maps can be displayed for advocacy or educational purposes (Boydell et al., 2020; de Jager et al., 2016).

Textile Arts

Textile arts like quilting have even been used as arts-based research methods. In fact, quilts have a long history of documenting identity, experience, and history through images, colors, symbols, and patterns while also serving practical and decorative purposes, and quilt making has historically been a collaborative, social process (Ball, 2008). Ball (2008) describes portraying survival stories in quilt blocks as a subversive but powerful means toward trauma recovery. Lawton (2010) engaged in collaborative quilt making as a "reciprocal learning relationship" (p. 7) between artists, preservice art teachers, and community members experiencing homelessness to collect life histories and create public art to challenge stereotypes.

Music

As we have done throughout this chapter, it is important to consider existing traditions within the communities in which we work to see how their everyday forms of knowledge can be utilized to counter dominant narratives and forms of research. Professor of ethnomusicology Angela Impey (2002) has documented how songs, dance and rituals are

> . . . rich repositories of local knowledge about the environment, and are particularly relevant signifiers of local meaning systems in a context where these systems may no longer

be learned through apprenticeships or oral tradition, due to geographic displacement and rapid socio-economic transformation. (p. 9)

In her project, Impey worked alongside youth researchers in Dukuduku Forests in northern KwaZulu Natal region of South Africa, to create an archive of Indigenous knowledge. Youth co-researchers were able to go out into their communities to record songs, dances, and rituals. This not only created a repository of traditional meaning making but allowed youth to learn from elders about many traditions that are not often taught or practiced due to competition from what is considered "modern" or "developed." As an advocacy project, Impey and co-researchers sought to create a dialogue about the connections between traditional meaning making such as music, and broader topics such as environmentalism and community (re)development. Through this project, the collective was able to encourage self-representation. By showing "how people transform landscapes into places of human action, and how nature is imbued with meaning by, and for social praxis and identity" (Impey, 2002, p. 14), it countered dominant policy narratives of how the community should develop and become more modern.

Soundscape

Chilean political exile Pilar Kasat (2014) used soundscape—a kind of audio collage—with Aboriginal Noongar people in Australia as a means of working through community trauma, grief, and conflict. In collaboration with a Noongar partner, Kasat recorded conversations with community members, identified segments representing main themes that had come through in the conversations (avoiding offensive or damaging statements in order to protect the speakers), and combined them into a cohesive and powerful audio narrative which was played at a community event. Again, depending on the interests, desires, and goals of a CPI collective, we could imagine doing something similar in projects about education, public health, youth development, and more.

Dance

Like theater-based approaches, dance offers infinite possibilities for creative and evocative depictions of experience and emotion that blur lines between data collection, analysis, and sharing findings (Wang et al., 2017). It incorporates music, visual art, performance, and storytelling (Leavy, 2009) and instead of depending on spoken or written text puts the body, the "locus of experience" (Blumenfeld-Jones, 2008), at the center of inquiry. For example, Boydell (2011a, b) used dance to embody research findings about young people's experiences of psychosis to a broader, non-academic audience and "in an accessible, creative, and thoughtful way, but also to provoke and perhaps disrupt the everyday assumptions individuals hold about mental health issues" (p. 13). Na et al. (2016) describe a community-based dance program for women defectors from North Korea living in South Korea designed to improve self-awareness, physical, emotional, and psychological well-being, and interpersonal interactions. Choreographing meaning into movement serves as an interpretive and communicative act, brought to life by the dancers through "space, time, shape, and motion" (Blumenfeld-Jones, 2008, p. 176). The audience also takes part in constructing meaning, as Blumenfeld-Jones (2008) states, "the best dances help us think about a phenomenon without telling us what to think about the phenomenon" (p. 181).

Combining the Arts

Arts-based forms of inquiry can, of course, be combined and adapted to the interests, goals, and talents of the collective, as Skinner and Masuda (2013) demonstrate in their work with Aboriginal Canadian youth focused on urban health inequity, in which youth co-researchers transformed findings of a place mapping exercise (Travlou et al., 2008) into various art forms in their repertoires, including photography, poetry, hip hop dance, and rap. As is always the case, we encourage CPI collectives to make these decisions based on what they deem valuable.

CONCLUSION

Return to the mural at the start of this chapter. Now that you have read about several examples of visual arts-based inquiry, how could you gather and make meaning of everyday pieces of art in your community? Just as we saw in the mural, there may be illustrations that are present in the foreground as well as symbols that we would need to make sense of through reflection and dialogue. By drawing on everyday art in our data gathering and analysis processes, we are able to privilege the existing knowledge created by the communities that we work alongside.

Data collection and analysis are almost always blurred, occurring simultaneously. In our everyday lives, we rarely take in information without trying to make sense of that information in some way. The traditional research process has artificially separated these processes to make research seem more technical and separated from our everyday lives. In this chapter, we illustrated that the knowledge creation process is an everyday process and is not reserved for a select few people who happen to work at universities or in other relative positions of power. Gathering data, or evidence, and making sense of it is a process that we all know and understand because it is how we live. We offered several ways in which participatory knowledge creation can be amplified through the arts.

RECOMMENDED PRACTICE 7.1: HOW WILL YOU COLLECT AND MAKE MEANING?

As proposed in the last recommended practice box from the last chapter, meet with your co-researchers to talk about how arts-based methods could be used to collect data and make meaning. Make sure to go back to the inquiry plan to note what counts as evidence, what type of evidence matters, and your priority areas of concern. Write out one area of concern on a piece of flipchart paper. What type of arts-based methods from this chapter would produce the type of evidence that your collective needs? What would motivate community members or decision makers to act? Repeat this process until method(s) are selected for each area of concern. If the methods in this chapter will not produce the evidence you need, consider those in the last chapter (e.g., interviews, focus groups) and next (e.g., digital and multimedia approaches).

SUMMARY OF KEY POINTS

- Any art form—visual, written, or dramatic—can be used for and as participatory data collection and analysis. It is important to consider the collective, the moment, and the audience in deciding which arts-based methods are appropriate, necessary, and helpful for your inquiry.
- In CPI, these decisions should be rooted in a critical approach to empowerment that seeks to amplify and honor the expertise of those typically excluded from research. This orientation to research shifts ideas about impact and can result in certain risks for university- and community-based researchers.
- Arts-based inquiry—paintings, murals, street art, storyboards, poetry, memoir, narrative, Theatre of the Oppressed textiles, music, dance, and so on—offers countless possibilities for generating knowledge, visualizing change, and returning findings to co-researchers and community members, practitioners, policymakers, and other stakeholders in accessible and effective ways.

SUGGESTED ACTIVITIES

1. Reconsider the first reflexivity question in this chapter. How could you employ art to document, develop, or analyze knowledge?
2. Choose a piece of art (a painting, song, poem, memoir, etc.) and analyze it for potential messages. What meanings are communicated? How? Who is the intended audience? How could this art translate to inquiry?
3. Identify a form of art that you or your potential co-researchers would find enjoyable or meaningful and brainstorm ways that you could incorporate it into your inquiry.
4. Try out one of the arts-based methods on your own or with a small group of classmates or fellow practitioners. Choose a method and theme, spend an hour or so creating individual or collaborative art, and then reflectively discuss the meanings. Consider displaying your artwork in your home, workspace, or a common area.

KEY TERMS

body mapping
rigor
testimonios
Theatre of the Oppressed

8 GATHERING DATA AND MAKING MEANING: DIGITAL AND MULTIMEDIA APPROACHES

LEARNING OBJECTIVES

By the end of this chapter, you will be able to

- Describe how digital and multimedia data collection and analysis approaches may have a positive impact on individuals, communities, and academia.
- Identify and describe digital and multimedia methods of data collection and analysis that are in line with a commitment to critical participatory inquiry.
- Explain ethical concerns of using digital and multimedia methods of data collection and analysis.
- Describe how to mitigate any negative impacts of using digital and multimedia methods of data collection and analysis.

FOCUS ACTIVITY 8.1: USING SOCIAL MEDIA FOR REFLEXIVITY—AND DATA COLLECTION

Create a personal social media collage from your accounts. The collage can be just like the collages you might have made as a child out of pictures or words from magazines, newspapers, or other craft supplies. Here, the idea is to examine your social media for clues about what is important to you, who you are, what relationships you value, and so on. You can be creative in the ways you organize pictures or words, what is placed at the center versus further away, how big it is, and more. Once you finish, you may ask yourself the following questions, or you may request others' help in discussing them:

1. What do you notice? What is most obvious (foregrounded)?
2. What is least obvious or apparent (backgrounded)?
3. What repetitions or patterns do you see?
4. What do you not like? What do you want to change?
5. Who would you show this to? Why?
6. Who would you *not* show this to? Why?

At this point, you have been introduced to and perhaps tried out various dialogic, textual, and arts-based approaches to blurred data collection and analysis. This chapter focuses on how you can engage in participatory data gathering and meaning making through digital and multimedia formats. Remember that as you make your data collection and analysis decisions, it is crucial to consider the needs of the collective, the moment, and the audience. Continually ask yourself as well as your inquiry collective: "What is appropriate? What is necessary? What is helpful?" As you ask and answer these questions together, you will be in a strong position not only to choose appropriate approaches, but also to tailor the examples and ideas we offer here to speak directly to the context in which you conduct your critical participatory inquiry. As always, we start off exploring key concepts and definitions of terms to anchor our guidance on approaches.

CONCEPTS AND DEFINITIONAL ISSUES

More than any of the other chapters in this book, the ideas and guidance offered in this chapter may be outdated in a few years because of the world's constantly changing digital landscape. With this in mind, we want to start this chapter with a few key concepts that can anchor your data collection and analysis decisions, no matter when or in what context you are working. As you review the guidance we offer later on in this chapter and as you find new digital opportunities not covered here, we urge you to continue to root your critical participatory inquiry (CPI) in these ideas. While we return here to discussions around validity and ethics, we urge you to constantly consider dialogue, respect, humility, openness, trust, and other touchstones, as they remain central components of ethical and valid critical participatory inquiry.

Memory and Validity

Look back at the collage you created for the opening focus activity in this chapter. If you have not already done so, ask yourself the questions we have listed or others as they come to you. Does the collage elicit any memories? Could you imagine yourself elaborating on the pictures and words you included in your collage in an interview or other opportunity for dialogue? Memories can be a wonderful way to reach toward intersubjective understanding of and with others. However, often we call our memories into question because, well, they are memories. We might tell ourselves, "It happened so long ago, what if I'm not remembering the *correct* things? What if it's not *the truth*?" Methodologists might refer to these types of questions as they consider the *reliability* of memory.

Think back to Chapter 3 when we discussed validity as strength and health. For critical inquirers in general, and practitioners of CPI in particular, validity is not equated with so-called truth (i.e., the idea there is one absolute truth). The supposed facts of some particular interaction or occurrence matter less to us than how a person experienced that interaction, because that experience is what will help lead us toward greater intersubjective understanding of another's ways of knowing and ways of being. So, when we invoke memory and memories through our data collection and analysis, remember that the goal of this approach to inquiry is deeper, more nuanced understandings of others' experiences, ways of being, and ways of knowing. Will our inquiry lead to a stronger and more trustworthy understanding of others' experiences? Will it lead to healthier ways of being and respect toward different ways of knowing?

Knowledge Sharing and Ethics

Some disciplines and fields refer to knowledge translation, the practice of making knowledge or research understandable or useable by people or organizations outside of a particular discipline, when discussing the sharing of participatory knowledge creation. We are uncomfortable with this framing as it seems to stress another's use of expert knowledge and has a focus on outcomes that does not always consider the ways in which the process itself is (or is not) participatory. Knowledge sharing, on the other hand, has a process orientation, reflects a collaborative and collective epistemological emphasis, and focuses on outcomes that seek reciprocity or balanced power and democratization. Then again, knowledge sharing can have particularly complicated implications as digital and multimedia forms open up opportunities to share knowledge in creative and accessible ways with people you may not be able to reach through more traditional methods.

Constant developments in digital technology offer us endless possibilities for creative, accessible inquiry methods; however, they also introduce new logistical and ethical dilemmas. For example, when Melissa was forced to shift her dissertation data collection with Syrian refugees in Turkey from in-person to virtual methods during COVID-19 lockdowns, she needed to consider their unique vulnerabilities—legal, economic, and otherwise. With input from her Syrian key informant, this led her to reduce the level of involvement requested from participants, since reliable internet service is costly and particularly difficult to access in refugee settlements. Instead of gathering a collective from one university to meet regularly and shape the direction of the research, she met once with each participant for an interview via their preferred platform—Zoom, Skype, or WhatsApp calling. Though Zoom offers video recording and automated transcription, she opted not to use these tools because of the political risk to participants, the poor quality of transcription for accented English, and the lack of capability for Turkish and Arabic, instead recording audio on a separate handheld device.

When Giovanni conducted a participatory inquiry project with former political prisoners in Burma/Myanmar, most of these individuals' activities were still being surveilled by security forces. For this reason, it was necessary to consider how each aspect of project design—from sampling, selection, and recruitment to consent forms to presenting findings—could affect those participating in the project. Although the core inquiry collective was interested in reaching as many potential participants as possible to take a feedback survey and invite to a community consultation, it would not have been safe to advertise this openly on social media or via email lists. In this case, one of the nonprofit partners in the collective was able to directly contact individuals, extending a personal invitation to those in their network and asking them to pass the word. While this personal touch took time, it led to nearly 80 individuals providing feedback through the survey, and nearly 40 individuals contributing to the community consultation and participatory data gathering and analysis. Additionally, as the collective was concerned with how the data they gathered and analyzed could be shared and used, time was spent to co-create a group agreement or consent form at the start of the community consultation (see Chapter 5 for a step-by-step guide). This was important because it laid the ground rules for interaction, confidentiality, and trust over the next several days. As the group created the consent form, participants agreed that they would not take photos and share on social media during or after the sessions. Additionally, the group agreed that photos of individuals would require follow-up whenever they were to be used after the session. This type of contextualized consent (differentiated from wholesale consent) meant that a participant could approve a request for their image one day but deny another the next. Although these individuals had already been released from prison, many continued their political activities and could continue to be unjustly prosecuted. This ensured that there was not an expiration date when it came to authorizing use and sharing the knowledge they created. While this could constrain sharing, it improved dialogue, trust, and openness during data gathering and analysis. It also forced a sense of humility on the research process, showing that the core inquiry collective did not wholly "own" the words and images created during this project.

During Meagan's dissertation in Idaho (U.S.), she knew she wanted to do something different, or more creative, than a typical dissertation product. She wanted to co-create something with her research collective that they valued. She knew a several-hundred-page manuscript that ended up sitting on a shelf somewhere and was never accessed by anyone except a few other scholars with shared interests would not be valued by her research collective members, all of whom were high school students at the time. They decided to create a website together that would act not only as an archive of all of their work and findings but also as a celebration of their democratized knowledge creation process. Meagan received approval from her dissertation committee and the graduate school at her university to create a **born-digital dissertation**. However, when the research collective began adding text, pictures, and videos to the website, they realized they would not be able to include much of what they had created. For example, they had recorded some of the students' experiences with racism, but they were worried that because they lived in such a small community, including those recordings on the website would allow others to identify their voices and expose them to a risk of retribution. In the end, they decided to ask Latinx students at Meagan's university to re-record their stories so that people who listened would still hear voices and emotion rather than read a sanitized version of those stories on a screen. The decision was difficult and meant that some important data could not be included on the website, but the collective felt that protecting the students' and their families' identities was more important.

As you have similar dilemmas in your own CPI, we urge you to continually reflect on your own commitments, engage in dialogue with your collectives about their own needs, commitments, and concerns, and ensure you are staying within the bounds of the legal and ethical requirements of your own government as well as any host government, professional organizations, employers, and ethics review boards.

Digital and Multimedia Approaches to Gathering Data and Making Meaning

Digital and multimedia platforms can open up a world of opportunities for gathering data and making meaning with research collectives. In 2009, Gubrium and Harper wrote in their introduction to a special issue of *Practicing Anthropology* that "New visual technologies are changing the ways [we] do research and opening up new possibilities for participatory approaches appealing to diverse audiences" (p. 2). Exploring methods including digital storytelling, photovoice, virtual ethnography, digital archival research, and participatory geographic information systems (GIS), Gubrium and Harper suggest that these approaches have democratized the research process in new and exciting ways. Because of recent and continued developments in digital and multimedia technologies, research collectives can now be spread across the world, working through apps, devices, and other technology both synchronously and asynchronously to learn about each other's lives, communities, and worlds. We acknowledge that some of the approaches we cover here may quickly go extinct, but we urge you to take these suggestions and make them your own, applying and adapting them to your own contexts, interests, commitments, and constraints.

Virtual and Online Ethnography

Ethnography is a methodological approach to gaining a deeper understanding of a culture (Scott-Jones, 2010). Through methods like observation and interviews, ethnographers document how people live, how they communicate with each other, how they interact with their environment, and more. To participatory inquirers, it may at first seem like ethnographic approaches stand in direct contradiction to participatory ones. In general, ethnographers are often presented on the sidelines of the interactions they are documenting and describing. They are observing, not participating. However, ethnographers do often participate, say, for example, through participant observation, which is one form of ethnography that requires them to actively engage and spend time with a group, often living in an area and learning a language. Although participant observation requires a great deal of reflection and reflexivity, it is possible that a conscious or intentional effort at democratizing the research process has not been made, such that participants—or subjects—of their inquiry are elevated from acting as traditional field subjects to co-researchers. So, why consider **virtual and online ethnography** in a book about critical participatory inquiry?

Gubrium and Harper (2009) argue that the social sciences—including anthropology, public health, education, nursing, and social work—must "catch up" with digital methodologies that "offer opportunities to open up the ethnographic research process" (p. 2) to people who have, to date, been seen as passive subjects of the research enterprise, rather than full-fledged members, owners, and creators of valuable knowledge in their own right. In this day and age, virtual and online spaces can offer unique possibilities for CPI collectives. While much has been written about online interviewing, and while many in the world now have significant experience connecting through platforms like Zoom, in this section, we offer several possibilities for engaging in critical participatory ethnographic methods that move beyond the online interview or virtual focus group and that remain tethered to the ontological and epistemological commitments of CPI.

It is important to note that moving into digital and virtual spaces does not mean we will not have to grapple with the same ethical quandaries we do in in-person settings. Whether your ethnographic work is in person or in a virtual setting, it is important to consider that ethnography, as Scott-Jones (2010) notes, is rooted in reflection, reflexivity, and representation. We must continue to engage in reflexive praxis as we learn about and engage with communities, build relationships, and act in humility and openness. If anything, this becomes more complicated in virtual and online spaces because we may not be communicating in real time or most likely will not be seeing each other face-to-face. This can inhibit our ability to build a sense of mutual understanding. In addition, you should consider questions of digital access among the communities you intend to engage as well as established practices for digital participation (Mayorga, 2014). Those with whom you hope to build inquiry relationships for purposes of data collection and analysis may simply be unable to do so because of a lack of reliable digital access or infrastructure or may feel uncomfortable participating virtually. For example, if your collective's interest is in learning more about seniors' healthy eating habits, you may not choose to collect data through online questionnaires, as seniors may have limited access to the internet or internet-ready devices and may not feel comfortable filling out lengthy forms online. So, as you read through the examples we have in this section, we encourage you to consider how you will stay true to the ontological and epistemological commitments of CPI in a digital world.

REFLEXIVITY QUESTION

How have you created relationships of trust online or in virtual spaces in your everyday life? Have you had experiences when that trust was broken or challenged in the digital world? How might those experiences translate to an inquiry setting?

Social Media, Websites, and Blogs

Much has been written in business and other fields about the use of social media for the collection and sharing of data. Most of these approaches, of course, do not fall in line with the commitments and goals of CPI. As your CPI collective begins to weigh options for data collection and analysis, we urge you to consider leveraging social media not to spy on peoples' habits but to make connections across time and space. We believe that digital environments – including social media—have the potential to meaningfully address concerns about (in)equitable access to knowledge creation opportunities. Many researchers have used social media to creatively collect and analyze data because these platforms open up possibilities for involving more people in knowledge creation, from students who are so often silenced in and through research (Akom et al., 2016) to seniors (Trentham et al., 2015), working parents, or refugees and migrants who may be assumed to be too hard to reach or too busy for participation. Facebook, Instagram, Snapchat, WhatsApp, Twitter, and other apps that allow groups, communities, and families to connect are perfect opportunities for research collectives not only to observe others ethnographically but to connect with people that may not typically be seen or treated as knowledge creators.

Edwin Mayorga (2014) writes about the *Education in our Barrios* project, or *#BarrioEdProj*, which "was conceived as an open wall where data would be shared and conversations could be had" (p. 9). The purpose of this project was the exploration of public education in the East Harlem neighborhood of New York City in the context of racial capitalism (Robinson, 2000), that is, how race has historically been and continues to be central to structural hierarchies within capitalism. Mayorga reflects that initially digital spaces did not seem to work for the project. After considering other data collection approaches that would move the project outside of the digital space, the team instead decided to center digital, participatory archiving as part of their research design. Engaging in critical, reflexive praxis, the participatory collective used social media "to deepen and solidify [their] engagement with people in East Harlem (El Barrio), and [they] wanted to encourage more public engagement among people in East Harlem and across New York City" (p. 2). They have included excerpts of interviews on their website (http://barrioedproj.org) and have collected images of East Harlem using Flickr and Instagram. They also embedded RebelMouse, a "social media tool that brings together various social media feeds from many social media platforms" (p. 7), on their website. One important aspect of this collective's work was their commitment to using digital tools that would allow for multiple languages, thereby increasing access to and use of the data and findings they sought to share broadly.

As another example, in 2021 Meagan's *Courageous Conversations* group invited high school students to share pictures or original art that represented how they felt "seen but not heard" in the context of COVID-era virtual schooling. *Courageous Conversations* was being held online through the host school's virtual learning platform, but students felt nervous about collecting data there because students could easily be identified and, potentially, targeted in response to their submissions. In addition, the group was worried that it would be difficult to attract many participants because the school's learning platform automatically created a closed group and people had to be manually invited in. The group decided to collect data through various social media platforms and then showcase the data on the school's learning platform. This addressed both of the students' concerns: Social media offered easy access to their peers during the COVID-19 pandemic, and it allowed people to submit photos and other artistic creations semianonymously.

As you think about the use of social media and digital platforms, consider how data gathering and meaning making might become blurred, rather than distinct activities. As an example: Consider if your CPI collective was interested in learning about first-generation students' experiences at large universities to raise awareness and promote equitable actions in admissions and student services. Co-researchers may be interested in developing a hashtag campaign, on a platform like Twitter or Mastodon, to gather data from a wide group of individuals. It is possible that co-researchers in the collective may start the campaign with stories of their own experiences and use the hashtag to generate interest in the topic. After individuals outside the collective begin to submit their own stories, it is possible for co-researchers to comment on others' posts, in essence, engaging with these individuals to collectively make meaning and build off one another's experiences. Commenting on another individual's post not only generates additional data, but the dialogic and relational aspects of social media (something we can often forget about behind our screens) also create opportunities for meaning making. If done responsibly, this can move co-researchers and participants toward critical self-consciousness, mutual understanding, and action.

Radio and Podcasting

As a widely accessible form of media, radio presents opportunities for participatory creation and sharing of local knowledge, even in low-resource or more remote settings. McKenzie's (2008) inquiry work about natural resource management with fishing communities in Nicaragua demonstrates this potential, in which the collective broadcast culturally relevant music, interviews, storytelling sessions, poetry, and scripted sociodramas portraying community concerns and solutions through a local university radio station.

A more contemporary version of radio is podcasting, which requires relatively affordable technology, has the potential to reach large audiences, and opens up possibilities for more equitable access to public engagement in knowledge creation. A local Boys and Girls Club in Virginia (U.S.), where Meagan lives, has created a podcast to celebrate and amplify (quite literally) the voices of their teen members on issues that are important to them. In preparation to launch *Manacast*, the teen members of the club learned about the technology needed to create and edit podcasts, made a list of topics and prioritized them, conducted research online and among peers on those topics, and then rotated hosting responsibilities among themselves, all with an eye toward connecting with teens across the world. The podcast was started during the COVID-19 pandemic to help teens connect with others, but it has continued to inspire the Virginia youth and those with whom they connect on issues as varied as mental health, family relationships, sports, entertainment, and virtual schooling. Keona Staton, the Club's podcast organizer, reflects that the podcast has "helped the youth gain more respect for others in the world and helped them see that their opinions really do matter compared to the messages they receive" (personal communication, June 25, 2021).

A CPI group in Toronto has used podcasting with "racialized newcomer youth" co-researchers who had recently migrated to Canada to "explore connections between sport and social development" (Smith et al., 2021, p. 128). The group reflects on various challenges and limitations, including a lesson on including youth co-researchers in creating consent tools but ultimately finds that digital technologies like podcasting "can facilitate opportunities to co-create knowledge and experiences about [sports for development] that may not be available or achievable within a traditional research framework" (p. 129). Even though tensions emerged around the responsibility to share stories in an authentic way while also producing stories suitable for an audience, the research collective finds power in sharing stories through short self-interviews and other methods. The co-researchers discuss a launch party to celebrate the podcast and the achievements of the group as particularly successful. Overall, they reflect that the choice to use podcasts to facilitate participatory knowledge creation was a relatively good one, despite the challenges, and that it helped to encourage greater participation, encouraged shifts in power dynamics among co-researchers, and allowed for ongoing reflexivity. In reference to our earlier emphasis on the need for increased attention to the ethical and epistemological considerations of and with participatory digital methodologies, the research collective notes that "the podcast project was not achieved or completed because of any inherent characteristics of podcasts, but rather because of the quality and reciprocal nature of the relationships that were built during the process" (p. 140). Again, relationships are central to the ways in which specific methods and methodologies can be deemed successful—or, in our terms, in keeping with the underlying epistemological commitments of CPI.

Digital Storytelling

The oral tradition of storytelling is one of the oldest methods of sharing knowledge and experiences with others. In a digital form, however, it provides an alternative and compelling medium that not only continues this sharing tradition, but it also provides an opportunity to engage with different audiences that we may have never reached before. For instance, think about what you would do if you were interested in finding a good restaurant near your home. In the past, we may have called a friend or neighbor to ask them about their recommendations, and they would have likely told a story about their experience: what to order, what to avoid, times to go. While this still happens, of course, we may forego that step and go straight to a crowdsourcing website (e.g., Yelp) to see what others are recommending. While these types of digital platforms are helpful, they are not available for everything that we would want to learn about within a neighborhood or community. If you were interested in learning more about what community members see as assets and resources that can be used to address problems—that is, community asset mapping or assets-oriented community assessment (Sharpe et al., 2000)—there may not be a dedicated website for this. That said, you could take inspiration from a crowdsourcing website and begin to digitally elicit stories from community members.

Take, for example, this participatory project where the team worked alongside community members in Los Angeles, California (U.S.) to map places that they deemed to be positive communication assets, that is, places where they felt they could interact and converse with others that would lead to community building and improved health outcomes (Villanueva et al., 2016). In this case, Villanueva et al. (2016) redefined assets beyond the physical notion of space (e.g., a community center), extending it to the communicative dimensions of interaction, including "communication hot spots," where residents gather and "engage each other in everyday conversation" and "comfort zones," which refers to business and institutions that residents are familiar with and have "an ongoing affective connection" (p. 2709). By working alongside neighborhood residents, they were able to digitally map the environment, showcasing spaces "that could potentially be accessed for building healthy communities" (Villanueva et al., 2016, p. 2712). As we mentioned before, when conducting a project like this, it is important to understand digital accessibility. Consider this: Do potential co-researchers or participants have access to the technology you are going to use? In what ways will digital platforms inhibit inclusion and participation? In this case, the team first printed maps and had residents identify the communication hot spots and comfort zones in their neighborhoods. They then worked with residents to create a digital map where users could click on a geo-coded pin, which would then show them the location, photo, and description of the community-identified asset. Box 8.1 offers another take on digital storytelling, called *storyworlding*.

BOX 8.1: STORYWORLDING

A feminist research collective in Indiana (U.S.) created a new digital methodology, **storyworlding,** to center the stories they have collected through the WomenWeLove Project (Dennis et al., 2020). Framed as a feminist ethnographic method, migratory storyworlding allows the research collective to honor the lives of six "ordinary" women across the world as they study women's lives in the context of geopolitical heterosexism and patriarchy.

Relationships between researchers and participants take center stage in this digital ethnographic approach.

The authors explore love as a methodological orientation. While this may seem bizarre to many socialized to believe distance between the researcher and the researched is of paramount importance, at this stage in the process of learning about CPI and its epistemological roots, we should feel comfortable enough to argue for close, trusting—even loving—relationships as central to ethical and valid participatory inquiry. Storyworlding as method is founded on hours-long life-story in-depth interviews in the context of relationships that the researchers expect to last lifetimes. These dialogues are augmented by various artifacts, including baby books, yearbooks, photo albums, local archival data, memories, informal conversations, and more. The collective collaboratively created a website to house the data. Importantly, "other sources are drawn upon so that interviews do not stand alone, but are set within their own contexts for understanding" (Dennis et al., 2020, p. 751).

This storyworlding approach to participatory ethnography highlights a collective nature in its process and outcomes, as participants contribute fully and with the respect and love of those in the traditional role of researcher. The data collection and analysis are anchored by dialogue and relationality. The analysis and resulting website, which uses the storymapping software ArcGIS, are both anchored by contextual complexity.

As you can see, utilizing **digital storytelling** through the lens of community asset mapping demonstrates the strengths and qualities that could potentially be used to promote health, as well as map areas where problems should be addressed. Just as we explored in previous chapters, the use of a strengths-based approach provides a counterstory or counternarrative that critiques dominant views (e.g., master narratives) of a group, neighborhood, or culture (Solórzano & Yosso, 2002). By using digital platforms like Google Maps and turning community-generated data into infographics—whether printed or left solely online—communities have the space to document their lived knowledge and lived experiences, which can then be used to advocate for social change. Collaborative critical discourse analysis is another way to analyze data from a strengths-based perspective. Box 8.2 offers a step-by-step guide to this analytic approach.

BOX 8.2: STEP-BY-STEP: COLLABORATIVE CRITICAL DISCOURSE ANALYSIS

Any of the analytic approaches mentioned in previous chapters, from thematic to narrative analysis, could be used to systematically make meaning from digital data. Using the example of the hashtag campaign in this chapter, we will review how critical discourse analysis (CDA; Wodak & Meyer, 2001) could be used by a CPI collective to explore how language and power are related when analyzing the experiences of first-generation university students.

Step 1. Organize co-researchers virtually or in person once the campaign has ended. If the collective were interested in exploring how power asymmetries and social hierarchies manifest in the experiences of first-generation students, it would be possible to analyze the text from social media posts. In addition to this, to analyze the language of those who hold more power, it would be helpful to bring in official university documents—those related to diversity, equity, inclusion, and first-generation policies—where participants or co-researchers are enrolled.

Step 2a. As Wodak (2001) mentions, CDA is used to analyze three interrelated concepts: "the concept of power, the concept of history, and the concept of ideology" (p. 3). If interested in understanding and exploring how these concepts figure prominently across texts produced by first-generation students and universities, a series of open-ended questions could be used to explore what co-researchers interpret. Here are a few examples of open-ended questions using Roy Bhaskar's (1986) explanatory critique approach, as outlined by Fairclough (2001):

- *Problem identification*: How do problems for first-generation studen ts manifest in the language they use to narrate their experiences? (How) Does it differ from the language used in universities documents and policies?
- *Diagnosis*: How does language (of students, of universities) demonstrate how life and society are structured in ways that make these problems difficult to resolve?
- *Negative critique ("needs" the problem)*: (How) Does the university system (i.e., social order) need the problem to sustain itself? (How) Does discourse sustain power asymmetries, domination, and oppression?
- *Positive critique*: In what ways can we observe contradictions or gaps in discourse, especially that which is produced by those in power? How can these contradictions or gaps by used to realize or create sites of possibility?
- *Critical reflection*: How accurate is our analysis? How can our analysis be used to move toward emancipatory aims.

Step 2b. As mentioned in Chapters 6 and 7, make sure several co-researchers are taking notes.

Step 3. (Re)presentation can be approached in a series of ways. The conversation from the hashtag campaign can be archived on a website along with analyses, as a form of advocacy. Excerpts from the text generated by first-generation students could be used in academic journals, reports, and policy briefs. Students' words could be flanked against university policies, demonstrating the contradictions that manifest through power asymmetries as well as the recommendations proposed by the students themselves. Students could be invited to speak their own words to decision makers at the university level or locally elected officials.

REFLEXIVITY QUESTION

Could you see yourself engaging in participatory ethnographic approaches? What feels uncomfortable for you about these methods? What feels exciting or possible for you?

Photographic Methods

Photography has gained popularity in participatory inquiry in recent years, especially with the expansion of access to smartphones with digital cameras, and has been incorporated into numerous approaches. For example, Toroyan and Reddy (2005) engaged South African youth in a participatory process of developing educational photocomics to promote HIV/AIDS awareness, using a medium popular with the target group. Similarly, Hidalgo (2015) reports on the creation of Augmented Fotonovelas, "visual counter-stories that center the experiences of People of Color" (p. 301) based on the culturally relevant fotonovela medium, as a pedagogical and social justice tool for Latinx populations in the United States.

Photovoice

Caroline Wang developed the **photovoice** method (originally called photo novella) in the early 1990s as a tool for rural Chinese women to conduct a reproductive health needs assessment and inform policy and service provision (Wang & Burris, 1994). The approach was explicitly grounded in Freire's (1972) problem-posing education, feminist theory, and documentary photography techniques in order to foster participants' critical consciousness about community assets and needs and communicate their perspectives and demands for change to policymakers (Wang & Burris, 1994, 1997). In practical terms, the process consists of four steps:

1. Collaborative identification of a theme or topic;
2. Taking and selecting photographs;
3. Discussing the selected photographs in group discussions or interviews; and
4. Drafting a descriptive text.

To guide the discussion and drafting steps, Wang and Redwood Jones (2001) suggest photo-elicitation questions using the acronym SHOWeD, which can easily be adapted:

1. What do you **S**ee here?
2. What is really **H**appening?
3. How does this relate to **O**ur lives?
4. **W**hy does this problem or strength **e**xist?
5. What can we **D**o about it?

The resulting photographs and accompanying descriptions can be shared with community members, policymakers, and other stakeholders to represent community knowledge and inform decision making (Wang & Burris, 1994; see Jarldorn & 'Deer,' 2017). Photovoice has become popular in participatory research, especially with children (e.g., Oh, 2012; Zenkov et al., 2014), immigrants and refugees (e.g., Berman et al., 2016; Sahay et al., 2016), Indigenous peoples (e.g., Wright et al., 2016), and other marginalized and vulnerable groups. While we have also employed photovoice to document the experiences and viewpoints of children, immigrants, and refugees, we caution you to carefully consider the political and ethical implications, particularly in schools and other hierarchical institutions (see Call-Cummings, 2017; Call-Cummings et al., 2019; Hauber-Özer & Call-Cummings, 2020). In addition, discussing and displaying photographs can potentially bring up distressing memories (Berman et al., 2016), expose participants to legal or social repercussions (Dumbrill, 2009; Sahay et al., 2016), or even resemble cooptation of participants' experiences (Hugman et al., 2011). As a result, decisions about what kinds of photographs to take, who "owns" the data, ethical procedures for ensuring informed consent and confidentiality, where and how to display photographs and narratives, and whether to use photovoice at all require the collective to think deeply about these factors (see Hauber-Özer & Call-Cummings, 2020 for a fuller discussion).

Virtual Photovoice

Although typically done through a series of in-person workshops and ideally in the context of established relationships, a handful of researchers—Meagan and Melissa included—have adapted photovoice to a virtual format. Our colleague Ahmet Tanhan has conducted several large-scale online photovoice studies on mental health and well-being using a web-based survey containing a consent form, detailed instructions, links for more information, and steps for uploading photographs and descriptions (see Doyumğaç et al., 2020; Tanhan, 2020; Tanhan & Strack, 2020). Tanhan's approach reduces confidentiality issues and expands participation but does not operate from the same explicitly critical and participatory ethic that we espouse. For example, community members are not involved in analyzing or sharing the photographs and texts; rather, participants provide themes for their submissions which the university-based research team uses to analyze and interpret the data.

During the COVID-19 pandemic, we (Meagan and Melissa) developed a few different approaches to virtual photovoice. First, in the spring of 2020, we partnered with the Knowledge Democracy Initiative of the Action Research Network of the Americas to gather images and texts representing solidarity and connection during the early months of social distancing and isolation. While not research, strictly speaking, the project webpage features submissions in multiple languages from Sri Lanka, the Netherlands, Turkey, Canada, Germany, the United States, South Africa, England, Scotland, New Zealand, Colombia, and Indonesia (Call-Cummings et al., 2020) and demonstrates the potential for asynchronous, virtual photovoice.

After the interview phase of her dissertation research, Melissa invited the participants to an online photovoice workshop, which she had originally planned as a series of collaborative discussions to determine the theme, discuss ethical considerations, take and discuss photographs, and write and edit narrative descriptions. To conserve internet usage and respect participants' time and energy during an extremely stressful period, she condensed the process to a one-hour session on Zoom, sending instructions in advance to bring photographs representing their university experiences and setting up Google documents for participants to upload their pictures and descriptions. However, she did not anticipate the difficulties participants would encounter using Google Drive on their mobile phones, as most did not have computers at home (university campuses and dorms had been emptied to reduce contact) and switching between applications. Melissa had to adapt on the spot, receiving participants' submissions on her cell phone via WhatsApp and then sharing them on behalf of the participants with to discuss using the following photo-elicitation questions:

1. I want to share this photo because . . .
2. What is important for people to understand about this photo?
3. What does this photo tell others about me or my community?

They took 10 to 15 minutes to write short descriptions (example in Figure 8.1) or sent the text separately by WhatsApp if they needed more time.

FIGURE 8.1 ■ My Way of Life: I took this photo from my university in Turkey. It represents my way of life. If I lost my way, or see a lot of difficulties which I can't deal with it, then I try to choose another way, there are many directions and methods in the life that we can choose it and achieve what we want. We just need to look around us.

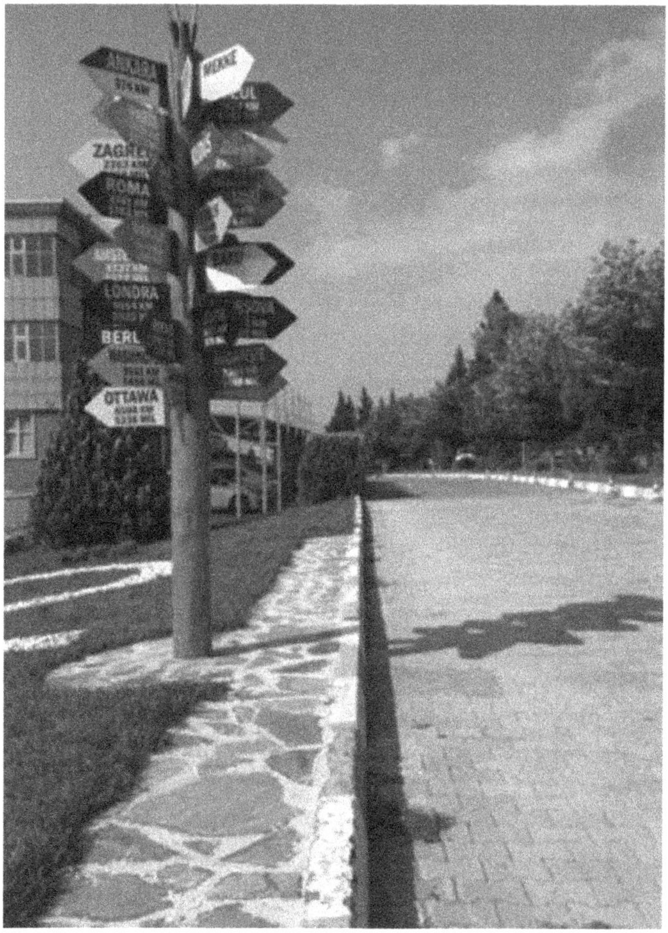

She also held a second workshop and added an asynchronous option to send submissions to her without attending the workshop for participants who had to work or attend to family responsibilities or did not have a strong enough internet connection. This highlights some of the unanticipated challenges that can pop up in virtual research, especially with marginalized populations. Melissa incorporated the texts and captions into individual narrative portraits (Smyth & McInerney, 2013) she constructed from participants' interview data and, as mentioned in Chapter 5, created an online gallery[1] to display their creations. She shared this gallery as an art exhibit at the 2021 virtual CIES conference to draw attention to their messages of resilience and resistance.

Meagan has used photovoice with her school-based *Courageous Conversations* collective several times, including an online version around the theme student co-researchers identified for the 2020–2021 year, "seen but not heard." In response to school district requirements that students keep their video cameras on and their microphones off during virtual schooling, the collective invited fellow students to anonymously send in photos, drawings and narratives representing their views on this policy, which were shared in a gallery on the school's distance learning platform. One student chose to submit her own original artwork created for the project instead of a photo, and connected her thoughts on being seen but not heard in the context of school with how she feels seen but not heard as a woman who identifies as Black. As a caption for the drawing she writes,

> This piece is about Racial Injustice and how it affects the surroundings of certain individuals, specifically minorities and the youth. I myself am a minority and a teenager so I wanted to do this piece sharing how everyday moments can cloud your mind with certain cases and situations. Hence, the portraits of Breonna Taylor, Michael Brown, George Floyd and so on in the background. I also decided to include some literature that not only touch[es] on the issue of Racial Injustice but also educates on it as well.

Even, or perhaps especially, in virtual spaces, photography offers countless options for capturing and communicating participants' experiences, dreams, and calls for change. We encourage you to think about ways to incorporate this powerful but often risky medium into your future inquiry.

RECOMMENDED PRACTICE 8.1: DO A MINI PHOTOVOICE WORKSHOP

Choose a photograph that has particular significance to you and share it with a small group of classmates or co-researchers in your collective. Use the SHOWeD photo-elicitation questions to discuss the image and its meaning. Then, based on the ideas elicited, draft a short (5–7 sentence) narrative describing the picture to share with your group.

Collage

Collage is an art genre that dates back over a thousand years, popularized in the 10th century in Japan and used worldwide thereafter. Many of us may remember primary school days, cutting up magazines or other print materials and sticking papers together to express ourselves on a topic, but in addition to this fairly common cutting-and-sticking format, collage can be used by stringing objects or beads together (Kay, 2013) or in other ways that are contextually and culturally appropriate. Collage helps us reflect on and illustrate the ways in which we view ourselves, our world, and the relationship between those two.

Look back to the collage you created from posts in your social media accounts for the opening focus activity. What did you learn about yourself through this activity? Did it spark any thoughts about how you might use this method in your own CPI? While sometimes considered an arts-based inquiry approach, we highlight it in this chapter as it may be used effectively and creatively in digital and virtual spaces as well. While we did not actually find academic examples of virtual, collaborative collage in our searches, we offer a few examples and discuss how they could be adapted in a virtual setting.

Our first example is from a community-based research project that used a collage technique within a larger project that aimed to explore wellness in a remote northern Canadian Inuit community, Hamlet of Arviat (Dutton et al., 2019). While the research group used various qualitative methods throughout the lifespan of the project, they used collage as a participatory method to build cross-cultural relationships, offer opportunities for reflection, and serve as an elicitation technique. As Dutton et al. (2019) note, "Like the use of other creative strategies to foster relational connections and knowledge sharing between people, the act of creating collage in a group dialogue setting can be transformative" (p. 2). The group found that the collage process motivates self-reflection and reciprocal, relational dialogue.

Another example uses beads and found objects to tell personal narratives (Kay, 2013). Kay (2013) tells of her own journey stringing beads into a collage that would facilitate her own self-reflection. She worked for 6 hours "gathering, arranging, ordering, stringing beads and miscellaneous found objects" (p. 1) and realized she could use similar methods as art therapy with her students at the special education school where she worked. Kay tells of one student who crafted a bead collage that represented special people in her life. The bead collage helped this student tell her life story because it helped her link "her feelings and memories" (p. 4). This student, who would traditionally be seen as a receiver of knowledge, saw herself as a creator of knowledge in her own right through this simple yet profound experience.

Although these examples of the collage making were conducted in an in-person context, it could easily be adapted for the virtual space, either synchronously or asynchronously. One could offer asynchronous instructions similar to those found at the beginning of this chapter and engage in analysis by posting individual collages on a shared workspace (Google Drive, for example) and engaging in interpretive practices by leaving comments. Working synchronously, a group could meet on a platform like Zoom, share their screens as they take turns creating their own collages or collaboratively create a collage on a theme the group chooses. Again, they could make meaning (analyze) dialogically in the same session or in subsequent ones. Box 8.3 includes another example of how one could use multimedia arts in CPI.

BOX 8.3: PARTICIPATORY MULTIMEDIA ARTS

For her dissertation focusing on youth literacy practices, PhD candidate Bethany Monea developed a participatory media project with a collective of Latinx students in Northern Virginia who met in a college bridge program. In a series of videos posted on their YouTube channel, LatiNXT GEN, the student co-researchers documented their experiences transitioning from high school to college as members of the first generation in their families to attend higher education. In the videos, co-researchers offer intimate glimpses into their disappointments, hopes, and dreams; explore cultural identity, language, and family relationships; and deliberate about college decisions and navigate their first year during a pandemic. During the course of the project, they also created multimedia visual artwork, including paintings, collages, poetry, and word art, "to validate, embrace, and learn from the fullness of students' creative, critical, and linguistic repertoire in the fight for justice within and beyond schools" (Monea et al., 2020). They collaboratively made meaning of the visual, audio, and textual data they gathered, co-authored articles, and presented their work at scholarly conferences, seeking to prioritize youth perspectives at every step of the way. This project demonstrates the potential for digital and multimedia approaches to engage youth in meaningful reflection, self-representation, and activism.

CONCLUSION

Rapid developments in technology offer an increasing and ever-changing number of opportunities to engage in digital and multimedia approaches to inquiry but simultaneously introduce new ethical dilemmas about privacy, confidentiality, and the impact of engaging in them. In this chapter, we covered a variety of digital and multimedia opportunities, from virtual ethnography to photovoice to collage, for gathering data and making meaning with your CPI collective. These are just the tip of the iceberg. Always anchor your decisions on the needs of the collective, the moment, and the audience. Remember to continually ask yourself as well as your inquiry collective: What is appropriate? What is necessary? What is helpful? As you do this, we urge you to explore which methods might help you and your co-researchers to increase mutual understanding and share knowledge beyond the collective.

RECOMMENDED PRACTICE 8.2: HOW WILL YOU COLLECT AND MAKE MEANING?

As you did in the last two chapters, meet with your co-researchers to talk about how digital and multimedia methods could be used to collect data and make meaning. Consider your inquiry plan and discuss the types of evidence that matter and priority areas of concern. Write out one area of concern on a piece of flipchart paper. Discuss if and how various digital and multimedia methods from this chapter could produce the type of evidence that your collective needs. Do any of the digital and multimedia methods in this chapter offer potential opportunities (e.g., broader distribution, reaching different audiences) that those in other chapters do not? Do they encourage community members or decision makers to act? Are there any potential risks if you use these digital or multimedia methods? If the methods in this chapter will not produce the evidence you need, consider those in the last two chapters (e.g., interviews, focus groups, arts based).

SUMMARY OF KEY POINTS

- Digital and multimedia approaches to data collection and analysis as well as sharing findings have the potential to reach larger and more dispersed groups of both participants and audiences than traditional methods.
- Approaches such as virtual ethnography, photovoice, and digital storytelling can facilitate deeper understanding of others' experiences, ways of being, and ways of knowing and can serve as powerful, evocative forms of community self-advocacy and activism.
- These methods also require careful consideration potential ethical issues regarding access, privacy, confidentiality, and safety. It is imperative to consider the collective, the moment, and the audience in deciding which digital and multimedia methods are appropriate, necessary, and helpful for your inquiry.

SUGGESTED ACTIVITIES

1. Journal about digital and multimedia approaches to inquiry: Which approaches caught your attention? Which came to mind that we did not include? Which have you used before, and which ones would you like to try?
2. Identify a digital or multimedia approach that you or your potential co-researchers would find enjoyable or meaningful and brainstorm ways that you could incorporate it into your inquiry.
3. Explore one of the online galleries or channels mentioned in this chapter and envision how you might display your collective's creations. What kinds of virtual or community-based platforms could be useful for data gathering or sharing findings? What ethical issues might you need to consider?

KEY TERMS

born-digital dissertation
digital storytelling
photovoice
storyworlding
virtual and online ethnography

ENDNOTE

1. https://melbeth27.wixsite.com/melissahauber/gallery

9 TAKING ACTION

LEARNING OBJECTIVES

By the end of this chapter you will be able to

- Discuss what it means to take action with co-researchers and others.
- Identify multiple opportunities to take action within academia and beyond.
- Analyze the various implications of taking action for social and organizational change in solidarity with co-researchers and others.

FOCUS ACTIVITY 9.1: MAKING DECISIONS TO TAKE ACTION

On any blank piece of paper, on your computer, or on Post-it Notes on your wall, create a balance board listing goals, needs, and risks. Don't worry about how it looks or if it makes sense to others. Consider the following and create a visual representation that will help you make decisions about the actions you can and should take based on your inquiry.

1. What are your goals and needs as a researcher?
2. What are the goals and needs of your research collective?
3. What are the community's (or audience's) goals and needs in this moment?
4. Who, and what, is at risk and in what ways?

At the beginning of each of the last three chapters, we have reminded you to focus your data collection and analysis decisions by asking yourself three questions: "What is appropriate? What is necessary? What is helpful?" These questions are offered to help guide you and your research collective toward intentional decision making rooted in the needs and goals of the community with whom you are working. They are also intended as opportunities to reflect on how you are framing your inquiry: Are you coming at the research with an appreciation for the strengths of the community, rather than in a deficit, damage or problem-centered orientation?

Are you guided by a deep understanding of what is valued by the community? Are you centering the voices, perspectives, and experiences of community members and co-researchers in your inquiry? As you and your critical participatory inquiry (CPI) collective move toward taking action, these questions should remain central to your decision making.

In this chapter, as in previous ones, we start by pinning down some concepts and definitions that are key to grappling with what is often a complicated process of taking action through and in inquiry. We conclude this section with thoughts on what it means to "fail" in CPI, acknowledging we often feel like failures when, in actuality, it may be more productive to consider the constraints we are navigating and, hopefully, changing a bit. The second section offers several ideas for ways you and your CPI collective can take action and call for change. We also discuss options for sharing findings both within academia and outside of it, recognizing that as critical participatory inquirers we often have to do a double share of work to make sure that findings are recognized in many spaces and among varied audiences.

RECOMMENDED PRACTICE 9.1: NEGOTIATING GOALS, NEEDS, AND RISKS

In the focus activity at the start of this chapter, we asked you to reflect on your goals, needs, and risks. While it is important to reflect on these questions, it is absolutely necessary to discuss and negotiate these terms with all co-researchers in your collective. As you meet, discuss the questions together and create a visual, such as a Venn diagram to show where goals, needs, and risks do and do not intersect. Or perhaps your visual looks like a three-columned balance sheet where you can account for each goal, need, and risk to show how they balance out. You can even use some of the techniques we discussed in previous chapters to facilitate dialogue.

CONCEPTS AND DEFINITIONAL ISSUES

Sharing findings and taking action related to those findings can be tricky in any community-oriented research context but can be especially difficult to navigate when engaging with co-researchers who are considered full owners of both the CPI process and any products to come out of that process. In this section, we offer some thoughts on what it means to share ownership in critical participatory inquiry.

Ownership

Academic literature and development discourse are full of examples of researchers' or practitioners' attempts to "share" **ownership** of research processes and products with people who are directly affected by them. Kilroy (2011) writes about the challenges of "participation" that he saw while studying the reintegration of ex-combatants in Sierra Leone. Kilroy notes that programs for the disarmament, demobilization, and reintegration (DDR) of ex-combatants need to be both flexible and responsive to local contexts because "re-integration ultimately takes place in the community" (p. 127) and each community's experience is unique. Because of this, Kilroy suggests a "partnership" or participatory approach to DDR is most appropriate because it "aims to engender a higher level of ownership of the programme by the community" (p. 128) and builds capacity and sustainability. Kilroy identifies a central concern around the unequal power dynamics inherent in these types of development programs, as well as the short timeframe they are allotted for implementation. Reviewing several additional contextual constraints, including "the needs of donors for quick, measurable results" and "divergent interests, agendas, and cultures among the many agencies involved" (pp. 142–143), Kilroy raises questions about the agency of the ex-combatants involved in the DDR process, concluding that one of the essential (and missing) ingredients in this case was the relationships between ex-combatants and those in positions of power.

We can learn several lessons from this example. First, we are reminded that CPI collectives and participatory processes will always operate in the context of varied constraints. In the example of DDR in Sierra Leone, these numerous constraints are both obvious and subtle. Kilroy notes the desire of financial donors to receive quick, measurable results of so-called success as well as divergent agendas of the many stakeholders involved. These are common constraints for development contexts and are often difficult, if not impossible, to maneuver around or through. What could have perhaps been addressed, though, were the relationships between ex-combatants and people who were implementing the DDR. This goes back to one of the core commitments of CPI, relationality, and connects to one of the constraints Kilroy identifies: short time frames. We strongly encourage those interested in or committed to participatory inquiry to make sure there is enough time to develop the trusting relationships necessary for open dialogue and equitable participation.

A second lesson we learn through this example is the imperative to decommodify inquiry. That is, to be set up for a greatest likelihood of success, in terms of reaching toward the goals of all co-researchers with an emphasis on the goals of those who are directly impacted by the focus of the inquiry, CPI collectives must reduce the importance and power of financial incentives. When inquiry is treated as a commodity by donors or funders, institutions of higher education, or local governments, uncomfortable power dynamics instantly pop up. Gone unchecked, these unequal dynamics fester until they destroy any chance of equitable participation and inquiry-based social change.

Finally, we learn through Kilroy's example that the process of knowledge creation must be decolonized. This lesson is particularly poignant in Kilroy's case as well as numerous examples from the development arena. The need to decolonize knowledge creation cannot be clearer than seeing donors from the Global North invading countries in the Global South with money, ideas, and power in the name of fixing local problems. This is the definition of a deficit orientation and is often replicated in research and evaluation.

For those working in research settings where institutional review boards (IRB) must approve consent forms and data collection protocols, this can further complicate the concept of ownership. This can relate to the fact that consent forms may need to be branded with university logos, which may diminish trust among community members who would otherwise be interested in completing a survey sent to them by one of their neighbors who is serving as a co-researcher in a CPI collective. Additionally, if interview protocols were co-created with community members and then sent to IRB for approval, the collective would then need to reconvene and discuss revisions if the IRB requests changes. On the other hand, a researcher may decide it makes more sense for the community to "own" the protocols and data. In this case, if the co-created protocols are administered by community members, and data are stored by this group, then IRB approval may not be needed. Although ownership relinquishes some control to communities, it can equate to more work (e.g., securely storing data, responsibility for data collection). For those working in settings where IRB approval is necessary, we recommend you contact your office as officials may have ideas on how to organize documents to comply with your institution's policies as well as your commitments as a CPI practitioner.

So, what does this all have to do with ownership in the context of CPI? Even using the word *ownership* implies something that *can* be traded, purchased, exchanged, or given. When we conceptualize inquiry as some*thing* to be shared or co-owned, we are already on a dangerous precipice propped up by power and positional blindness. Interrupting the automaticity with which we jump to the alluring idea of co-ownership is difficult. Focusing on building and strengthening relationships among members of the CPI collective and anchoring our work in humble dialogue, however, can help us navigate this. As we develop strong relationships, co-researchers who may not be in traditional positions of power because of profession, identity category, or experience will have agency (something the ex-combatants in Kilroy's example were lacking) to offer opinions or suggestions or to say no to others' opinions or suggestions. When Meagan hears the question, "When do you know you're doing 'good' participatory inquiry?" she often responds, "When co-researchers say no to me." Remember that critical participatory inquiry is a practice rooted in dialogue and deliberation, so when co-researchers feel comfortable disagreeing with us, it may indicate that we are moving toward more equal relationships.

Implications of Being "Community Led"

In addition to the concept or practice of "co-ownership," as CPI practitioners we often throw around dreams of projects being "community led" without much attention to what this actually means or looks like in practice. Through the example of their own participatory action research (PAR) project conducted in a working-class neighborhood school they call Ruby Bridges Elementary, Dworski-Riggs and Langhout (2010) help clarify how power relations can play out in the context of CPI and what can be done to address tensions and unintended consequences of the social norms of the community in which CPI is being conducted.

Dworski-Riggs and Langhout's project related to parent, teacher, and principal concerns about the social climate at the school. Results from an initial survey found that the main problem that needed to be addressed was that "the social-political climate [of the school] did not facilitate a more consensus-based model of governance" (p. 218). Given that this concern is directly in tension with PAR's commitment to equitable stakeholder participation throughout the inquiry process, Dworski-Riggs and Langhout explore the implications of this tension in the practice of participatory inquiry. They conclude that "the school's social norms regarding decision making discouraged most community members from participating" and that opportunities for participation that the PAR group sought to create "were in fact constrained by local social norms" (p. 222) as well as by the perception on the part of school staff that that social reality was fixed (p. 223). Dworski-Riggs and Langhout questioned whether it was appropriate (or ethical) to directly or indirectly question or challenge these social norms, given their deeply held commitment to "community-led" inquiry.

We often hear questions related to this type of quandary: What if the community members are uninterested in the type of participation that CPI espouses? What if they are too busy? What if they honestly do not care? What if, structurally, community members are somehow constrained or limited in their ability to participate, whether because of established social norms, as was the case at Ruby Bridges Elementary, or because of other reasons? We typically fall back on those core CPI commitments to open dialogue and humble, trusting relationships. If those relationships are in place, open dialogue about interests and limitations can occur. A teacher could, theoretically, explain to Meagan her hesitancy about participating in a CPI project. Students could express to Melissa why they feel vulnerable taking pictures for a photovoice project. Or a community member could clarify to Giovanni why they do not feel comfortable participating in ways Giovanni assumes are useful or important.

However, sometimes dialogue and trust cannot overcome or even address structures and norms we may not be fully aware of ourselves. We can envision our students asking, "What do we do then?" We readily acknowledge that we do not have all the answers. We may offer advice for one context or the next. Jenny Cameron (2008), a professor of geography and environmental sciences in Australia, notes that PAR can be conducted for various and multiple aims (e.g., for liberatory purposes, researching with or for institutions, or a combination of these). As Cameron mentions, critical inquirers must be able to identify, manage and mitigate institutional challenges, which can help us to focus on action. The important thing is that we are aware of these possibilities and that we acknowledge CPI is not a panacea for all that ails inquiry. It is a radical way of thinking that helps us to call out and push against injustices.

Moving Through Constraints and Limitations

With all of these thoughts on how CPI may not work out the way we envision it, we often think (and write) about the ways in which we have felt constrained in reaching the full potential of many of our CPI projects. Indeed, sometimes we think of this as **failure**. This is not always self-inflicted. As CPI is most often conceptualized as action oriented, when we are interviewed for podcasts or classroom visits, we are often asked to reflect on the changes our inquiry has made. Meagan often tells of a question she gets asked about her dissertation, which usually sounds something like, "So, what are the concrete steps that were taken through this project that explored racism among White teachers in rural Idaho?" Meagan typically responds that, in many ways, she felt like her dissertation was a failure because of an inability to address issues like racism in tangible ways. She had been trained in critical PAR by people who had gotten policies changed and projected findings on the sides of buildings (literally!). What did her project actually *do*? Students visited a school board meeting and talked about their experiences with racism; they were metaphorically patted on the head and . . . that was pretty much it. She failed, didn't she?

Well, there is, of course, a problem in that framing. It was not *her* project to begin with. She didn't own it. It was a collective investigation, exploration, and process. By conceptualizing failure in this way, we are buying into a neoliberal definition of worth and success—something that is concrete or tangible; something we can point to and celebrate and perhaps even monetize but definitely count or rank. We urge practitioners of CPI to avoid this trap. This approach to inquiry is not built for a neoliberal agenda; rather, it is intended to expose the fallacies and dangers of it.

It is important to remember that we are not failures just because we have experienced constraints or limitations in our inquiry. We have found that the commitments we make as CPI practitioners to democratize the inquiry process "create a unique view of what may count as 'failure'" (Ross & Call-Cummings, 2019, p. 107) and that we must attend to the differences between our commitments and the backgrounded, taken-for-granted norms that limit our ability to reach or achieve those commitments. We must resist the deficit orientation that the concept of failure embodies and remember that CPI is connected to the constraints we experience in the context of our inquiry, be they structural, institutional, or contextual. The important part is how we maneuver through those constraints.

REFLEXIVITY QUESTION

When have you felt constrained in your own research or inquiry-based practice? Consider what limitations you experienced. How did you attempt to navigate those? Were they beyond your control? Looking back, how might you act differently in the future, given similar circumstances?

TAKING ACTION, CALLING FOR CHANGE

When it comes to various forms of CPI—whether critical participatory action research (CPAR), youth participatory action research (YPAR), or community-based participatory (action) research (CBPR)—we often think about three separate components of the process: participation, research, and action, usually in this order. However, thinking about CPI in this way can be unhelpful as it establishes a linear and hierarchical order and makes it seem that all participation and research will lead to concrete forms of change. In this section, we highlight several ways to think about action, from self-transformation to mutual understanding to collective action.

Transformation

As we begin this section, we feel it is important to start with the changes that we may forget about or lose sight of due to larger and loftier goals, such as impact on policy. However, within the process of a CPI project, all changes are important, even those at very personal and individual levels. You may recall that in the first few chapters of this book, we talked about different levels of change, including *conscientizaçao* (critical consciousness). In our own research on the impact of CPI projects (Call-Cummings et al., 2021; Call-Cummings et al., 2022), we have explored various levels of change and how co-researchers identify and define these forms of **transformation**.

Consider Figure 9.1, which provides an overview of the types of change that could occur within a CPI project. As in Chapter 1, we apply the work of community psychologist Urie Bronfenbrenner (1979) to the context of human development across the CPI lifecycle. Moving around each concentric circle, you can see examples of each level of change presented with parentheses (e.g., mutual understanding as an example of interpersonal transformation). We can see how this idea of human development does not solely focus on cognitive changes, though. For instance, experiencing an interpersonal change where we understand an individual who may think differently from us requires cognitive, behavioral, and emotional forms of change on the part of two individuals.

Depending on the situation, there may also be a connection across these levels. An individual may need to experience some level of intrapersonal change (e.g., self-actualization); recall Freire's (1970) concept of *conscientizaçao* (critical consciousness), which leads them to understand their historical and socioeconomic position in society and how this affects their everyday life, especially with regard to how they experience or perpetuate oppression. Take, for example, an instance we depicted in our own research with community co-researchers in a high school

FIGURE 9.1 ■ Ecological Map of Change

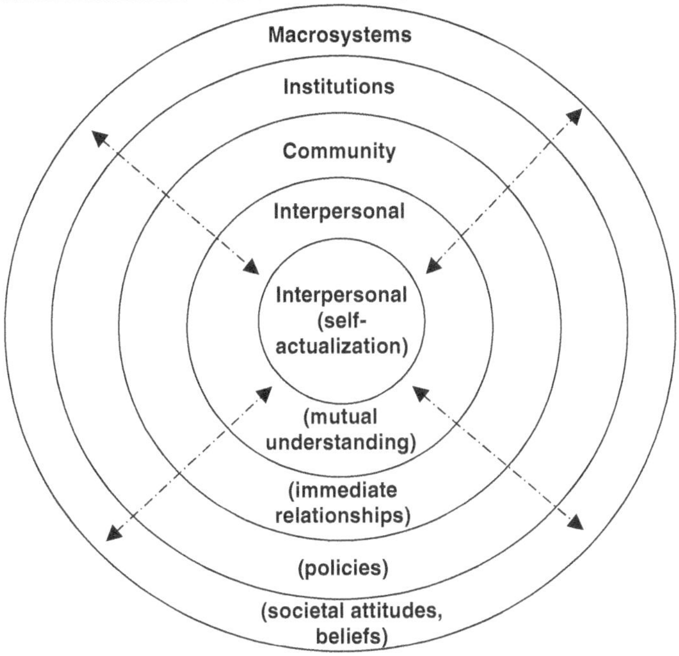

Adapted from Bronfenbrenner's (1979) The Ecology of Human Development and Freire's (1970) conceptualization of transformation.

in the United States (Call-Cummings et al., 2021). Through this project, we were interested in understanding how high school co-researchers experience change and transformation, so we asked them about their experiences. During our participatory reflection and analysis sessions, high school co-researchers talked about how performative activities (Conquergood, 1985, 1998; Madison, 1998) like *Theatre of the Oppressed* (Boal, 1979) or spoken word poetry (Endsley, 2014; Fisher, 2007), which were used to collaboratively gather data, provided an opportunity to share and to learn about what others were experiencing in their high school.

What we generally found during our discussions with high school co-researchers, however, was that they were less likely to explicitly mention self-understanding as a form of transformation; rather, they spoke of mutual understanding and forms of action such as policy changes. This is not to say self-understanding did not occur, but it is a point to be further explored and one that we encourage you to question in your own CPI projects. Is the idea of self-understanding—or a critical self-awareness—simply too abstract? As Freire (1970) outlines in his work, must it occur before an individual is able to understand another and experience transformation, empowerment, and liberation? Nonetheless, although the idea of self-understanding was not always explicitly mentioned, university and high school co-researchers did allude to self-understanding and mutual understanding occurring as more cyclical or concurrent events. Co-researchers mentioned how participatory activities opened space for communicative action (Habermas, 1996), in turn allowing high school students to connect on a deeper level with their peers and providing spaces for them to then reflect on their own unique experiences.

Action

In the previous section, we highlighted how transformation, both as a process and an outcome, can occur across the entire ecological map, from self-understanding to mutual understanding. However, we want to differentiate between these types of change rather than compare one with the other. Comparing interpersonal changes against policy reforms does not provide a useful comparative measurement, as they are at different units of analysis and serve different purposes. For this reason, we wanted to separate transformation and action to provide a helpful heuristic for how we can think about change in a CPI project, writ large. The difficult part comes with a simple question: What counts as action?

In a project working with college students and incarcerated individuals studying together in a classroom, sociologists Yasser Arafat Payne and Angela Bryant (2018) articulate how they frame action around four dimensions, including (1) local history, (2) audience, (3) people, and (4) an action plan. In these four components, which they refer to as "Community and Advocacy," they note that the project should be grounded "in the spirit, interests, and culture of the local correctional facility" (p. 462). Their logic, however, can be extended to any environment in which we work, as these areas hold true to an orientation in CPI. Like any methodology framed in a critical inquiry, Payne and Bryant (2018) start with a historical analysis, working alongside their community co-researchers to learn about the local and historical context of oppression. Much like we would see in an advocacy or communications plan, they then highlight their target audience, that is, those they would like to inform or educate through their research. In the next dimension, they reference the work of McDougal

(2014), who notes that it is crucial to understand "how well the research allows members of the setting to gain a better understanding of their social conditions" (p. 273). If we think about this, we see an intersection between this section and the previous one, where we talked about how individuals often need to experience and work through their own critical consciousness before they can take liberatory actions. Last, in their framework, they note that action or social activism is a requirement. By forming an action plan, which outlines the type of action and an associated timeline for each action, groups of co-researchers (note that not all co-researchers may be interested in social activism) can then take up specific action-oriented projects.

Action can include a number of things. By utilizing data from a CPI project or administrative data sets (e.g., government statistics), groups can form policy recommendations for decision makers, create informational flyers or art to post around the neighborhood to increase public awareness, or organize community projects to assist those in need. Remember that it is important to pair the action with the identified target audience. For instance, writing a policy brief with recommendations may be a helpful starting point, but you need to first identify who the specific decision makers are and where and how your recommendations will be presented. Additionally, it is necessary to understand where your strengths lie. Not all researchers will feel comfortable leading or facilitating social action, so it is necessary to reflect on your own personal and professional skills. As your collective determines what constitutes action, work alongside your co-researchers to identify where they can lead or if your group may need more support in this area. Last, it is also important to note that actions do not need to be on a massive scale; rather, they need to be of importance to the community you are working alongside.

When thinking about policy reform, you need to consider how your data can apply to any level. Policy reform and shifts in practice can range from how a school considers the racialized and gendered dynamics of its dress code and then changes it, as Meagan observed in her *Courageous Conversations* project; how changes were made in financial assistance and reintegration efforts for former political prisoners in Burma/Myanmar, as Giovanni saw in one of his projects; the partnership formed between the university and prison that led to the co-facilitation of four different programs, as noted by Payne and Bryant (2018); and working alongside other community-based organizations to advocate that the New York City Police Department's controversial stop-and-frisk (i.e., the ability of a police officer to stop, interrogate, and search an individual solely on the basis of reasonable suspicion) was unconstitutional, as seen in the Morris Justice Project's work (Stoudt & Torre, 2014).

SHARING FINDINGS

Although seemingly straightforward (as academics or practitioners we often default to an assumption that we "write it up and publish it"), the process of sharing findings can present its own challenges and can have complicated ethical, financial, and other implications. Whether you are a practitioner working for a nonprofit organization or government agency or an academic working for an institution of higher education, you will surely find yourself experiencing competing demands as you consider how you will share your findings. There are many ways to navigate those competing demands; in this section, we offer several ideas you could build on.

REFLEXIVITY QUESTION

If you were totally honest with yourself (and your collective), what is the most important or meaningful way you would want to be recognized for your critical participatory inquiry? Share this with your collective.

Navigating the Expectations of Academia

It can be challenging to commit to CPI, but with a bit of creativity, we have found that we can navigate the expectations of academia while staying true to our epistemological commitments. The CPI process—building relationships, opening ourselves up to transformation of our worldviews and goals, prioritizing different kinds of impact—can be difficult to align with academic productivity as measured by presentations at scholarly conferences and publications in top-tier journals. CPI can often demand that we double our workload—satisfying the demands of jobs that will allow us to provide financial security for ourselves and our families while at the same time satisfying our personal desire for the moral satisfaction that comes with taking a critical epistemological stance to stand against injustice. Making this commitment within academia may require you to "double write" (Call-Cummings, 2021), that is, to write for multiple audiences.

Like many CPI practitioners, we have all found ways to do this. Meagan's born-digital dissertation (described in Chapter 8), presented her dissertation study on a website co-created by the research collective with whom she worked. The website is much more dynamic than a typical dissertation would have been and allowed her to stay true to her epistemological commitment to participatory inquiry. At the same time, she was required to write three scholarly articles to submit alongside the website. Both sets of publications took hundreds of hours of writing, although the website was probably more time-consuming. While the articles garnered more recognition within academia, the website has attracted more educators as they have taken up some of the "lessons learned" highlighted there.

Along with writing for multiple audiences, we have found that publishing with community co-researchers as co-authors has been rewarding. Through these opportunities, co-researchers receive due recognition for their labor in tangible ways. We have also presented at academic conferences with co-researchers, including high school students, educators, and practitioners from public health and beyond. We are careful to not use these opportunities to show our co-researchers off like trophies. We are all equal members of a collective. We have also accepted invitations to attend conferences our non-academic counterparts value, such as professional conferences they may attend regularly. Just like in other phases of CPI, we anchor these decisions in humility, relationships, and dialogue. We learn what is valuable for and to our co-researchers and then work together to make sure we are all getting what we need and want out of the strategy we plan.

Sharing Findings in Policy Arenas

Publications such as white papers or policy briefs may be written in and for academic, nonprofit, and government settings. A white paper or policy brief may still be composed in a more academic or formal style, as it should provide sufficient evidence that decision makers or the public can use to learn about and assess policy proposals. While peer-reviewed journal publications may be 20 to 30 pages, policy briefs are generally shorter to appeal to decision makers with little time to consume longer pieces of research. Depending on the setting, these memos may be as short as one to two pages. Additionally, policy briefs tend to follow a structure more like journalistic writing, in that the most fundamental information, such as conclusions or recommendations, are communicated within earlier sentences or paragraphs rather than in the last section, as we would see in an academic paper or white paper. White papers, on the other hand, may be just as long as peer-reviewed journal publications or even much longer.

With any type of writing, though, there are positive and negative implications. For university- and community-based researchers, these types of publications may require a shift in writing style, but they can be highly effective in making policy recommendations to decision makers. Although effective in policy settings, for tenure-track faculty, however, these publications may be weighted less than peer-reviewed publications intended for academic audiences. It is also necessary to understand how others may perceive your research, as not all audiences appreciate or agree when researchers compose publications that are political in nature. In any case, when sharing your collective's research, it is important to understand your intended audience, the message you would like to convey, the best means to deliver it, and the potential positive and negative consequences.

Getting Creative in How We Share Findings

Each of us has explored different ways to return knowledge to community members and stakeholders who can create meaningful change. We have published blog posts (Dazzo, 2019, 2021; Hauber-Özer, 2020a, 2020b; Hauber-Özer & Call-Cummings, 2020) and been interviewed on podcasts and webinars (e.g., Dazzo, 2016; Hauber-Özer, 2020c; VanCleave, 2021) which have greater potential to reach nonacademic audiences, including teachers, policymakers, and other stakeholders. We have mentioned Melissa's web-based gallery of dissertation participants' photovoice products, which powerfully represent their experiences as refugees studying in Turkish universities through photographs and accompanying texts in Turkish, English, and Arabic. As you may remember from Chapter 5, Melissa also presented her findings about participants' experiences learning Turkish and gaps in services as a webinar for educators affiliated with the Turkish as a Foreign Language Education Association (YADOT) (Hauber-Özer, 2020c).

While these kinds of invitations to share findings through podcasts, interviews, guest speaking, or webinars may come, we have found that CPI practitioners need to create their own opportunities to share both processes and products broadly. For example, Meagan has family ties in Jamaica and mentioned to a friend who has connections with the University of the West Indies (located in Jamaica) that she would be interested in offering workshops in CPI or participatory methods for free. The Department of Social Work contacted Meagan about their students' interests and needs and they worked together to provide two separate workshops on CPI and photovoice. These kinds of opportunities usually happen because we take the initiative and network, which can happen at professional conferences as well as through personal connections. Think back to the relationships matrix you completed in Chapter 4. Maybe one of those relationships could facilitate sharing your findings more broadly than you may initially anticipate. In Box 9.1, we provide a creative example from the Morris Justice Project, showing how data can be used to inform the public and broadly shared with the communities with whom we work.

BOX 9.1: GETTING THE WORD OUT: MORRIS JUSTICE PROJECT'S "DEAR NYPD BAT SIGNAL"

In their CPI project of the New York City Police Department's (NYPD) controversial and unconstitutional "stop and frisk" policy, the Morris Justice Project (Stoudt & Torre, 2014; Stoudt et al., 2015) shared data with community members by projecting it onto the side of an apartment building in a busy area of the Bronx (Morris Justice Project, n.d.). The collective shared quantitative and qualitative data from a community survey, showing the type of data they collected to residents, law enforcement, and the media. In addition to projecting these data, they also hosted a musical performance, showed a series of related videos about public safety and the "stop and frisk" policy (The Illuminator, 2012), and followed it with a "know your rights" campaign.

As much of Giovanni's work relates to participatory forms of program evaluation, he often takes the opportunity to write blog posts about the process behind the methods he uses. These posts are generally no more than 450 words and provide a snapshot of how he conducted a study or utilized a particular method (Dazzo, 2017, 2021), which can be of interest to researchers and practitioners—within and outside academic settings—who may want to replicate a certain study design. As an example, Giovanni summarized his work with Kaqchikel co-researchers in Guatemala in one of these short pieces, highlighting the important ethical considerations that researchers should take when collaborating with individuals who have experienced trauma.

There are also websites that exist that are hosted as learning environments for practitioners. In one case, Giovanni incorporated his personal experiences and a literature review to develop a case study showcasing how trauma-affected communities have used art as a way to negotiate collective memories and contest dominant narratives (Dazzo, 2020). In these pieces, the writing may include components similar to a peer-reviewed article, such as a literature review, or may be similar in structure or length. However, the primary intended audience includes practitioners who may use the evidence in ways that change how they conduct their work, for example, nonprofit workers interested in novel or effective strategies. While the structure may be similar to an academic piece, it is important to note that these articles are often published on websites that are not hidden behind a paywall or subscription service; they are accessible to everyone (i.e., open access).

As previously mentioned, there are also opportunities to publish policy briefs intended for policymakers, nonprofit organizations, or residents at a town hall; however, in many cases, you would likely be asked to present this work in person or virtually. In these cases, it is important that your presentation follow a similar structure as your writing; in other words, make sure to provide the most noteworthy points upfront. In policy settings, starting off with the most important points is often referred to as "bottom line up front" (BLUF). You may also be asked to completely forego or limit how much space (e.g., one presentation slide) and time (e.g., a few minutes of a 1-hour presentation) you devote to explaining your methodological process. These points are often reserved for appendices in your written outputs. To end this chapter, we leave you with a list of examples (see Box 9.2) that will hopefully inspire some creative ideas for how you can share findings with the broader public and decision makers.

BOX 9.2: EXAMPLES OF CREATIVE SHARING PRACTICES

Websites, blogs, and social media: Websites can be used as an efficient way to share findings and share with a broad set of audiences. Depending on your resources and time, you can develop your own website. As an example, see the Public Science Project's website for the Morris Justice Project (n.d., URL in references) and a related video on YouTube (The Illuminator, 2012). If time or funding is limited, you can also contribute a blog post to an existing online community. For instance, the Institute of Development Studies site on "Participatory Methods" has its own "News & Blog" page.

Postcards, posters, and pamphlets: Through their Space & Places Eskasoni Project, a collective of co-researchers including university faculty, community service providers, and Mi'kmaq First Nations youth in Nova Scotia, Canada, used postcards to share their findings (Reich et al., 2017). The postcards and posters developed by the collective were distributed around the community and to local leaders. They also complemented these mobile practices with videos, slideshows, and a mural that showcased their findings.

Curricula, professional development: U.S. teacher educators Tara Brown and Louie Rodriguez (2017) each facilitated similar PAR projects with Black and Latinx high school students, Action Research into School Exclusion (ARISE) in the Mid-Atlantic region and Promoting our Will through Education and Research (POWER) in the Southwest region, respectively. The goal was to supplement (largely White, middle class) preservice teachers' knowledge for effectively serving students of Color. Youth co-researchers from each project presented their findings in teacher education courses at the nearby universities where Brown and Rodriquez taught; they highlighted the importance of "caring and supportive social and academic relationships" and issues of "low expectations, discrimination and favoritism" among teachers (p. 76).

Town halls, school assemblies, presentations to local organizations or policymakers: Local events can be an excellent way to share findings with those around your community. As an example, education scholar Melanie Bertrand (2019) shows how youth in her collective presented the findings of their project at a community center, which "attracted a full house of predominantly Latina/o and Black parents, teachers, educational administrators, and community members" (p. 9). Community events, if publicized well, can provide opportunities to share research not only with community members but decision makers as well.

Chalk-walks: One of Meagan's graduate research methods classes built a website to share their findings and then created a hashtag to bring people to the site. They used sidewalk chalk to write the hashtag and website address all over their university's campus, directing people to view their findings and contribute to ongoing discussions hosted on the site.

Wearable data: Printing snippets of data or findings on t-shirts, buttons, or other "swag" can be a great way to attract the attention of varied audiences. Your collective might all wear T-shirts with data printed on it to a community market or other event. You could give out buttons for others to wear for a kind of snowball effect. The sky (and funding) is the limit!

CONCLUSION

In this chapter, we explored several aspects of taking action in the context of CPI projects, including challenges related to the goals and needs of the collective and the potential risks and benefits involved. We illustrated that committing to CPI is not impossible within academia but may present unique challenges, including an increased workload in order to satisfy multiple, potentially competing, demands. We offered several ideas for creative sharing practices, including websites, blogs, social media, postcards, posters, pamphlets, curricula, professional development, various meetings, chalk-walks, and even wearable data! When making decisions about how, when, and where to take action, your collective should be open about each member's needs so you can all receive the recognition you deserve.

RECOMMENDED PRACTICE 9.2: SHARING STRATEGIES

Consider outlets where researchers, practitioners, community members, and so on, in your field get information, ideas, and resources. Start discussing strategies in your collective: Where could you potentially share your research findings so that the most relevant audiences would have access? Think beyond peer-reviewed academic journals. Are there community or organizational newsletters that are accessed by practitioners, community members, or decision makers? Professional development workshops? Create a table that outlines the outlet (e.g., journal, newsletter, email list) and the primary audiences that access it. In the last column, check submission or participation guidelines such as word count and formatting. As you plot these out, discuss how you can present your findings in ways that appeal to specific audiences.

SUMMARY OF KEY POINTS

- The CPI process should be guided by relationships and the objective of facilitating transformation through inquiry, but this outcome can look very different for particular groups, local contexts, historical moments, and so on.

- CPI occurs within varied constraints and realities that often conflict with expectations about timelines, participation, or measurable outcomes.
- The "action" or transformation resulting from CPI can take many different forms and occur at multiple levels, from the intrapersonal to the macro level.
- There are many options for sharing CPI findings both within academia—primarily through conference presentations and journal articles—and beyond, in practitioner-oriented and general interest outlets.

SUGGESTED ACTIVITIES

1. Journal about taking action: Look back at the focus activity and consider what goals, needs, and risks you (might) encounter in your CPI work. How do or will you navigate external constraints and disagreements within the collective? What might change look like at each level of the ecological map of change in your context? What existing relationships and opportunities could you leverage to get the word out about your collective's findings?
2. Create an action product for your (proposed) project based on one of the ideas in the chapter or one of your own (e.g., a blog post; a flyer for a performance or town hall; a blurb advertising a podcast episode or webinar; or an abstract for a white paper, conference presentation, journal article, or dissertation). Share your action product in class and elicit feedback.

KEY TERMS

failure
ownership
transformation

10 STAYING COMMITTED AND IN SOLIDARITY

LEARNING OBJECTIVES

By the end of this chapter you will be able to

- Articulate what it means to stay committed to and with co-researchers and others.
- Identify opportunities to stay committed and in solidarity with co-researchers in ways that they and the community in which you conduct CPI value.
- Analyze the various implications of staying committed or agreeing to move on.

FOCUS ACTIVITY 10.1: RETURNING TO POSITIONALITY, HUMILITY, AND OPENNESS

Go back to the work you did in Chapter 5, when you clarified your own needs, interests, and goals. What did you say at that point? Has anything changed? Consider the following questions as you reflect:

1. After building relationships with your co-researchers and within the community, have your personal or professional goals shifted at all? In what ways?
2. Have your personal or professional priorities shifted? In what ways?
3. How have your co-researchers indicated their ongoing needs or priorities during your CPI? How do those needs and priorities fit with your own? Are there conflicts or opportunities for alignment?

As you reflect on and answer these questions, we encourage you to be as open, humble, and honest with yourself as you can. As potential concerns or exciting alignments come up, we urge you to engage in dialogue with your co-researchers and other community members to think through next steps in your CPI and beyond. Next steps may present as an expansion of your inquiry or other work that is not oriented to an inquiry stance.

At this point, your ontological and epistemological commitments to critical participatory inquiry (CPI) have most likely come a long way, perhaps from a sense of being vaguely drawn to participatory methods to being firmly committed to critical participatory inquiry as an epistemological stance—one that will (hopefully) impact your future professional and personal work. This is exciting! It can, however, also be daunting, even overwhelming. Don't worry; you are not alone! Each of us has felt that sense of heaviness on our shoulders at one point or many as we have endeavored to stay true to our critical, participatory epistemological commitments. It can be difficult, if not almost impossible, to maintain these commitments within academia, schools, government agencies, and other institutions. As we have detailed in previous chapters, these hierarchical institutions were not built to support participatory, democratic, decolonizing structures, to amplify the voices and experiences of those who have been ignored or injured by unjust social systems and hegemonic norms, or to disrupt an inequitable status quo. Similarly, social systems across the globe most often privilege the loudest voices and deepest pockets above all else. As academics, social inquirers, activists, practitioners, and organizers, we are not typically rewarded for bucking trends and questioning the way things have always been. So, what do we do?

This chapter will work through some of the key concepts that are often invoked in discussions about staying connected to and with the people with whom and communities where we conduct our inquiry. After teasing these concepts out, we will focus on the ethical implications of sticking around and the practical implications of doing so. We offer specific, concrete recommendations for how to stay connected in ethical ways that prioritize the needs of the community and that are transparent about your own needs.

CONCEPTS AND DEFINITIONAL ISSUES

This section is dedicated to thinking through some words and concepts that are often used when researchers discuss maintaining or building on the relationships they have created with members of a community in which they have conducted research. Our goal in this section is to address how these are commonly used and to trouble the underlying assumptions of those uses.

Reciprocity

In many introductory (and advanced) research methodology classes, we hear a refrain of reciprocity: What's the give-back? What do participants get out of the research? Some suggest as university-based researchers who are getting paid (either through salary or in grant funds), we should pay participants for their time. Others encourage us to share our own experiences as they share theirs, so there is a kind of informal give-and-take. Still others may urge university-based researchers, who may be in a position of relative power or influence, to offer letters of recommendation, networking opportunities, or help with social organizing. These are all laudable ideas for ways to ensure community-based co-researchers feel valued and honored in the CPI process. Indeed, we do not believe any of these actions are in themselves bad. We do, however, believe that these types of incentives that revolve around a transactional relationship have the potential to pit researchers against participants. There is an underlying us-and-them to these approaches that leaves us feeling uncomfortable.

Reciprocity is often framed in this way: I, as a university-based researcher, have conducted research with you or in your community so in some way have taken something from you (knowledge, time, energy, experience). By practicing reciprocity, I seek to give something back to you that in some way will make up for or at least address this extraction. This approach, while stemming from good intentions, actually reproduces an extractive, colonial approach to research. Reciprocity, when seen or practiced as a give-and-take, maintains the binary of knower/known or researcher/subject that is the antithesis of critical participatory inquiry (Call-Cummings & Hauber-Özer, 2022).

REFLEXIVITY QUESTION

Have you ever thought about or practiced reciprocity in your personal life? In what ways have you tried to "pay someone back" either through your time or other resources? How did that act make you feel? How do you think they felt?

As you know from previous chapters, Melissa conducted her dissertation in Turkey with people who had been forced to migrate from Syria because of civil war. The project explored how young adult Syrian refugees overcame barriers to success in the Turkish higher education system. As a relatively privileged, White, American woman living in Turkey by choice, Melissa felt unsure about how to address inherent power dynamics in her project or how to push against the extractive nature of research. She did not feel free to frame her study as fully participatory because of the political context at the time—she would have been risking her safety as well as the safety of her participants if the project were seen as in any way criticizing the political or social status quo. Also, because Melissa did not have existing relationships with the people who would participate in the study, she was concerned that power dynamics would not allow for open, honest dialogue early on. Melissa's friend, Samar (pseudonym), worked as her research assistant and key informant. It is important to note that although Melissa did not have any official position at the university, her husband was a lecturer there, and Samar had been a student in his class, potentially introducing complicated power relations. However, because they had an established trusting relationship, Melissa asked Samar what would be most valued by the study participants. This led Melissa to incorporate participatory methods such as photovoice in her project so that the participants could communicate their stories through multiple modes. In response to participants' wishes to share their experiences beyond the dissertation, she also worked to share their findings in settings such as a practitioner conference[1] designed to facilitate refugee self-representation and a multilingual, interactive online gallery. Because Samar had expressed interest in graduate studies, they presented findings as co-authors at several conferences, and Melissa has provided research design support to another participant, Maqsood, who was working on his master's thesis. Finally, after Melissa had built closer relationships with the participants during months of working together, she gladly wrote several letters of recommendation for jobs, scholarships, and graduate school applications. More than a year after the official end of the project, she maintains a natural flow of contact with the participants through social media and WhatsApp, exchanging updates and Eid greetings. She follows her artist participant Nasir's Instagram account, both enjoying and supporting his work. Each of these "acts" occurred organically through the working relationship they had built.

Again, no one incentive or act of reciprocity is inherently good or bad. If you do happen to have the funds available, asking participants how they would like to be compensated in a quantified way may be important (Limes-Taylor Henderson & Esposito, 2019). The goal is to anchor the decisions we make in the relationships we build with our co-researchers and the open dialogue that comes in and through those relationships. Building on the work of Jamesson et al. (2011), Zuchowski et al. (2017) discuss the differences between *thin* and *thick* reciprocity: **thin reciprocity** is based in goals of mutual benefit through the exchange of resources while **thick reciprocity** "emphasizes shared voice and power and insists upon collaborative knowledge construction . . . and encourages all partners to grow and to challenge and support one another's growth" (Jamesson et al., 2011, p. 264, as cited in Zuchowski et al., 2017, p. 84). Zuchowski et al. (2017) engage this *thick* conceptualization of reciprocity as transformational as opposed to transactional. They conclude, as do we, that "there is clearly a need to avoid processes that strengthen professional imperialism and paternalistic framing of the Other" (p. 84). Before making decisions about how we work toward transformational collaborations, we must first understand how our co-researchers frame transformation.

Thus, it is when we build authentic relationships that allow for openness and sincere, honest dialogue that we create an environment that can foster an epistemological ethic, which requires us to question "why we do research, who is (should be) doing research, how we relate to the researched" (Guishard et al., 2018, p. 16). Through dialogue, we can establish what is important to co-researchers across our collectives. Rather than assuming there is something tangible or concrete that we can give back, a transformational view of reciprocity and an epistemological ethic requires critically engaging with co-researchers to discuss and negotiate what is valued and what would be appreciated. Rather than thinking about reciprocity solely from a transactional view, a transformational collaboration would be valued by the strength and health of relationships with co-researchers. Recall in Chapter 3 where we talk about validity in this way, as dependent on the health and strength of our arguments. This form of building reciprocal relations (Schensul & Berg, 2004) allows us to see how a give-and-take becomes more about measuring our sense of community rather than solely assessing the exchange of goods.

This idea of building a healthy community, however, is not solely one that lives in academic theory; it is also seen across many Indigenous definitions calling for self-determination (AIATSIS, 2020; Caldwell et al., 2005; Native Governance Center, 2021). As noted by the Native Governance Center, wealth is often defined as "living reciprocally," "being a good relative," and as a "form of community care . . . that prompts participants to consider what matters most to their communities" (Native Governance Center, 2021, p. 1). So, to live and research in reciprocal ways also requires us to understand how various communities determine how something is shared. If we solely focus on capitalistic notions of wealth, we may think that it is appropriate to provide monetary payments to individuals, but for some Indigenous communities, this may go against shared notions of wealth and living in community (Native Governance Center, 2021), which can then result in negative consequences in existing relationships.

Solidarity

Solidarity is a word that is often used without critical thought about its underlying assumptions. Like the term *reciprocity*, solidarity (or actions taken under its banner), is not in and of itself a negative thing. What *may* be problematic are the assumptions we make as we claim solidarity. Meagan remembers the first time she saw a respected colleague's automatic email signature read "In Solidarity," with her name below. Meagan felt a vague sense of discomfort but was not able to pinpoint why until she began talking with her friends and colleagues, Peiwei Li and Karen Ross. In conversations that spanned over a year, they worked together as critical friends to think through what is taken for granted or assumed when a claim of solidarity is made. In a co-authored manuscript (Ross et al., 2022) they describe how solidarity is often a one-sided claim that can be paternalistic or condescending, similar to how claims of empowerment may unintentionally indicate that one person or group has power that they are in a position to "give" to someone else. Solidarity, while not really being "given" in the same transactional way, has the potential to reproduce similar (neo)imperialistic, hegemonic hierarchies of power. Meagan, as a White woman, may claim to be in solidarity with, for example, her co-researchers, all of whom are youth and many of whom identify as Black or Brown. While intending to show her commitment to the priorities these youth identify as important, Meagan's claim of solidarity may lead to unintended consequences that actually build barriers of hegemony rather than bridges of understanding.

In addition to these possible unintended consequences, Ross et al. (2022) also found that claims of solidarity can lead to static or fixed understandings of power and power differentials among social identity groups. In Meagan's example, her claim of solidarity positions her as always in a position of relative power and as the students who are her co-researchers as in a position of having or exercising less power than she. Solidarity is something that Meagan "has" and that she is in a position to claim, as opposed to these youth co-researchers, who are framed as passive recipients of Meagan's claims. Overall, these uncritical claims of solidarity can be problematic.

Ross et al. (2022) suggest that solidarity must be treated as fluid and dynamic, built on relationships, which are always in a state of constant change and evolution. They also argue that a praxis of solidarity must foreground action but should always recognize its contingent nature; that is, solidarity reflects social relationships that are tenuous and always in the process of creating something new rather than reproducing static identity categories. Similar to our conclusions around reciprocity, Ross et al. (2022) conclude that solidarity is intersubjectively constituted and must center relational action oriented toward **mutual recognition** and liberation.

REFLEXIVITY QUESTION

Whom do you feel solidarity with in your personal or professional life? How do you show that? How have you seen mutual recognition show up in that relationship?

Sustainability

Another concept to consider is whether our research projects support or lead to sustainable systems. **Sustainability** can be defined in a number of ways depending on the discipline (e.g., ecology, economics); however, for the purpose of this chapter, we acknowledge the definition articulated in a report commissioned by the United Nations, titled *Our Common Future*: "Sustainable development is development that meets the needs of the present without compromising the ability of future generations to meet their own needs" (WCED, 1987, p. 41). From this definition, we can note a few important topics. When we are sustainable, we hold ourselves accountable to future generations. Sustainability also requires us to live modestly, or in relationship with the systems we live in, considering there are social, economic, and environmental limitations for present and future needs.

What does this mean for us, as critical researchers, and the CPI projects we organize? If we think back to the idea of reciprocity and pair it with sustainability, it requires us to partner in ways that have transformative effects for the communities we work alongside. We may engage in dialogue with our collectives around several reflective questions:

- Do co-researchers hold themselves accountable to future generations when deciding how research will be used, or will it solely serve their purposes and reduce equity for others?
- Do those in the collective determine their strategies based on the systems in which they live?
- Do they consider social relationships between generations or how limited economic and environmental resources will meet the needs of future generations?

In Giovanni's CPI project in Guatemala, the concept of sustainability arose as Kaqchikel co-researchers discussed their hopes for their community memorial site. For many of the Kaqchikel co-researchers, it was important that the memorial serve as a link to the past, acting as a tool to educate future generations about the country's armed conflict. Although the community had limited funds (economic resources) and land (environmental resources), they partnered with their Guatemalan nonprofit counterparts in the inquiry collective. By using the research from their participatory data gathering and analysis activities, the collective was able to secure funds and additional plots of land as a way to improve the security of the memorial so that visitors would feel comfortable visiting the site. For the collective, sustainability meant educating future generations. Through education, the violent conflicts of the past—which denied their generation of social, economic, and environmental benefits—could provide future generations with the information needed to learn how to live together in peace.

For additional insight on the topic of sustainability, we encourage you to read the case study showcasing the work of Dr. Tamarah Moss in the Appendix. In her case study, Moss reflects on her work with a nonprofit partner and survivors of intimate partner violence. In this work, sustainability was viewed from several perspectives: how she could partner with a nonprofit organization to work on funding proposals that would ensure the service work would continue, considering community members' feedback on the types of services provided, and listening to community members about the way in which services should be facilitated and provided in responsible and respectful ways. Through an iterative process of data collection and analysis that was done through the instant messaging platform WhatsApp, Moss and the nonprofit organization were able to consider community members' feedback throughout the process, contributing to a feedback loop that allowed them to continually reassess whether the program was meeting the changing desires and needs of the group. This not only ensured the program's financial sustainability but also assured participants that their views and needs were being considered to maintain and adapt the program.

ETHICAL CONSIDERATIONS

In Chapter 3, we provided the theoretical foundations to show how ethics and validity are so intertwined that it is difficult to think of them separately. In the examples throughout the book, we tried to demonstrate how our processes—from research design to data gathering and analysis to sharing findings—were adapted to local epistemologies. By engaging in dialogue and democratic deliberation with communities, co-designed processes require three considerations from the critical participatory inquirer: a *commitment* to the process and the relationships we build with communities; an *ethic of humility* to understand that communities are not beholden to us; and the responsibility of **witnessing** the private and lived experiences of those we work alongside.

Commitment

When we think of commitment, we understand this in two ways: being committed to the practice of critical participatory inquiry and being committed to the co-researchers with whom we work. As Erickson (2011) notes, validity in participatory inquiry can be assessed from this commitment to praxis and social change. If we are not committed to the acts of dialogue and democratic deliberation that form the basis of participatory thinking and methods, then it may be difficult to commit to the idea that knowledge is located in the lived experiences of the communities where we work. Thus, critical participatory inquiry requires us to think of both theoretical and ethical commitments as we untangle how social science can lead to social justice (Fine & Torre, 2004). Going back to Jürgen Habermas' (1996) idea of creating communicative space, this means that co-researchers must be committed to mutual understanding and arriving at consensus in way that is not forced. This type of democratic and deliberative communication and action takes time. As we have shown through examples and throughout the chapters, it is long-term work that challenges us to build relationships. It means that we continue to show up, as a community of co-researchers, to tease out and conceptualize the tough questions that require us to confront social realities.

Ethic of Humility

In the introductory chapters of this book, we talked a lot about all of the "-ologies"—epistemology, ontology, axiology, methodology—that are important to consider when conducting critical participatory inquiry. These theoretical notions are important, but to put it simply, an *ethic of humility* (Grenberg, 2005; Limes-Taylor Henderson & Esposito, 2019) requires us to check our privilege and recognize the time, value, and expertise that co-researchers bring to our projects. Following from the previous paragraph, this ethic of humility is a commitment to our praxis and notions of social justice. As we have stressed throughout the book, taking an equitable and a decolonizing stance in our work requires a radical rethinking of *self* and our identities as researchers: What does it mean to question our expertise? How do we "compensate" participants/ and co-researchers for their time? Do we need our participants and co-researchers more than they need us? (Limes-Taylor Henderson & Esposito, 2019) Yet, to do this work in an ethical way requires us to push beyond these theoretical questions and to cautiously confront them as a *humility in practice*. In Patricia Hill Collins' (2010) work on Black feminist thought, there is a critical confluence among the elements of care, compassion, and humility, as she calls on inquirers to follow an ethic of personal accountability and an ethic of caring as we listen and document. Māori scholar and educator Linda Tuhiwai Smith (2012) extends this notion of humility when she speaks of how insider researchers (i.e., those who are part of the communities they research) must conduct research humbly because of their more intimate relationships and positions within a community. Gaztambide-Fernández, (2012) who speaks of the politics of solidarity as a decolonizing response, asserts that we can redefine "human relations that are premised on the relationship between difference and interdependency, rather than similarity and a rational calculation of self-interests" (p. 49). As we untangle what it means to act through an ethic of humility, we can see that much of this scholarship, as well as the practice of CPI, is based on affirming our differences as a way to develop respect, trusting relationships and mutual understanding.

Witnessing

As a critical approach that questions the status quo, CPI requires us to build our human capacity to care as we listen, observe, and document, even in instances where the stories are difficult to hear. We are called on to bear witness, but what does it actually mean to bear witness in a critical inquiry approach that requires co-researchers (and this includes us as just one of many co-researchers), to share in the responsibilities of listening, documenting, and observing? In the *Vulnerable Observer*, anthropologist Ruth Behar (1996) questions our actions as distanced observers: "as a storyteller opens her heart to a story listener, recounting hurts that cut deep . . . do you, the observer, stay behind the lens of the camera, switch on the tape recorder, keep pen in hand?" (p. 2). Here, we can see our ethical and methodological dilemmas as inquirers. Do we stop recording? Do we continue in the effort to document the story to motivate change? More specifically in a CPI project where we are just one co-researcher among many, do we share our own difficult stories with those in our collective? In their critical participatory engagement with communities, Fine and Torre (2004) speak of the inquirer's duty to bear witness, but also note that our methodological and ethical practices must be fluid; that a "negotiation of power and positionality is an active and ongoing practice among the team" (p. 26). In cases where our work may be construed as challenging the status quo, community-based youth studies scholar Caitlin Cahill (2007) notes "our responsibility, and a process, to consider the political ramifications of making the invisible visible" (p. 367). Additionally, if we make a commitment to decolonize or question the Western roots of many of our practices, we are tasked with understanding how we witness and document. From the field of trauma studies, Stef Craps (2013) questions how the practice of bearing witness has often become politicized, as the trauma of minoritized groups is not often "acknowledged on their own terms" (p. 3) but rather documented in ways that ascribe to Westernized notions of storytelling. Thus, as we bear witness, we have a commitment to hold ourselves responsible for our actions, to remain accountable to those who tell their stories to us, and to question the evolving intricacies of our ethical and methodological positions. Education scholar Becky Ropers-Huilman (1999) offers several practical guidelines for us as we bear witness, including six obligations for social justice-oriented researchers:

- Recognize your engagement in active and partial meaning-making.
- Consider how your research may change or affect others.
- Be open to change.
- Share our experiences and perspectives with others.
- Listen to other witnesses' interpretations.
- Explore and promote multiple meanings of equity and care.

RECOMMENDED PRACTICE 10.1: OUTLINING YOUR SIX OBLIGATIONS TO HOLD YOURSELF ACCOUNTABLE

Consider Ropers-Huilman's (1999) six obligations for researchers as they bear witness. As part of your own reflexive practice, use these obligations as a guide and write out how you will hold yourself accountable through your CPI project. As you meet with your collective, take the opportunity to use Ropers-Huilman's guidelines to facilitate a discussion on how everyone, as a collective, will hold themselves accountable.

PRACTICAL CONSIDERATIONS

Throughout this book, we have emphasized the epistemological commitments and idealistic goals behind critical participatory inquiry as well as the practical, day-to-day practices and challenges you might encounter along the way. We want to close by reiterating a few crucial aspects to keep in mind as you prepare to embark on your CPI journey or perhaps wrap up your first foray.

Anchor in Dialogue

From the early days of action research (see Chapter 1), dialogue has been central to the inquiry process. Establishing a collective, identifying social problems of concern to the group, and working toward solutions must occur first and foremost through dialogue. Closing out a project (or, in many cases, transitioning to a new phase or focus) should also center reflective discussion and mutual understanding in order to celebrate successes, identify missed opportunities, or articulate shifts in goals. To facilitate these conversations, you can revisit initial mapping activities or needs assessments that you conducted (see Chapter 5). You may use these tools to consider with your collective what you have accomplished, what you may have missed, or whether priorities have shifted.

Don't Overpromise

By this point in the book, you have likely picked up on the fact that, despite its potential for challenging structures and systems of inequity, critical participatory inquiry can be difficult, all-encompassing, exhausting work. Even under the best of circumstances, the burden of trying to create change can feel daunting. As with any form of advocacy or activism, we want to offer fair warning that it can be easy to oversell the capacity for transformation and to neglect your personal and professional boundaries. Those in academia face demands to share findings, show "impact," and satisfy tenure or promotion committees (see Chapter 7) against the often slow, incremental, and less tangible results of social change-focused inquiry. For practitioners, the longer time frames associated with developing strong relationships for respectful participatory work may be complicated by the demands of funders and board members, as project timelines are generally short (and generally, once a project ends, so does interaction with a community) and requirements for tangible results (e.g., the number of people supported, evidence of skills gained, policy change) are many. As Jones and Whittle (2021) discuss, the neoliberal academy pushes academics to create knowledge and bring in profit in the form of tuition fees and large grants, goals at odds with the epistemological tenets and practical realities of CPI. This can be similar for practitioners, as nonprofit staff may spend the majority of their time writing proposals to secure grant funds (i.e., the never-ending proposal mill), rather than developing relationships with community co-researchers in an effort to stay committed to longer term social change. In this environment, whether working with nonprofit organizations, in academia, or for government, burnout is real. With that in mind, it is crucial to weigh your personal and professional goals and needs along with those of your co-researchers.

As you consider engaging in this type of inquiry as part of your role as an educator, social worker, community activist, student, program director, or policymaker, reflect carefully on your strengths as well as your limitations and the amount of time, energy, and effort you can realistically commit to it. Delving into other people's experiences and social ills can expose you to deeply upsetting information, lead to compassion fatigue, and, in cases of disclosed abuse or other discoveries, force you to make difficult ethical choices about what to do with this knowledge (Guillemin & Gillam, 2004; Vincett, 2018). If you do decide to engage in CPI, set aside time and space for self-care and encourage your co-researchers to do the same (Jones & Whittle, 2021; Vincett, 2018). Depending on researchers' positionality, CPI can also be risky—personally, professionally, and politically—so think through the risks you are willing to take and those that you are asking potentially more vulnerable co-researchers to take. Work to balance safety and well-being with needed and desired disruption of the status quo.

Create Sustainability

Staying committed demands not only respect and humility but also practical actions, such as creating processes and structures that encourage sustainable and transformative experiences for individuals, communities, and the organizations where we work. Although sustainability is often associated with maintaining consistent funding so a project can continue, we need to remember that much more is needed. In previous chapters, we have written about the importance of maintaining relationships, and this continues to be a vital point, along with creating the necessary procedures to establish coherent practices that continue to be in line with our commitments. As you begin thinking about a sustainability plan, it is important to answer this question: Even as the collective's members change (i.e., co-researchers leave for other opportunities or priorities), how can we maintain or refine our values? Staying committed to your values and principles, as a collective, will provide a map for where you would like your work to go and how you would like it to continue. In Table 10.1, we include a worksheet with several guiding questions that you and your collective can use as you determine your priorities for moving

TABLE 10.1 ■ Thinking About Sustainable Communications and Strategies

	Guiding Questions
Guiding Questions	• What do you want to achieve going forward? • What are your short- and longer term goals? • How have you communicated your work in the past? To whom? • What needs to change about how, and to whom, you communicate your actions and goals to others going forward?
Guiding Questions	• If co-researchers in the collective leave, do you have enough people to continue your work? • Do you have outlets to reach out to and recruit new co-researchers? • Do co-researchers have the skills (e.g., research, facilitation, communications) to move the initiative forward? If not, how can these be developed? • How can you establish relationships with the broader community to garner support for your work? • How can you establish relationships with decision makers so you can further promote your initiatives?
Guiding Questions	• Going forward, do you need to establish policies to structure how and when people meet? • Do your plans require funding? If so, how will you go about securing it through grants or in-kind support? • How can the collective use evidence to improve its own operations? • How can the collective use evidence to advocate for social change? • What actions should be phased out and which should be continued?

forward and for lasting change. This can be used to encourage dialogue, especially about questions around plans, people, and procedures.

As we think about the types of actions we should prioritize going forward—from planning research activities to framing advocacy messages—we also need to explore the risks associated with our work. Throughout the chapters in this book, we stressed the importance of establishing an ethic of humility (Limes-Taylor Henderson & Esposito, 2019) and an ethic of personal accountability (Collins, 2010), and with these orientations comes the responsibility of asking difficult questions. This includes asking what could go wrong: What are the consequences of our actions? How will our CPI project affect our individual reputations, relationships, our collective, and the organizations where we work? In Table 10.2, we present a series of factors that you and your collective can consider as you think about the types of risks associated with your initiatives as you move forward.

As you meet and discuss the points in this table, it is necessary to think about the types of risks that exist. By working with co-researchers, you have the opportunity to bring in diverse and varied perspectives based on previous research and lived experience. Remember that each co-researcher will bring in their own interpretation of what constitutes a risk, but this is a

TABLE 10.2 ■ Documenting Risks and Our Mitigation Plans

	Describe the risk.	How likely is this risk? (*improbable, possible, probable*)	What is the potential impact? (*minor, moderate, major*)	What actions will we take to mitigate risk?
Safety and security of individual co-researchers				
Broader community				
Communities where co-researchers reside				
Organizations where co-researchers work				
Intended processes and outcomes of the CPI project				

strength for your collective. Unlike Table 10.1, which would require you to reach some level of broad consensus on your short- and longer term goals as a collective, in Table 10.2, consensus is not needed; rather, it is best to list every risk that co-researchers bring up, no matter how small. To complete this table, first think about and list all of your planned actions as a collective. Then, move down the list one by one, discussing the potential risks that could occur for each action. While risks will never disappear, following this process provides for a more comprehensive view of the challenges that may present themselves and what needs to be done to reduce them.

CONCLUSION

Critical participatory inquiry is a big commitment. In this chapter, we covered the tensions that arise in deciding whether and how to remain committed to this epistemological stance, to communities, and to members of our inquiry collectives. These tensions are present in discussions around reciprocity and solidarity. We discussed both ethical and practical considerations of these decisions and offer tools to help you in the process. We encouraged you not to overpromise to yourself, your collective, or your audience, but to create concrete plans for sustainable social change.

RECOMMENDED PRACTICE 10.2: SUSTAINABILITY REVISITED

Back in Chapter 2 (see Recommended Practice 2.1), we asked you to consider Tilakaratna's (1991) description of sustainability and the four interrelated factors that lead to it: (1) the emergence of a group of internal animators, (2) practice of self-review by people's organizations, (3) the ability to move from micro groups to larger groupings, and finally (4) an expansion of the action agenda to move toward a total or comprehensive development effort. Meet with your co-researchers to discuss how you can refine your plans for sustainability: What types of actors (e.g., community members, administrators, decision makers) will you need to engage to move toward sustainable social change? As you list actors, be specific and include names and organizations. How can your agenda for action be taken up by others in the community? How will you adapt your findings and action plans in ways that resonate with others so they take up your message and work with you?

SUMMARY OF KEY POINTS

- Reciprocity has the potential of reproducing imperialist and paternalistic framing of the Other. No one incentive or act of reciprocity is inherently good or bad. The goal is to anchor the decisions we make in the relationships we build with our co-researchers and the open dialogue that comes in and through those relationships.

- Claims of solidarity can have negative unintended consequences. Solidarity is intersubjectively constituted and must center relational action oriented toward mutual recognition and liberation.
- CPI collectives should work together to create sustainability processes and structures that will allow a project to live beyond one project, individual, or group.

SUGGESTED ACTIVITIES

1. Ask someone who is in some way different from you how they would want an act of giving (of time, money, expertise) reciprocated. How do their thoughts differ from or align with your own? How might you have this kind of dialogue with a co-researcher?
2. Conduct a search of literature in your field with a focus on understanding how practitioners plan and strategize for sustainability. This search should move beyond scholarly publications to practitioner articles as well as media coverage, blogs, project websites, and more.
3. Reflect on and then record in your researcher journal a time when you witnessed something inequitable or unjust occur. How did you feel? What did you do in the moment? What did you wish you would have done? What did others do in the moment? What did you wish others would have done? How did you feel constrained or limited in your ability to act in that moment? How were others constrained or limited? How can you relate this everyday experience to how you should or should not act as a witness in your CPI practice?

KEY TERMS

mutual recognition
sustainability
thick reciprocity
thin reciprocity
witnessing

ENDNOTE

1. https://kiron.ngo/community/amplify-now-virtual-refugee-conference-on-world-refugee-day-20-06-2020/

APPENDIX 1: CASE STUDIES

Case Study 1

***Amigas de la Comunidad:* A Critical Case Study of Community-Based Participatory Research (CBPR) With Central American Immigrant Mothers**

Colleen K. Vesely[1], Bethany L. Letiecq[1], Rachael D. Goodman[1], Elizabeth DeMulder[1], Krishna Leyva[2], Marlene Marquez[3], Members of Amigas de la Comunidad

[1]College of Education and Human Development, George Mason University, Fairfax, VA

[2]Alexandria City Public Schools

[3]Alexandria City, Department of Community and Human Services

BACKGROUND AND CONTEXT

Our Community-Based Participatory Research (CBPR) project, *Amigas de la Comunidad* (Friends of the Community), is a partnership between Central American immigrant mothers of young children, many of whom are undocumented and all of whom are low income ("Amigas"); local community agencies, nonprofit organizations, and schools ("community partners"); and faculty and students at George Mason University ("Mason Team") that began in October 2014.[1] As an approach to research, CBPR is uniquely suited to engage immigrants and other minoritized and marginalized communities in research (Vaughn et al., 2016). CBPR is premised on the assertion that research *with* (and not on) people is critical to their liberation (Fals Borda, 2001; Fals Borda & Rahman, 1991; Freire, 1982; Reason & Bradbury, 2008; Wallerstein et al., 2018). Using a CBPR approach, we work as a collective to blur the lines and disrupt power hierarchies between university researchers and research participants (or co-researchers), such that the collective becomes co-producers of research for the direct benefit of the community (Cornwall & Jewkes, 1995; Letiecq & Schmalzbauer, 2012; Wallerstein et al., 2018). Essential to our CBPR work is the establishment of trust, shared power, and a collaborative spirit that engenders cultural humility, democratic engagement, and the surfacing of different ways of knowing (Reason & Bradbury, 2008). CBPR approaches should engage the community in all phases of research, and university researchers should engage in community-led action to improve people's lives (Letiecq & Schmalzbauer, 2012; Vaughn et al., 2016; Wallerstein et al., 2018).

Our work began when a local foundation expressed interest in funding a project focused on early childhood education (ECE), early literacy, and immigrant families. In response to this call, the Mason Team, composed of researchers with combined expertise in clinical mental health, ECE, family systems, and participatory action research approaches, pitched a CBPR project focused on building meaningful connections in the community through both research and action. The foundation trusted our vision, took a leap of faith, and funded the proposal. This was a leap of faith because the Mason Team could not lay out exactly where the project would go as they had not yet identified the community's agenda. However, the Mason Team could describe the participatory nature of a CBPR approach and how we would engage in the project, building inroads with the community and including both research and action components. As described below, the Mason Team started this project in earnest by spending time in the community and meeting with staffs of local schools, agencies, and nonprofit organizations serving the community. Those "on-the-ground" workers helped us identify community leaders and invited us to a consequential community meeting where we described the project and asked leaders to join with us to build a CBPR project. Those critical steps early on led to the establishment of a community advisory board (CAB) called *Amigas de la Comunidad*. While the funders and Mason Team came to the project interested in ECE and immigrant family physical and mental health, including stress, trauma, and resilience, Amigas and the community were primarily focused on housing, employment, and their children's education and well-being. We worked together to establish a collective mission, vision, and goals.

RESEARCH QUESTION/AIMS/GOALS

The goals of *Amigas de la Comunidad* emerged over time as the Mason Team and Amigas worked together to understand

- The needs of the community through research (e.g., surveys, in-depth interviews, on-going focus groups);
- The resources that already existed in the community (e.g., school-based resources, resources and supports provided by nonprofit, immigrant-serving advocacy organizations); and
- How *Amigas de la Comunidad* could best support and extend the reach of community-based resources without duplicating efforts and make a difference in the community.

Through data collection efforts and initial action steps, it became clear that the role of *Amigas de la Comunidad* was not that of a service agency in which we provided programming or interventions informed by the research components of the project but rather that the action component of our work was to serve as liaisons, providing institutions (e.g., schools), systems (e.g., health care), and community-based organizations with guidance regarding the unique needs of the Central American immigrant community while at the same time supporting the community in building navigational capital (see Vesely et al., 2017). Navigational capital refers to the resources, tools, and skills needed to maneuver within institutions and systems that typically oppress individuals of color and others who have been marginalized and disenfranchised by dominant groups (Yosso, 2005). Our collective research and action taking is guided by an overarching research question: *How can we partner with the Central American immigrant community members who have been relegated to the social and economic margins of society by anti-immigrant laws, policies, and practices to develop or carry out attuned, aligned, and responsive research and action steps that are meaningful and useful to the community?*

AMIGAS DE LA COMUNIDAD CBPR PROJECT: IMPLEMENTATION STRATEGY

We used a multipronged implementation strategy for this CBPR project (see Letiecq & Schmalzbauer, 2012; Letiecq et al., 2022) where we (1) identified community leaders, (2) established a CAB, (3) established community partnerships, (4) collaborated with CAB and community partners in research, and (5) implemented action steps. Throughout each of these areas of project implementation, we worked to develop critical reflection skills and processes regarding power dynamics, trust building, and democratic engagement that informs and guides all aspects of the work. This implementation strategy is not linear, rather each prong continues to develop over time as *Amigas de la Comunidad* continues to develop and evolve.

Identifying Community Leaders

At the beginning of the project, which was funder and university initiated rather than community initiated, the Mason Team identified community leaders by connecting with the local schools and community agencies that were already trusted in the neighborhood. Because the foundation that funded the work was a trusted local organization deeply connected with ECE in the city, they were also helpful in making initial contact with agency and school leaders. Leaders in these organizations helped make connections with the natural Central American immigrant leaders—mothers—in the community. As our work has evolved through various data collection and advocacy efforts, more women have joined. At least once or twice a year as we take on new work, the CAB actively recruits additional board members with the knowledge, skills, and abilities to continue to grow the leadership and depth of community knowledge among *Amigas de la Comunidad*.

Establishing a Community Advisory Board (CAB)

With the help of emerging community partners, the Mason Team invited these identified community leaders to come together to discuss possibilities for the project in the community. Over the fall of 2014 through regular and frequent meetings—about once a week—we formed the CAB, which would guide all aspects of the work. At the time, the Mason Team consisted of three White upper middle-class women with varying degrees of Spanish language proficiency, and the Amigas were women from El Salvador, Honduras, and Guatemala with varying degrees of English language proficiency. All of the Amigas were low income, and some were undocumented, often in mixed status families. Our community partners were a Latina woman and a White woman;[2] both were highly engaged, trusted in the community, and bilingual. These partners conveyed the importance of *familismo*, or the dedication, commitment, and loyalty to family, and *personalismo*, or the importance to Amigas of building trusted interpersonal relationships (Ortiz, 2020) and supported the Mason Team in building relationships within the community that were grounded in these cultural values. Both women assisted with Spanish–English interpretation and meaning making during the meetings. To build trust and engage in power-shifting work, we spent months getting to know each other and engaging in action taking. The Mason Team learned about mothers' needs while honoring their journeys, drawing upon their experiences while working together to build easier pathways to existing resources. In line with principles of CBPR, the Mason Team worked to "share the purse" or project funds with the community by ensuring at least 50% of funds were spent in the community. From the beginning, we have provided $20 to $25 gift cards to CAB members for their time and participation in CAB meetings. We have also compensated Amigas for their participant recruitment and data coding efforts, and, whenever feasible, we have directly hired community members as employees on the grant to serve as research assistants, transcriptionists, translators, or interpreters.

Throughout the course of this work, the Mason Team has engaged in critical reflexive processes to challenge power dynamics between the Mason Team, community partners, and Amigas. Specifically, as researchers, the Mason Team regularly and critically examined their assumptions regarding the experiences of Amigas, and the experiences of the broader community. Surfacing our blind spots as "outsider" researchers has been an on-going process (see Letiecq et al., 2022). Early on, the Mason Team also observed somewhat unexpected power dynamics among the CAB members as a function of country of origin, legal status, and language proficiency. At the start, we had assumed that our greatest trust-building task would be between the Mason Team and the immigrant community. However, during CAB meetings we noted a tense dynamic between Amigas on the CAB that reflected limited within-group trust and solidarity. In one extreme case, an Amiga seemed to be bullying another CAB member by dismissing ideas and sometimes laughing or making light of the other woman's painful experiences migrating and adjusting to life in the United States. As we worked to understand the genesis of these unexpected power dynamics among Amigas, our community partner from the local public schools, who at the time was pursuing a master's degree in social work, suggested that these internal dynamics may be due to experiences of trauma, time in the United States, and differences in legal status among the women. We had assumed that women who had been in the United States longer, but who had similar migration and adjustment experiences, would empathically connect and feel solidarity with other women who had recently arrived and experienced similar traumas. Rather than solidarity, however, some women who had been in the United States longer or held legal status were actively distancing themselves from women who had only recently arrived there or who lacked legal authorization to be in the United States. This observation is consistent with research exposing "toxic ties" within mixed-status immigrant families and within immigrant enclaves (e.g., Del Real, 2019; Menjívar et al., 2016).

To interrupt these internal power dynamics, the Mason Team and Amigas agreed to work on board commitments and processes. As a first step, Amigas suggested we develop ground rules or commitments to create an emotionally safe space for our CAB meetings and in our work together. The CAB spent a couple of meetings discussing the importance of these rules and brainstorming what agreements or commitments might be most important. We developed a contract that all CAB members would sign, agreeing to uphold the rules that the group created (see Figure A1.1).

FIGURE A1.1 ■ Community Advisory Board Contract

Amigas de la Comunidad

Membrecía de la junta consultiva de la comunidad

Community Advisory Board Membership

***Contrato* (Contract):** *Yo estoy de acuerdo de acatar las siguientes reglas en la medida de mis posibilidades. El no seguir estas reglas podrían ser razones para ser despedida de la junta consultoría de la comunidad.*

I agree to uphold the following rules to the best of my ability. Failure to meet these rules can be grounds for dismissal from the community advisory board.

Reglas (Rules):

1. *No lastimar.* Do no harm.
2. *No chismes.* No gossiping.
3. Ser honesto, no mentir. Be honest, no lying.
4. *No agarrar coasas sin permiso del dueño.* Do not take things that are not yours without permission.
5. *Comprometerse a enfocarse en el trabajo establecido del grupo.* Come focused to complete the work of the group.
6. *Compartir problemas o preocupaciones del grupo con el grupo.* Share concerns or problems with the group
7. *Hacer lo mejor possible.* Do your best.

***Firmado por:* (Signed by)**

____________________________ ____________________

Nombre (Name) *Fecha* (Date)

***Testigo por:* (Witnessed by)**

____________________________ ____________________

Nombre (Name) *Fecha* (Date)

With the creation of ground rules, we were able to redress the bullying behavior and negative interactions, particularly among the Amigas. The Amiga who had exhibited bullying behavior contributed enthusiastically to the creation of these ground rules but ultimately left the group as she moved out of the community.

During our first 6 months of work together, we also developed a mission statement and logo for *Amigas de la Comunidad*, as Amigas were keen on sharing about our work with the community. Our mission is *Somos un grupo de madres trabajando juntas por el mejoramiento y bienestar de nuestra comunidad y sus familias* [We are a group of women working together for the improvement and well-being of our community and our families.]. The Mason Team recruited an undergraduate design student, and as a collective (that included Amigas' children), we worked to co-create a logo that represented our work together. The logo reflects the importance of family, home, the environment, and women standing together in solidarity (see Figure A1.2).

Another key component of our development as a CAB was the leadership of our community organizer, Marlene Marquez (6th author). At the inception of *Amigas de la Comunidad*, Marquez (a Salvadoran woman who immigrated to the United States at age 12) was a social work student at George Mason University and was interning with Krishna Leyva, our community partner and staff member of the local school family and community engagement program. In addition, Marquez lived in the immigrant enclave and really straddled the community and university as an essential cultural broker. As Marquez's internship ended, she took on a larger role in the CAB particularly in terms of data collection efforts as well as action and advocacy in the community. When Marquez graduated with her bachelor's degree in social work, she secured a position as a family service worker at a local publicly funded ECE program. She later moved into a position within the community services branch of the city government. As such, Marquez connected all parts of the CAB, serving multiple, intersecting roles.

As Marquez's leadership and community organizing skills developed, and our work in the community became more established, the CAB decided to take an important step toward professionalizing the board: establishing bylaws and an executive board. This provided opportunities for all of us to better understand board governance and, importantly, to align the structures of the board in such a way that ensured our work was community driven. Per Amigas by-laws, only Amigas are eligible for executive committee positions on the board (i.e., president, vice president, secretary), and the Mason Team and community partners serve on the board in *ex officio* roles (i.e., as nonvoting members). The size of the CAB, particularly in terms of the number of Amigas, has shifted over the years due to women moving in and out of the community as well as time constraints due to employment and families' needs. Initially our board included 10 Amigas; today, there are five Amigas (one from the original group) who consistently engage in the work.

FIGURE A1.2 ■ Amigas de la Comunidad Logo

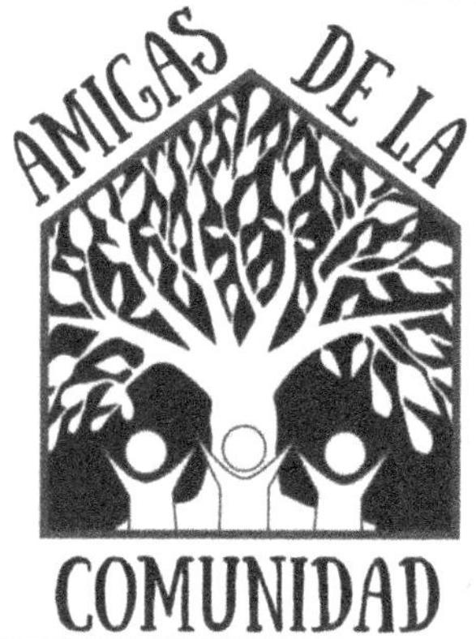

Courtesy Bethany Letiecq, Amigas de la Comunidad

Establishing Partnerships

Throughout our work with *Amigas de la Comunidad,* we have developed many partnerships with community organizations, systems, and institutions to carry out the goals of our project. Our community partners want to ensure the programs, resources, and supports they are offering are attuned, aligned, and responsive to community needs and desires. One of the most salient partnerships has been with the local public school system, and in particular, the Family and Community Engagement Office (FACE). Krishna Leyva (5th author) is the manager of the FACE office, and she provides a critical link between *Amigas de la Comunidad* and the schools. Over the years, Leyva has been an active member of the CAB, supporting both research and action steps. Leyva's and the Mason Team's shared values, vision, and strengths-based approach to community engagement has ensured smooth collaboration. This partnership has included direct liaising between *Amigas de la Comunidad* and the school system as well as collaboration in publications, presentations, and other efforts to share findings.

The partnership with our funder has been extremely important to achieving the goals of the work as well. The funder, who described *Amigas de la Comunidad* as among the most meaningful of their funded projects, has not only financially supported our efforts in the community but also has been an important thought partner and helped connect us strategically to various city leaders throughout the project. Indeed, *Amigas de la Comunidad* informed citywide strategic planning, inclusive of the youth master plan, and participated in several early childhood working group meetings that informed ECE programming in the city.

Several community organizations have also been instrumental to our work throughout the years, including a local housing advocacy nonprofit organization located in the heart of the community. From 2014 until 2020 (when the COVID pandemic sent us to virtual meetings), the nonprofit provided *Amigas* with a space for our CAB to meet, often on a weekly basis and always free of charge. We have also partnered with local health organizations, labor unions, free legal aid nonprofits, worker-rights advocacy organizations, as well as publicly funded ECE programs to carry out the work of *Amigas de la Comunidad.*

Collaborating With the CAB and Community Partners in Research

Our work examines undocumented Central American mothers' family experiences and their working and living conditions in the context of "illegality." Immigration scholars describe "illegality" as a national project to target, criminalize, detain, and deport immigrants, especially men from Mexico and Central America (De Genova & Peutz, 2010; Golash-Boza & Hondagneu-Sotelo, 2013). While this national anti-immigrant project primarily targets men for removal, it also threatens and constrains women. For example, illegality challenges Central American mothers' ability to generate resources and supports, access quality housing, and meet the needs of their children (Letiecq et al., 2019). The context of illegality can also expose mothers and their children to discrimination, predation, toxic relationships, and other harms to their health (Abrego, 2014; Asad & Clair, 2018; Del Real, 2019; Enriquez, 2015; Logan et al., 2021; Parrado et al., 2005).

In this context of illegality, *Amigas de la Comunidad* has worked to document the stress, trauma, and resilience of Central American immigrant mothers as they navigate early childhood systems and negotiate relationships and parenthood in the United States. Since 2014, our collective has been engaged in multiple aspects of data collection (i.e., qualitative in-depth interviews, focus groups, surveys). We co-created data collection tools including an interviewer-assisted survey as well as an in-depth interview protocol. At this point, we have collected 134 interviewer-assisted surveys with undocumented Central American mothers focused on housing, employment, mental health (see Letiecq et al., 2019), physical health, parenting, immigration experiences, deportation concerns, and social support, as well as 55 childcare history interviews, 10 in-depth interviews focused on navigating life in the United States as immigrant parents, 12 in-depth interviews focused on housing, and 23 in-depth interviews focused on families' experiences during the COVID-19 pandemic.

Our work has been highly iterative, deepening our understanding of mothers' experiences over time. For example, during initial in-depth interview and survey work in people's homes, we observed a number of families whose living arrangements were challenging and stressful. Multiple family units (two, three, and even four families, self-described as "strangers" to each other) were living together in two- or three-bedroom apartments. We discussed with the CAB how families managed to rear children and do family in these environments. These conversations led to an expanded in-depth interview protocol that focused specifically on how mothers "did family" while living in these multifamily apartments (see Letiecq et al., 2022). Importantly, the CAB partnered with us in the coding of these data. Together, we developed a community coding process where the CAB engaged in coding, analyses, and dissemination efforts with the Mason Team (see Vesely et al., 2019 for an overview of these community data analysis processes). Since then, Amigas have partnered with us in all of our qualitative data analytic efforts, including those focused on childcare (see Vesely et al., 2021a) and experiences of COVID (see Vesely et al., 2021b).

Another area of interest that emerged during our time in the community was deportation planning. Based on feedback from the CAB as well as what we were finding in the interviewer-assisted surveys, we became sensitized to how families were thinking about deportation and planning for this as a family. This new knowledge guided additional analyses of survey data related to deportation worries and additional data collection efforts to understand families' deportation plans, how parents were speaking with their children (or not) about the possibilities of detainment and deportation, and how to best support families regarding these concerns. Most recently, as the COVID-19 pandemic ravaged the community in the summer of 2020, Amigas implored us to collect in-depth interview data to record families' experiences such that community organizations and schools could best respond to families' on-going housing, food, and education needs related to the pandemic.

Dissemination of our action research findings within and beyond the community has been an important component of our work together. After our first major data collection effort using surveys and in-depth interviews, the CAB organized a community event to share and discuss the findings. The event, hosted by *Amigas de la Comunidad*, was held in a building owned by a local, trusted, immigrant-serving community organization. The Mason Team prepared several data slides in Spanish that were hung around the community meeting room. Amigas invited friends and neighbors to the event, and in small groups led community members on gallery walks to explain the findings. We then engaged in a community meeting to discuss, based on the findings we shared, what actions the community members and CAB leaders wanted to take. As we shared study findings beyond the community, Amigas co-authors preferred to remain anonymous given their documentation status and vulnerabilities in the context of illegality.

TABLE A1.1 ■ Message From *Amigas de la Comunidad*

We know how to parent.
We value our children's education and all that schools offer.
We are frustrated that we cannot be the parents we dream to be.
Our circumstances are difficult.
Our lives here are better than in our home countries, but we did not anticipate the challenges we face.
Thank you for your understanding and support.

Thus, in presentations and publications, we include "Amigas de la Comunidad" as co-authors rather than listing members' names. Also, Amigas created a message for those who engage with our work such that whenever the Mason Team and our community partners share about *Amigas de la Comunidad*, Amigas are present, if not in person, in their words (see Table A1.1).

Implementing Action Steps

Our work together as a CAB consists of both research and action steps, which are hallmarks of CBPR (Wallerstein et al., 2018). As such we worked with the community during and after data collection to develop both short- and long-term actions or advocacy steps in the community. Among our earliest action steps was a community-based school registration event. During the community meeting and gallery walk discussed above, community members described struggling to complete forms required by schools and organizations because of language barriers. Given our partnership with the local public schools, we were able to offer a school (and preschool) registration day in which families, in the safety and comfort of their local neighborhood, could register their children for school while also receiving health physicals necessary for school entrance. In addition, local health clinic officials and child development specialists were available to screen children and answer any questions that community members had.

Like the registration event, the CAB has driven many community actions based on our research findings and the direct experiences of CAB members and their neighbors. During CAB meetings, we have worked intentionally to make space to ask about individual and collective concerns emanating from the community. Sometimes, these critically engaged conversations derail whatever agenda was set for the meeting. For example, during one meeting, we learned about a community member's son who tragically drowned while crossing the Rio Grande en route to reunify with his mother and two sisters. Together, we decided to raise money to help cover the costs of the son's burial. We also have planned and implemented donation drives to provide community members with basic necessities, like winter clothes, diapers, and household goods.

Amigas de la Comunidad has also worked to address the contextual and structural stressors experienced by the community. For instance, in the context of rising fear about deportation and detention, we partnered with lawyers, notaries, immigration advocates, and Spanish-speaking volunteers to provide Know Your Rights and legal assistance clinics. During these clinics, participants learned about their legal rights and how to respond if detained. Parents also were assisted in completing the paperwork necessary to give a trusted adult the legal authority to care for their child(ren) should the parent be detained or deported. Throughout the project, as we have also worked to educate service providers and educators about immigrant family life in the context of illegality and how they can better support immigrant parents and their children, Amigas have served as cultural brokers. For instance, members of our CAB met with the superintendent of the local school district and her assistants to inform them about our research findings and request specific policy changes that would benefit immigrant families directly.

CONCLUSIONS

For too long, research has been extractive and harmful, taking from the community for the betterment of researchers and universities rather than directly benefiting marginalized and minoritized communities. CBPR holds promise as an approach that is transformational, shifting power hierarchies and building trusted community-university partnerships to produce research that is justice based and liberating (Fals Borda, 2001; Wallerstein et al., 2018). Importantly, as Collins (2019) wrote, CBPR and other action research projects should be led by people "penalized by colonialism, patriarchy, racism, nationalism, and similar systems of power" whose "experiences with oppression are often the catalyst for critically analyzing these systems and taking action within them" (p.12).

Since 2014, we have built this CBPR project in partnership with Central American immigrant mothers. Together, we have developed an implementation process that ensures, whenever feasible, that Amigas are guiding our collective research and action agenda. As we discussed, we have had many successful iterations of conducting research and taking action steps for the betterment of the community, and we are proud that the project is sustaining even without additional funding. However, we also acknowledge several limitations that continue to challenge our work. For example, the cultural and structural divides that exist between the Mason Team and Amigas are ever-present, and the Mason Team depends on interpreters to communicate with Amigas and ensure we are co-producing knowledge that is meaningful and valid to the community. This is no easy task, and we acknowledge that our limits and blind spots may at times get it wrong. Our partnerships are critical to catching errors in appraisal, measurement, and interpretation, and we are grateful for the commitment of the collective to overcome this challenge.

The Mason Team is also challenged by the structure, policies, practices, and expectations of the university. CBPR approaches do not fit nicely within university systems that demand researchers be the experts of their disciplines, generate a constant flow of external grant funds, and "publish or perish" to maintain their positions within the academy. We are encouraged that over time, university systems and funders are changing, embracing community-engaged research approaches, and adapting policies and practices to promote new translational research methods that improve the lives of our community partners (Letiecq et al., 2022).

Lastly, our collective work has also been challenged by the context of illegality that was hardened under the Trump Administration yet continues unabated under the Biden Administration. Until U.S. laws, policies, and practices cease to threaten, criminalize, detain, deport, and separate immigrant families, CBPR projects with undocumented immigrants must operate with caution, ensuring the most vulnerable among us feel safe and empowered to lead. The Mason Team is grateful to Amigas for their trust and courage to serve their community while knowing the risks. It is our collective hope that our work arcs toward justice and liberation of the oppressed.

Case Study 2

Empowerment as a Guide to Expanding Notions of Critical Participatory Inquiry

Tamarah Moss, Scholar-in-Residence, The Bahamas Crisis Centre and assistant professor, Graduate School of Social Work and Social Research with Bryn Mawr College

Sandra Dean-Patterson, founder and executive director, The Bahamas Crisis Centre

As an introduction, my name is Tamarah Moss and I am a Bahamian American academic and community-engaged researcher and evaluator. Through my years as a dually trained practitioner in public health and social work, I continue to learn and grow from my engagement with community and the practice of participatory inquiry, which continues to evolve. While initially seeming unnecessary, the ability to identify areas of positionality and intersection with the community being served is essential for effective and culturally responsive research.

I begin this case study utilizing reflexivity as an approach for sharing on a case study, relevant to an expanded notion of critical participatory inquiry. It is hoped that in taking this approach and "in order not to be a mere technician but competent practitioners of research [we] should be able to reflect in a deep way" (Mortari, 2015, p. 1), in the development of my reflective case study as a research and evaluator as well as an inside/outsider in some regards to the country setting of Nassau, The Bahamas.

This type of reflexivity in practice is a great opportunity to share perspective from the "me" in collaboration with my co-author Dr. Sandra Dean-Patterson, in pursuit of community engagement for the most effective and responsive participatory inquiry. The participatory components of this case study serve to demonstrate a helpful approach to expand our thinking of participatory inquiry. We have moved beyond the thinking of engaging community at the stage of implementation, but also thinking about the pre-stages of implementation and the iterative process of evaluation to inform the next cohort of activity. The anticipation is that this perspective will enhance program or intervention content to be more culturally responsive to the needs and strengths of community participants. I will focus on three stages of this research–evaluator–community relationship as a form of community–campus partnership. By community–campus partnership, I am referring to the partnership that a community-based organization has with an academic institution, in this case me as an academic based at Bryn Mawr College, and The Bahamas Crisis Center (henceforth The Crisis Centre) as the community organization partners. Academic/academic institutions and community-based organizations may come together to promote issues related to health and mental health promotion, interventions, and related resource equity. This case study is focused on partnership, most interested in overall health and well-being for survivors of gender-based violence and intimate partner violence. Now, back to the stages of engaging community, my activities included pre-implementation, implementation, and evaluation and learning lessons.

For the purposes of this case study, community refers to the adult cis-gender women survivors of physical, mental, and sexual violence. The initial relationship between me as the researcher–evaluator and the community organization is one to promote the health and well-being of adult women survivors violence who are able to participate in a 6-week psycho-educational support group, via an online platform, in Nassau, The Bahamas. There were discussions about possibly hosting a second cohort of women in person, but our planning team decided to wait to assess the issues of safety, as groups would be implemented during the persistent global pandemic of COVID-19.

BACKGROUND AND CONTEXT

Preimplementation Stage of Community Engagement

As mentioned earlier, it is important to be able to identify and describe areas of positionality as a researcher and evaluator. It should be noted that historical context is also important. As with all community-based participatory activities, the critical nature of providing a historical context of not only the agency or organization but also the relationship of the researcher–evaluator with the agency partners may be said to sustain the undertaking of activities. In this case, requests for funds and program design and implementation along with evaluation span the stages of pre-implementation and implementation.

The Bahamas Crisis Centre was founded in 1982 by Dr. Sandra Dean-Patterson. Initially named The Women's Crisis Centre, it is a nonprofit organization created to provide intervention, prevention, and advocacy for women and children who have experienced domestic or sexual violence. Originally sponsored by the Bahamas Psychiatric Hospital (Sandilands Rehabilitation Centre), the organization held a single room within both the Psychiatric Social Work Department and the Community Mental Health Centre at Knowles House, which is adjacent to the Princess Margaret Hospital. The Princess Margaret Hospital (PMH) a nonprofit publicly funded facility was built in 1952 and falls under the Public Hospitals Authority of the Commonwealth of The Bahamas. The PMH provides primary, secondary, and tertiary health services. The facility is currently a 402-bed complex in four major blocks or wings, namely, (1) medical, (2) surgical, (3) ambulatory care, and (4) administration, with subdivisions in wards, units, and departments.

Clients of The Crisis Centre had opportunities to attend afternoon sessions twice a week and an evening clinic once a week. The services were free and included couples and family therapy, walk-in crisis counseling, support groups, and legal advice. The Centre quickly expanded after a 6-month trial due to demand, and in 1988 The Lyford Cay Foundation funds enabled The Crisis Centre to have additional office space and employment of a paid administrator. There began to be an increase in volunteers, and service grew to reach the community through services and programs on the effects of all forms of sexual and family violence.

It was in 1995 that the Crisis Centre changed its name from The Women's Crisis Centre to The Bahamas Crisis Centre, also known as The Crisis Centre. This was done to be responsive and reflect the growing need to engage men in the work of eliminating violence against women and children. In addition, men and boys were increasingly coming to the Centre as victims or witnesses of domestic or sexual violence with a need for an intervention. Knowles House was demolished in 2010, and the work of the Centre became situated into two rooms within the outpatient area of Princess Margaret hospital. It was not until 2013 that the Crisis Centre was able to relocate to larger accommodation, given the generosity of the Ministry of National Security.

The Crisis Centre is now in a nearby location and no longer on the physical premises of the public hospital since recent renovations and development of the PMH took place.

The first staff members of the Crisis Centre were social workers, psychiatrists, and counselors offering their services on a voluntary basis. Primarily run by volunteers, the number of volunteers continues to grow, and the Centre offers trainings to volunteers on a biannual basis to enable volunteers' capacity in sensitive topics of rape survival, domestic violence survival, child abuse, depression, sexually transmitted infections, and others. Monthly meetings are held and services are currently provided on the 24-hour crisis hotline, rape survivor advocacy, domestic violence survivor advocacy, court watch, education outreach programs, support groups and trainings as well as a children's holiday party. My in-residence time with the Crisis Centre was in 2022, the year of the organization's 40th anniversary of offering free counseling and other crisis intervention activities and education in The Bahamas. It should be noted that The Crisis Centre continues to be acknowledged nationally and internationally for efforts to support women, men, and children facing violent or abusive situations.

RESEARCH AIMS AND GOALS

As a longstanding volunteer working on various activities, I was invited to support The Crisis Centre in applying for funding from an international foundation based in The Bahamas. I worked along with the team of the founder and executive director, Dr. Sandra Dean-Patterson; the administrator, Mrs. Cleopatra Christie; and lead volunteer, Mrs. Leila Greene, to develop and design a program proposal. The program was to focus on empowerment of adult women survivors of physical, mental, and sexual violence. Critical to the design was the evaluation of the program to ensure cultural responsiveness and relevance of the length of the psychoeducational groups and topics for this proposed 6-week group format program.

As a cautionary step to have clinical support readily available should the need arise within the group and for appropriate referrals, the lead facilitator was one of the clinician volunteers. In addition, there would be at least one rapporteur from a legal and advocacy background to provide counseling and education and summarize the experiences of each cohort of women over the 6-week period. We were successful in achieving the funds for between 80 to 100 women to complete the program. The criteria of inclusion for participants were to be an adult woman, 18 years and older, who had experienced gender-based violence and/or intimate partner violence. Women, thus far, have been former clients of The Crisis Centre and referrals from partner organizations in the business of recovery and healing for adult women.

WOMEN'S EMPOWERMENT PROJECT: IMPLEMENTATION STRATEGY

It should be noted that the inclusion of the term *empowerment* became important to the naming of this particular support group, given the emphasis on supporting and informing adult women survivors through a holistic approach that not solely focuses on the women's experiences of violence and abuse but also their experiences and readiness for recovery and healing as part of the process of empowerment. The theoretical framework of empowerment resonated as this term was voiced by the community organization on behalf of the community being served.

Rappaport (1981, 1984) described empowerment as a construct of involving the three components of individual strengths and competence along with a natural helping system and proactive behaviors related to social policy and change. The theoretical framework of Perkins and Zimmerman (1995), with their description of empowerment, aligns well with The Crisis Centre approach. Women's psychoeducation is focused on connecting mental health and mutual aid with the creation of a community response. The emphasis is on wellness, competence, and strengths. Along with being trauma-informed, this intervention of the Women's Empowerment Project is an empowerment-oriented intervention focused on the enhancement of wellness "to provide opportunities for participants to develop knowledge and skills and engage professionals as collaborators instead of authoritative experts" (Perkins & Zimmerman, 1995, p. 570). Our role as the planning and implementation team, as engaged professionals, continues to be co-creators with the program participants. Participatory inquiry, from inception to funding and naming of the project, centering community, and embracing community perspectives happened from the beginning.

The trauma-informed approach is based on the six key principles outlined by the Substance Abuse and Mental Health Administration (n.d.) The principles are (1) safety; (2) trustworthiness and transparency; (3) peer support; (4) collaboration and mutuality; (5) empowerment, voice, and choice; and (6) cultural, historical and gender issues. When it comes to trauma-informed interventions like the Women's Empowerment Project at The Crisis Centre, the approach is survivor centered. An environment of respect, hope, and connectedness is critical to recover, the link between trauma and symptoms is understood, and the work and activities are carried out in collaboration with the survivor.

Outside of sharing personal stories with the aim to reduce shame and stigma amongst the participants, topics of healthy relationship in terms of an intimate partner as well as with children and relatives. Discussion also addressed continuing education, including for high school diplomas, vocational pathways, and those seeking first-time or continuation of degree-seeking opportunities. Finally, the focus is on overall women's wellness in terms of physical health, mental wellness, and spiritual health. As a part of the last session, participants shared about their thoughts about empowerment. While being a part of the conceptualization team and writing for the program proposal, I was also the program monitor and evaluator. I was in close communication with the facilitator, provided a template for rapporteurs, and later engaged with participant cohorts who had completed the 6-week program.

The participatory context of this stage is engagement from conceptualization. The power of development, design, and anticipated application were shared between the researcher–evaluator and the organization from inception. The framework of perspectives and their overlap was to maintain the mission of the organization and, in this case more specifically, enhance the well-being of adult women survivors. This was through dialogue based on open communication at all points, from identifying the purpose of the support group, to the naming of the initiative and deciding on the engagement of staff and steps for sustainability. It is at this stage that the co-creation, collaboration, and participatory inquiry was activated. It should be noted that prior to the groups starting, I worked along with the facilitator, who was a clinical counselor, and we developed the Participant Preamble, which was read to the participants at the first session to ensure that participants understood the voluntary nature of participation along with their right to discontinue.

Establishing Community Goals and Priorities

The planning and implementation team decided on the name of the *Women's Empowerment (WE) Project Program*. It is sometimes referred to as a project or program, and sometimes both. The WE Program was certainly an initiative of The Crisis Centre. As a team, we decided on three specific goals which the WE Project Program would strive to achieve within the 6-month timeframe. The following anticipated results were threefold, along with indicators of measurement:

1. To offer 6-week trauma-informed and survivor-centered empowerment groups to between 80 and 100 women survivors of domestic and intimate partner violence between September 2021 and March 2022 (6 months), through the Women's Empowerment (WE) Project Program.

   Measurements: Participant attendance, pre-check-in phone calls to determine the topics of interest for the participants so that the approach is survivor centered, utilization of the child-care services during group sessions by women with school-age children, Development of a trauma-informed, survivor-centered workgroup (support and psychoeducational), for the WE Project Program's future funding opportunities and activities.
2. To improve the knowledge and understanding of at least 50% of WE Project Program participants on topics related to general women's health and mental health well-being.

   Measurements: Debrief notes from the counselor or facilitators, and the use of brief pre- and posttest group session evaluations to assess knowledge and understanding.
3. To develop a cohort of between five and 10 women who would become peer leaders for women's empowerment and inform future WE Project programming, including cofacilitation and related activities at The Bahamas Crisis Center.

   Measurements: Motivation for leadership surveys for participants during the final session of each 6-week group to signal interest in peer leadership, debrief notes form the counselor or facilitator on persons emerging as peer leaders, posttraining evaluations from the cohort of five to 10 women initially recommended for peer leadership with the Women's Empowerment (WE) Project Program, and participation of peer leaders in the final 2 weeks of the 6-month program.

The following areas were the anticipated outcomes based on the results previously indicated.

1. To develop a cohort of between five and 10 women by March 2020. These WE Project Program participants would become peer leaders for women's empowerment and inform future WE Project programming, including co-facilitation and related activities at The Bahamas Crisis Center. These women may also be considered as part of

a community advisory board that informs the continued development of programs, the WE Project Program Workgroups Curriculum, and funding opportunities.

2. WE Project Program Workgroups Curriculum by June 2022: development of a trauma-informed, survivor-centered workgroup (support and psychoeducational), for the WE Project Program's future funding opportunities and activities.

When it comes to the actual implementation, due to protection orders during the COVID-19 pandemic, the thought of an in-person activity was completely diminished. The start of the groups was delayed as our planning team discussed the environment of COVID-19 protective orders of curfew, availability of staff to coordinate as a result, and uncertainty related to actual participant motivation. Our planning team worked with partner organizations, our first cohort of five women was identified, and the group started in September 2020 with a 7-month delay from our original March 2020 plans. Our anticipated plan was to have 10 participants, but we remained genuinely excited to have the women who were able to attend, and they were enthusiastic about getting started.

Data Collection and Analysis

The clinician facilitator contacted me as the program monitor and evaluator immediately following the first week of meetings to discuss the roll-out of program content in relation to the priority of this first cohort of women. Along with the director, we discussed the pros and cons of moving from a structured format to one that was semi-structured. We came to the conclusion that it was important to provide knowledge and information for understanding and accessing resources, and it was as important to have the women take the time to share their personal stories. The issue of internet access also emerged in term of ongoing communication within the group and not solely relying on Zoom meetings to connect. Immediately the assistant administrator and the clinician facilitator created a cohort group on the WhatsApp platform (an internet-based application used for sending messages, images, audio, and video).

In my role as program monitor and evaluator, I then followed up with the first cohort participants in November 2020 via WhatsApp to ask questions related to their experience with the program. The perspectives included requests about their decision to participate in this type of program, what went well in the program, what areas of the program could be strengthened, recommendations for future planning, any list of words or a statement that would capture their experience, their age (as the only criteria related to age was to be at least 18 years old, which is the age of majority and adulthood in The Bahamas), and, finally, if they had any additional questions or comments. Once this phone evaluation was completed, participants were then provided with a hardcopy certificate of participation and small monetary gift that could be picked-up in person at The Crisis Centre. Prior to beginning these feedback calls, each participant was reminded that their name would not be tied to any findings and that their participation in this part of the program was also voluntary. Permission was requested to continue with the evaluation questions where I would be taking handwritten notes of their responses.

Utilizing Community Feedback to Adjust Priorities

During the writing of this case study, we were beginning the process of the third cohort of survivor participants. Our planning and implementation team had decided to make considerations for a full revisit of the Women's Empowerment Project Program, once we reached between 40 to 50 participants, which would be our 50% mark of the 80 to 100 adult women survivors we had hoped to reach. Thankfully, the funding organization has remained responsive and supportive in the need to expand the timeline of the activity, given the context of COVID-19 and emerging variants that may present barriers on varied levels for women to be able to participate. The implementation of the engagement stage actively informs the logistics of the group for responsiveness to participants' needs, and the collection of feedback is ongoing. This stage demonstrates that participatory inquiry can be a gradual process as well.

LEARNING LESSONS FROM COMMUNITY ENGAGEMENT

Although potentially awkward to read, this final stage is titled learning lessons instead of lessons learned. This is critically important, as during the time of writing this case study, the program was currently being administered. As our planning team continues to collect feedback on the length of the program, the topics of discussion, the continuation of a series of groups for cohorts, we continue to learn about participatory inquiry and the relevance for trauma-informed, empowerment-based psychoeducational groups for adult women survivors of gender-based violence or intimate partner violence. While writing this case study, I had a conversation with a colleague who was seeking to understand community research and how to go about it. My repeated priority was for my fellow research colleague to consider the priorities of the community first. The philosophy of "not about community, without community" illustrates the critical nature of community-based participatory inquiry: Start there and see where it takes you as a researcher in terms of your contribution to the inquiry, informed by community priorities, feasibility, and sustainability.

ONGOING WORK: POSITIONALITIES, RELATIONSHIPS, POSTURE

As socio-cultural-political-environmental situations change, so do communities. While not an exhaustive list, the following are my top three "learning lessons" for community-based critical participatory inquiry for consideration, based on my experience with The Bahamas Crisis Centre. In terms of what order to address the list, it depends on one's self-awareness as a researcher to identify areas of strength and areas that serve as opportunities for growth and strengthening. Approaches and strategies include the following:

Awareness of Positionality: As insider/outsider (in this case my ethnicity and connection to The Bahamas) along with my long-standing volunteer status, these identities of positionality may inform the ability of the organization planning and implementation to embrace my participation as the program monitor and evaluator.

Acknowledgement of the importance of relationships: Many times in research, the relational nature of collaboration is not acknowledged or fully understood. In the case of critical participatory inquiry, the degree of connectedness of the planning and implementation team, along with the co-creation of program environment through community engagement, is essential. On a basic level, without participants, there is no program.

Holding a posture of community strengths and collaboration: Sometimes as researchers, even those of us with the best intentions, we take an approach that is more deficit-oriented than strengths-based. We take an inappropriate authoritative expert stance that lacks culturally responsiveness and is certainly not trauma informed.

CONCLUSION

"Empowerment [single word to describe this first cohort member experience]. I felt empowered regardless of what I went through . . . there is hope for me. I am confident in myself."

-WE Project Program, Cohort #1 participant

This quote from the first cohort group in response to using one word or a statement to describe her experience in the psychoeducation group. Her quote provides a synthesis of the impact of the program on this participant's life, an indicator of anticipated outcomes, and motivation for continued sustainable work with the Women's Empowerment Project Program for The Crisis Centre as we engage in critical participatory inquiry as an emergent process, through ongoing community (organization and program participants') feedback.

ACKNOWLEDGMENTS

Many thanks to the commitment, skills and passion of Mrs. Cleopatra Christie, Mrs. Leila Greene, Ms. Rodisha Rolle, Ms. Sharmaine Knowles, and Ms. La Gloria Davis, and special thanks to Mrs. Kavita Garikaparthi, who serves as our clinician facilitator.

Case Study 3

How Can Research Include? Including the Experts: Critical Participatory Inquiry of Inclusion with Young Adults with Intellectual and Developmental Disabilities

Alexandra S. Reed, Academic Coordinator, Mason LIFE, George Mason University

Early on in my graduate studies it became worryingly clear that the research process and PhD requirements were not going to be a simple set of tasks for me to achieve. With a background in special education, I was familiar with the "See, test, fix" process of intervention methods and the fact that historically educational research with students and individuals with disabilities focused on a similar results-based process. While colleagues and mentors were led by data-informed, groundbreaking, or trendsetting research questions, any connection to strong research questions seemed to fade away. What continued to thrill me was the power and potential of research to cultivate conversations, community, and platforms for individuals with disabilities in my life. It is perhaps this lack of needing to answer a question or fix a problem and instead a deeply rooted belief that researchers (I) should be listening and working together that led to seeking out critical participatory inquiry (CPI).

This balancing act between conducting good and ethical research and producing work likely to be recognized and publishable led to the design of a participatory inquiry study focused on including participants in each step of the research process while discussing concepts of inclusion, belonging, and college. Including participants, however, in a benevolent effort to give "the voiceless a voice," called ethics immediately into question. A White, currently nondisabled graduate student and teacher organizing a group of former students and individuals with disabilities to engage in participatory "equal" research sounded great on paper, but would it be a reality? The concept of calling out the research–participant relationship and using others in the nicest way possible (Limes-Taylor Henderson & Esposito, 2019) consistently helped and helps me through the balancing act of engaging in CPI.

BACKGROUND AND CONTEXT

Our participatory inquiry project emerged out of my dissertation, which intended to include participants in a meaningful way (i.e., how each person chose to participate) in order to learn about inclusion. Research on special education and intellectual and developmental disability (IDD) has a long and dark history. Individuals with IDD have been systematically prevented from participating in research and knowledge construction as valued participants, and instead have either been ignored entirely, exploited and forced to participate without proper consent, or used as subjects (McDonald et al., 2012; Strnadová & Walmsley, 2017; Turnbull & Turnbull, 2000). Protections and safeguards which have emerged in response to past murderous deeds (involuntary and forced participation, lack of consent or assent protocols, forced sterilization or medical procedures, actual murder), often prevent participation of individuals with IDD in research due to IRB and legal documentation (i.e., requiring legal guardians to speak on a person's behalf or deeming this population too vulnerable for research). What little research does exist often "includes" persons with IDD through proxies or a systemic "you say, I take" (extractive) approach. Simply following institutional [review board] safeguards (IRB) may protect an institution legally but does not always ensure ethical research methods.

As in other contexts of life, the inclusion of individuals with IDD in research can acknowledge them as valued, worthy members of society. This acknowledgement is necessary in addressing the historical marginalizing and devaluing of this population. At the individual level, creating an opportunity for individuals with IDD to represent themselves in education research can help increase self-esteem and worthiness, demonstrate capabilities, and contribute to the production of knowledge that is reflective of their experiences (McDonald et al., 2016). At the societal and academic levels, incorporating inclusive practices and developing research with individuals with IDD may further humanize the research process in an area where research has been incomplete and downright dirty or violent. In our current climate focused on fighting for and celebrating inclusion and diversity, there seemed no better time to investigate inclusion by including individuals with IDD as experts in my research process.

RESEARCH CONTEXT

I sought to learn about inclusion from a group of young adults with IDD who have gone to college programs labeled "inclusive." This research topic has both excited and haunted me throughout my career as a special educator, as I have often made decisions based on "inclusion" without asking my students what they believed, wanted, or even how they felt—because I was "the expert." Initially this study was focused on the following questions: (1) What are experiences of inclusion held by individuals with IDD at college? (2) What are the recommendations and expectations of inclusive college experiences held by young adults with IDD? and (3) How do we navigate and reconcile imbalances of power and equity and the dilemma of creating a research community that did not ask to be created? As our group met and worked together, we would stray from these questions and instead found ourselves speaking about a number of topics, usually whatever was on our hearts and minds each day!

Incorporating new or nontraditional ways of knowing into research design and methodological decision making became necessary in order to remain true to my personal epistemological beliefs (see Chapter 1 of this volume) as well as the research collective of which I was a member. The development of this CPI project emerged from my desire to engage in work that is equitable and inclusive as well as from the onto-epistemological belief that individuals are experts on their lived experiences. Here, I share the story of our research collective, *Everyday Friends Research* (EFR) group: how we formed, our work, our lessons learned, and our thoughts for next steps.

FORMATION OF THE COLLECTIVE

The EFR group initially formed out of my personal desire to understand inclusion from the perspectives of young adults with IDD through an inclusive research study. These (my) individual goals are noted here only to highlight and acknowledge the tension in creating a group that did not ask to be created. I note the tension not as a limitation but as a critical part of the CPI process.

I personally reached out to all potential participants via email, text, and social media messaging. Each potential participant and I had personal relationships through the classroom (teacher–student), Special Olympics (coach–athlete), or community organization (member–member). Due to these relationships, there was an immediate recognition of power dynamics and imbalances that needed to be acknowledged but not necessarily critiqued. The nature of this research involved discussing life experiences and concepts of inclusion, belonging, and exclusion—intimate and, at times, heavy topics. This was at the forefront of my mind when forming the research group. It was important to me that I engaged with people who knew me, trusted me, and who had knowledge of my role related to our topic: education, postsecondary programming or college, and inclusion. Eight individuals responded to me with interest in joining the research group and followed the university procedures (IRB requirements) as well as research group participation agreement procedures (or collectively created requirements). These requirements did overlap with some of the IRB requirements but were explicitly separated. I felt IRB protections offered the bare minimum, and it was important to me that our group was protected *and* a safe community. A few examples of our collective requirements are as follows:

- What we say in our group stays private.
- We can turn off our camera or microphone any time.
- Listening is also participating.
- Our parents are not part of this.

INTENTIONAL DESIGN AND RESEARCH GOALS

Once individuals agreed to participate and signed consent forms or provided assent, each person met one-on-one with me to review in detail what the study was and to brainstorm what it could be. Through these individual meetings, I aimed to continue developing our relationship and to strive for purposeful transparency: I was a PhD student in need of a study, but I was also (and am still) attempting to be an ally and a community member and to remain in a positive relationship with each person. Additionally, through these meetings I was able to listen to each participant's concerns, fears, hopes, and interests before directing us towards my own research agenda. In order to remain true to our collective, I will refer to our research group as our chosen name, *Everyday Friends Research* (EFR) group, and refer to participants as co-researchers. A few co-researchers have chosen to use their real names or pseudonyms which will appear throughout the text.

As the principal investigator of this study, I intended to explicitly and transparently delineate my role as a researcher, leader, and decision maker within the research group or collective, but I also deeply wanted to create and allow space for co-researcher roles and input to emerge throughout conversations and experience sharing. Guided by Freire's (1970) "trust through dialogue," where discovery and knowledge emerge from the sincere desire to understand reality, this research sought (continues to seek) to understand the reality of inclusion for individuals with IDD through individual and group conversations. Social science and educational research, particularly with historically marginalized populations, is often focused on the documentation of damage or highlighting oppression (Tuck, 2010) which may be benevolent in hopes of instilling change. However, this is also seen as voyeuristic and exploitative of individuals' experiences (Tuck & Yang, 2014). Therefore, this research sought stories that are desire-based not pain-based narratives: I tried not to focus on what *hasn't* been inclusive but rather wanted to know the positive experiences in an effort to not (consciously) exploit participants or their experiences.

EFR GROUP STUDY

Due to the COVID-19 pandemic and social distancing protocols, our study was conducted virtually in accordance with university IRB procedures over the course of seven months. Study procedures were developed based on the CPI expectation that participants are active co-researchers involved in each step of the research process (Fals Borda & Rahman, 1991; Fine & Torre, 2004; Kemmis & McTaggart, 2005.) As such, our data were collected in multiple ways based on group member's needs, wants, and interests. Most importantly, these data collection procedures were focused first on EFR co-researcher preferences, and varied. In fact, traditional research terms like *data collection* or *protocols* were rarely, if ever used except to satisfy institutional requirements. Instead, we met as a group to share, be together, and listen. We engaged in individual and group discussions and interviews. Adapted photovoice interviews were also used. Co-researchers led group discussions and analysis procedures. It was essential that co-researchers shared what they wanted, how they wanted and I made that methodological choice explicitly. This also resulted in our study shifting directions from *my* research questions to *our* research group interests.

We shared our experiences through individual interviews, structured group interviews, unstructured weekly group meetings, photography, word collages, drawings, and email exchanges. We also created a private Facebook group to share ideas and keep conversations going outside of the meeting, but only six posts were made to the group over seven months. We much preferred to chat in person through our screens.

CONVERSATIONS

Individual interviews took place throughout the study, and were referred to as "One-on-ones" or simply, "conversations." While not an unfamiliar term, the word *interview* seemed to elicit emotions related to performance and work completion (e.g., "Did I answer that correctly?" or visibly frowning while struggling to answer), so I consistently used "one-on-one," "group meeting," and "conversation" instead. Co-researchers who preferred group discussions only participated in two one-on-ones, and those who preferred one-on-one conversations participated in up to four individual interviews. I developed a semistructured interview protocol to be used as a roadmap for conversations. Many EFR co-researchers seemed to prefer this way of sharing—it was familiar to wait for a question, reflect, and share an answer. This was one area I consistently found myself "checking" my ableism. I kept thinking, "This is too 'researchy.' This is not inclusive." I had to remind myself that this format is what my co-researchers were asking for, and I needed to hear and accept that!

GROUP MEETINGS

Group meetings and discussions also served as primary data sources as well as analysis procedures. It was through these meetings that some of our most powerful and community building work was done! In order to develop a safe group environment, EFR met initially to practice group discussion dynamics through the computer (e.g., muting, sharing screens, raising hands, use of emojis, the chat box function). Group meetings initially followed a semi-structured protocol with open-ended questions. Meetings began with general rapport building through greetings and welcomes and then an ice breaker (e.g., your favorite TV show, your best meal in the last week) followed by versions of conversation prompts related to inclusion, college experiences, and favorite memories. All co-researchers were invited to lead group discussions and develop individual research questions to lead conversations. Interested EFR co-researchers took turns leading group meetings and prepared discussion topics and research questions to pose to the group, which added to our study goals, research questions, and future directions. I provided facilitator support as needed (e.g., screen sharing, rewording questions, or supporting the co-researcher in calling on co-researchers to share answers). At times group meetings were focused on a topic related to research and inclusion (Figure A1.3). Other times, we spent our time together venting about work and roommates or sharing happy news and future plans!

FIGURE A1.3 ■ World Cloud as Data Collection

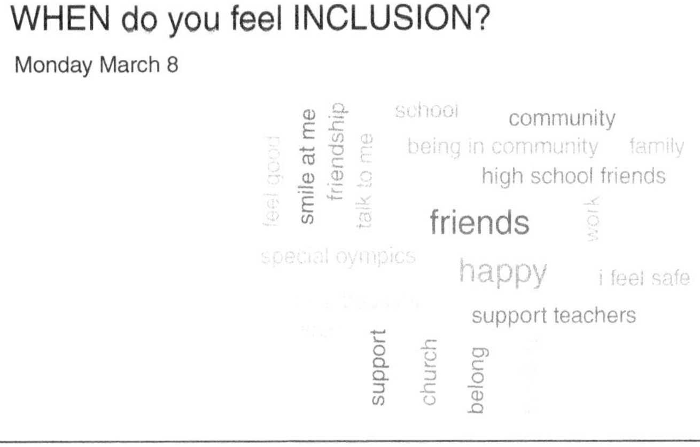

Note. Figure A1.3 is a finished word cloud which was generated during group conversation about when we feel inclusion, an example of when we strayed from the protocol, and just shared as a community.

Visual Data

Participatory photographic research methods support individuals engaging in research who may require visual support or prefer to communicate other than spoken word (Jurkowski, 2008). Photovoice is one participatory approach to data collection and analysis which can support amplification of historically marginalized populations (Wang & Burris, 1997). This approach is used to visually record and honor the voices, experiences, and knowledge of individuals and issues impacting their lives (Call-Cummings et al., 2019). The use of photovoice with individuals with IDD has been proven an effective way to collect data and increase participation of individuals in the research process (Cheak-Zamora et al., 2018; Jurkowski, 2008; Povee et al., 2014; Prohn, 2014). Typically, photovoice encourages participants to take photos, assign captions to the images, and share photos as part of analysis procedures (Wang, 2006). In light of the health crisis and social distancing measures, our visual support procedures instead invited co-researchers to share a picture that reminded them of or represented inclusion in their lives. Additionally, co-researchers were also offered the option to draw inclusion. Five of the eight co-researchers shared photographs as part of the interview process. This adapted photovoice interview drew from Wang's (1999) SHOWeD photo elicitation process to discuss the visual data source. Adapting the SHOWeD method was necessary to support understanding (Francis et al., 2020) and as such, rewording questions resulted in a new acronym. The SHIMeT protocol emerged during individual interviews and group conversations in which co-researchers discussed two example photographs:

1. What do we **S**ee here?
2. What or How is/was this **H**appening?
3. What makes this **I**mportant for Inclusion?
4. What is the **Me**mory behind this?
5. What can this **T**each/Tell us about inclusion?

This protocol, while used as an interview technique, also served as an analysis tool when discussing inclusion and experiences shown or represented in the visual data source.

Data Analysis and Meaning Making Procedures

In CPI, the expectation that participants are involved in all steps of the research process includes the analysis of data gathered. This was a particularly exciting but difficult step in our research study. EFR co-researchers had not previously participated in formal research and certainly had not been invited or instructed to follow analytical steps like coding. As the primary researcher, I was looking for ways to analyze data that fit our group—not necessarily the research methods textbook procedures which left me straddling traditional research methods and inclusive and accessible methods. Ultimately, I felt compelled to support EFR co-researchers in the analysis phase and questioned the fairness of expecting immediate participation in "analysis," a concept all eight had not recognized by name. What I found was through discussion, modeling, and basic human conversation (how novel!), our collective was able to summarize hours of data and conversations into important takeaways and to truly make meaning from the data.

Preliminary Analysis: Meaning Making

Meaning making was initially researcher generated, "behind closed doors" and not participatory. I wrestled with this choice and continue to do so, but I always return to my responsibility to the EFR group and what my role as a group facilitator required. I followed general open coding and thematic analysis techniques often found in grounded theory analysis and narrative inquiry (Clandinin & Connelly, 1990; Strauss & Corbin, 1998) to identify and develop major themes or ideas emerging from perspectives of EFR co-researchers. This analysis process was shared with participants during later group meaning-making conversations, and so the methodological decision to use plain language when describing each step was purposeful and important. Initial thematic analysis followed this process: (1) open-stage codes formed by reviewing participants' vocabulary, expressions, and input to develop potential categories for group discussion (e.g., emotions, places, people, situations); (2) generated a list of interesting "themes" based on the categories from interview data, which may turn into overarching themes in group analysis. Primary analysis followed during the group-work stage, where I share these initial interpretations with our research collective.

Primary Analysis: Our Meaning Making

Primary meaning making was group generated, participatory, and most importantly, voluntary. This was another place where I consistently checked my power and ableism in response to how my co-researchers chose to participate. The expectation of a unified "according to the text" analysis procedure wasn't equitable or, frankly, respectful of my co-researchers, and though that concerned me from an institutional lens (i.e., getting published or deemed "good" work), it actually opened up what analysis could and should be!

Our analysis work took place during group discussions and individual discussions based on co-researcher interest and preference for analysis. As the facilitator, I modeled identifying themes and repetitive words heard throughout discussion and shared the preliminary interpretations gleaned from the first analysis phase. For example, I read or replayed an excerpt of a conversation with a participant (with permission) and asked the group to share one or two ideas or phrases they heard throughout the recording. At the end of each shared excerpt, audio clip, or viewing of visual data, co-researchers would engage in analysis through one or more of the following steps: (a) share words or phrases that seemed important to them, (b) agree or disagree with statements heard, (c) respond using the statement "This person is saying ___ is important," and (d) state "This teaches us ___ about inclusion." Additionally, we returned to the phrase, "What is important from this story?" Using group analysis procedures such as priority sorting (participants identify top two or three points of significance from a story or shared experience) or retelling "the most important part," the group identified major themes. We also engaged in visual analysis using the SHIMeT protocol while discussing photographs or drawings. Table A1.2 shows an example of a meaning-making discussion table. This was often what was shown on the screen, and we discussed what we heard, saw, and learned from the excerpt.

TABLE A1.2 ■ Example Group Meaning-Making Discussion and Response Table

Our Stories	What We Heard and Learned		
S: What about any other things that you really liked about the program? Rikki: Meeting new friends. They know about my disability and they help me with it, like whenever I'm having problems or having a seizure, they know kind of what to do.	I like meeting friends. My friends help me when I have seizures.	Friendship was important part of program. I trust and rely on my friends from the program.	Having friends like me is more important than the classes or setting. **Friends that understand disability is important.**
"Because my friends are very important because it's socializing with people that you love very much and people that you can hang out with and play with and do all sorts of things."	Having friends and socializing is important.	I love my friends. I love hanging out with them and doing the same things.	**Inclusion is when I am with my friends no matter where we are.**
Rikki: Like classmates said at lunch about like, "Oh, do you want to sit with us?" S: So you were with students from [program] and you were eating lunch. How did it make you feel? What were you feeling? Rikki: I felt happy that they let me sit with them at lunch.		It was important to belong with friends from the program.	Having friends outside of class is more important.

Note. Table A1.2 shows a group meaning making discussion table. After rereading or listening to our discussions, co-researchers shared what was important, and responses were recorded verbatim. Bold responses indicate majority feedback or agreement.

Table A1.3 shows another version of our meaning-making discussion tables. This discussion was centered around the idea of inclusion being a feeling (later this was one of our major themes).

TABLE A1.3 ■ Group Meaning-Making Discussion Example

Story or Memory	What is important from the story?		
So: I feel included at work. SR: What do you think makes you feel included? So: Everyone is nice to me at work.	People are nice at work and include me.	I can tell when I am being included, it feels nice.	
Because everyone is very kind to me. And there are no bullies and very kind to me in the George Mason University.	Everyone is kind to me.	I feel good when everyone is kind.	

TABLE A1.3 ■ Group Meaning-Making Discussion Example (Continued)

Story or Memory	What is important from the story?		
Inclusion means not being lonely and understanding each other and doing things together. I feel happy and comfortable when I am included.	I feel happy about inclusion.	I feel inclusion when I am not lonely and I can do things with people.	Inclusion is something you can feel.
I just know I'm always included. I just feel that I'm always included. I just always felt included. I don't have a memory. I don't remember. I just felt included.	I know I'm included.	Inclusion is a feeling that you know when you feel it.	It is hard to explain what inclusion is, you just feel it.

Note. Table A1.3 is an example of group meaning-making discussion surrounding the idea of "Inclusion is a feeling."

OUR RECOMMENDATIONS AND THEMES

Two major areas of findings emerged from our work together: (1) general themes and recommendations regarding inclusion at the college setting, and (2) lessons learned for doing research together. EFR summarized six main themes to help describe and define inclusion or inclusive experiences for students with IDD at college: (1) Inclusion is People > Places, (2) Inclusion is Friends that "Get Me," (3) Inclusion is Choices, (4) Inclusion is Opportunity and Permission, (5) Inclusion is Help and Support, and (6) Inclusion is that Feeling: You Just Know It. The following briefly summarizes the six themes and recommendations with additional data collection and analysis examples.

People > Places

EFR group shared that inclusion and memories of inclusion were tied to people and groups, not physical places or settings. Stories reflected the importance of being with friends when feeling included, regardless of setting.

Friends that "Get Me"

EFR group described inclusion as being around friends who are similar to them, who have disabilities, and who understand their experiences. This was one of the most powerful discussion topics because so often this group of co-researchers were told to believe inclusion was being with those without disabilities. Here, our group could share what makes them truly feel comfortable and included. One co-researcher shared, "I remember I was [finally] making friends that [also] have a disability, which actually amazed me because I never thought that I was making new friends since I moved to college for the first time." Table A1.4 shows another example from a group meaning-making discussion which led to this theme.

TABLE A1.4 ■ Group Meaning-Making Discussion Table

Our Stories	What we learned and heard. What is important?		
I don't know. I just kind of really wanted to go college and meet a bunch of people that kind of, I don't know different. I would say not normal. I don't know.	I wanted to go to college to meet new people.	It was important to meet new people who are like me.	**Inclusion is being with people similar to me.**
Em: Hanging out with your friends and people would just try and be nice to each other. S: Cool. Is it important to you to be with people who have disabilities? Em: Yeah. I can hang out with people that might understand my disability and help me out with that.	It's important to me to be with people with disabilities.	**Friends understand my disability.**	Inclusion is when I feel safe with people like me.

Note. Table A1.4 shows a group meaning-making discussion table. After reviewing our discussion and transcripts, EFR co-researchers shared what was important, and responses were recorded. Bold responses indicate majority feedback or agreement.

Choice

EFR co-researcher's stories and memories were filled with individual experiences of making choices and feeling included because of that option to choose. This was such a dominant theme throughout our work that choice was also the top recommendation for colleges, professionals, and families: let us choose. Choosing how to spend time, where they learned, lived, or played, and who they were with was extremely important to feeling included. Table A1.5 and Figure A1.4 share some data collection and analysis examples from our work together.

Table A1.5 provides another example of a meaning-making group discussion table which informed our preliminary theme of "choice." Figure A1.4 is a visual representation from a young girl. She was sharing a memory of hers related to choosing who she sits with to each lunch on campus, "I just did a drawing of lunch. Here are people and then that's me. Then one of the friends at the table says 'You can sit with us,' so I can choose to sit with them."

Opportunity and Permission

EFR co-researchers shared about opportunity and permission being linked to inclusion. Co-researchers described inclusion as being able to join organizations or activities without needing permission or fighting through barriers (see Table A1.6).

Help and Support

Our conversations also centered around the idea that inclusion requires help and support, and does not always happen naturally despite physical or personnel supports.

TABLE A1.5 ■ Group Meaning-Making Discussion Table

Our Stories	What we heard and learned		
I felt included when I had spoke up for myself, and I have to audit some classes off campus. I knew that, so I spoke to [Staff], and I went ahead and I did it on my own, where I had audited some two or three regular classes outside of the program, where I did public speaking, and two different communication classes. I loved those classes a lot, and I passed all those classes.	I liked taking audit courses.	When I spoke up for myself and made choices I felt inclusion.	It is important to have a say in where we are included and want to belong.
I just did a little drawing of at lunch. Here are people and then that's me. Then one of the people at the table says, "You can sit with us." I can sit with them.	I like choosing my friends and what I do.		

FIGURE A1.4 ■ Visual Data Representation

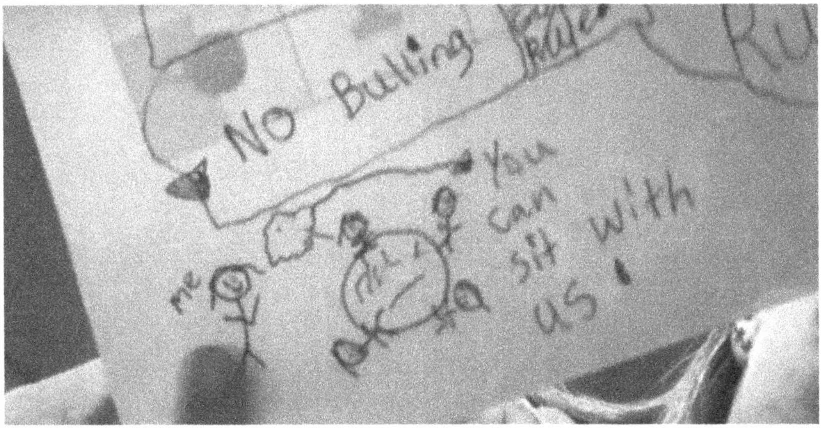

A Feeling: You Just Know It

The final important concept we talked through regarding inclusion was that is something you feel and know, like an intuition. EFR co-researchers shared that when they experienced inclusion, they just knew it when they felt it. Simply put by Sophia, "I just know when I'm included. I know it when I feel it."

The EFR group engaged in honest and critical conversations regarding inclusion, what it is, what it is not, and what it could or should be, particularly at the college settings and for those living in communities outside of the family home. Above all, these ideas are important in showcasing the expert opinions regarding inclusion. Very little research exists which centers the perspective of the young adult with IDD, and of those, proxies or secondary data sources

TABLE A1.6 ■ Meaning-Making Discussion Table

Our Stories	What we heard and learned		
Well, since the first years at they weren't allowed any [of us] students to join the student government as well, which is a big struggle because they weren't allow any us to join, and they only allow [general ed] students instead, which is a big struggle.	We were not allowed to join organizations.	It was painful to not be allowed. **It was hard.**	This was not inclusion for me.
I have one friend who got rejected from every single sororities, which got her very sad because she had Down Syndrome and I was really surprised. So they weren't allow any [of us] to join a sorority, fraternities, and they weren't being able to join the student government. It was just really hard. It was the program, said no.	We were not allowed to join the organization.	It was painful to be excluded.	**Inclusion is giving opportunities and permission to join events and activities.**

Note. Table A1.6 shows a group meaning-making discussion table. After reviewing our discussion and transcripts, EFR co-researchers shared what was important and responses were recorded. Bold responses indicate majority feedback or agreement.

are also included to confirm truths or reach an accepted level of" trustworthiness." Providing space for sharing stories and experiences, listening to those, and then believing and accepting as truth is important to acknowledge individuals with IDD as capable and valued experts who contribute to research.

ONGOING WORK

As I set out to create a research opportunity that was inclusive and participatory and shifts the power from the PI (me) to participants, I was immediately met with conflict and contradictions. These led me to adopt the refrain "This is hard *and* important." Too often the hard work with individuals with IDD leads to extractive, researcher-controlled projects. Barriers such as literacy level, speech intelligibility, and physical behaviors or limitations often results in research that is short, lacking in depth, or done through proxies. The EFR group includes individuals with varying literacy levels, speech abilities, and behaviors that would be deemed unexpected for a traditional research group. Taken together these could create a hard environment to conduct research, until the very idea of research is reimagined.

In the *Everyday Friends Research* group, we continue to reimagine research and who can construct, collect, and share knowledge with the tenets of CPI as our guide. While I continue to move forward with the EFR group in work that is good, safe, and inclusive, I return to my own struggle with ethic of humility (Limes-Taylor Henderson & Esposito, 2019) to consider how I am using co-researchers and gently remind myself that I need them more than they need me. This tension has resulted in shifting future plans of publication in journals to developing video and text-based public service announcements from the EFR group. Over the next year, we hope to release research group productions with advice, information, and messages of how to include.

ENDNOTES

1. "Amigas" refers to the Central American women who were community members and a part of the *Amigas de la Comunidad Community* Advisory Board (CAB). The "Mason Team" refers to George Mason University researchers, inclusive of faculty (Betsy DeMulder, Rachael Goodman, Bethany Letiecq, Colleen Vesely) and several undergraduate and graduate students who have worked on the project over the years. "Community partners" refers to staffs of several community agencies and the local public schools who have contributed to the project in terms of resources, connections, and support (including co-authors Marlene Marquez and Krishna Leyva). *Amigas de la Comunidad* CAB includes Amigas, the Mason Team, and community partners. Throughout, we use "we" and "our" when referring to *Amigas de la Comunidad,* including Amigas.

2. This person left her position and the community within a year of the inception of the project. However, her support of *Amigas de la Comunidad* in the earliest months of the project was instrumental to establishing the CAB.

APPENDIX 2: SAMPLE POSITIONALITY INVENTORY

1. What are all the identities I hold?

   White, woman, cisgender, mother, mother of children who identify as Black and biracial, wife to a Black man, researcher, university professor, friend, sister, sister-in-law, activist, teacher, church member (relatively conservative religion), Democrat, middle class, home owner, friend to several K–12 teachers . . .

2. How are these identities salient to who I am as a researcher?

   I prioritize relationships in my life. I'm less aware of privilege and power dynamics than others because of my social positioning. I strive to be aware but find I often fall short or make mistakes. Power dynamics around student–professor in CPI work.

3. How might some of these identities help my critical participatory inquiry?

   I understand some aspects of anti-Black racism in some ways but not in other ways. It's not embodied in the same way it is for my kids and partner but I do have a particular sense of the roles race plays in children's lives and educational experiences. I have established relationships with community members who are activists and could potentially facilitate CPI projects around race and racism in schools, specifically.

4. How might some of these identities hinder my critical participatory inquiry?

   It's that lack of awareness that comes with whiteness. This will always hinder portions of my work. I need to continue to engage in reflexive praxis and act in humility, building relationships of trust with others who can help and challenge me.

5. What can I start doing now to become aware of how my identities play a role in my inquiry and research?

   Use my researcher journal to capture moments of insight or confusion. Educate myself through literature and dialogue. Stay active but humble in activist spaces. Seek out opportunities in my community that align with my interests and experience and seek feedback anchored in relationships.

APPENDIX 3: SAMPLE SYLLABUS

Critical Participatory Inquiry

COURSE OVERVIEW

This advanced graduate-level research course focuses on a methodological approach to inquiry that actively engages participants in confronting and changing their life situations or patterns. It is community based in that it engages with already existing communities, privileging the terms, interests, complexities and challenges of the communities themselves.

In this class, you will learn the foundational history and principles associated with the many approaches that fall under the umbrella of critical participatory inquiry (CPI), with an emphasis on the epistemology, ethics, and practice of CPI. In the critical tradition, research works best when it is open to critiquing inequity in its findings, research practices, relationships, and purposes. It is not a neutral way of approaching research, nor does it enact a hierarchy of expertise with the researcher at the top. You will engage in reading and discussions as well as conducting a CPI project. Through these means, you will come to your own understanding of and appreciation for practitioner-centered research.

LEARNER OUTCOMES OR OBJECTIVES

This course is designed to enable students to do the following:

1. Articulate the historical and theoretical foundations of critical participatory inquiry
2. Describe the common characteristics of CPI
3. Discuss common practices associated with designing CPI studies
4. Outline ethical considerations common to the CPI process
5. Describe the various types of data collected in CPI studies
6. Design a CPI study
7. Carry out participatory and collaborative fieldwork, including multiple forms of data collection

8. Carry out participatory and collaborative data analysis
9. Describe ethical issues related to representation and sharing findings in CPI

Assignments	Points
1. Participation	30
2. Documentation of CPI process	20 (4 times x 5 points each)
3. Research Journal Entries	50 (10 times x 5 points each)
	100 total points

PARTICIPATION

Participation and attendance will comprise 30% of your grade. In keeping with the underlying epistemological commitments of CPI, this grade will ultimately be assigned through a process of dialogue and mutual understanding. On the first day of class, we will develop a list of community agreements and we will check in on those as a collective throughout the course. Some of these agreements will likely relate to how we aim to engage (participate) with each other and what it means to participate fully. We will also decide how this grade will be assigned at the end of the course.

DOCUMENTATION OF CPI PROCESS

The research project portfolio in total will comprise 20% of your grade. The goal of the course is to learn CPI theory through practice; thus, we will form a CPI collective together and will work on a small-scale CPI project that is of interest to all of us in some way. In the past, students have chosen to work on a CPI project that relates to our institution. As we work as a collective each person will each demonstrate and document their own participation in ways they feel are appropriate and helpful.

RESEARCH JOURNAL ENTRIES

Each student will have a private (between the student and instructor) online journal. Students are required to add entries as indicated in the main text and on the class schedule. You should add your work on "focus activities" in your journal prior to class meetings and responses to reflexivity questions during or after class meetings. You should choose one of the end-of-chapter suggested activities and record that work in your journal as well. Again, this is meant as an opportunity to engage in dialogue with the instructor in between class sessions and to engage in self-reflexivity throughout the course.

CLASS SCHEDULE

Week	Topic	Readings and Activities to be Completed Before Class	The Research Project	Post-Class Session Assignments
1	**Introduction** Introducing the course, making initial fieldwork and manuscript decisions and plans Creating class/course agreements, selecting additional readings	CPI Introduction and Appendix Cases (Read prior to our first class)	Dialogue	Journal: Explore your initial wonderings about CPI. What cases seem interesting to you? What initial questions do you have?
2	**The roots, goals, use, and process of CPI; researcher positionality**	CPI: Chs. 1 and 2 Complete chapter focus activities prior to class. Supplemental readings TBD depending on student interest or discipline	Dialogue and reflection	Journal: Choose one of the reflexivity questions or suggested activities from the chapters to answer or complete.
	Conceptualization and operationalization of ethics and validity in CPI	CPI Ch. 3 Complete chapter focus activity prior to class. Supplemental readings TBD depending on student interest or discipline	Dialogue and reflection	Journal: Choose one of the reflexivity questions or suggested activities from the chapters to answer or complete.
3	**Building (On) Relationships:** Insider/outsider research, inclusion and power dynamics, ethics of "entering the field"	CPI Ch. 4 Complete chapter focus activity prior to class. Supplemental readings TBD depending on student interest or discipline	Identify potential project and make contact or prepare to make contact with the community.	Journal: Choose one of the reflexivity questions or suggested activities from the chapters to answer or complete.

(Continued)

(Continued)

Week	Topic	Readings and Activities to be Completed Before Class	The Research Project	Post-Class Session Assignments
4	**Getting Started:** Identifying stakeholders, key informants; identifying and dealing with power structures; engaging ethically and reflexively	CPI Ch. 5 Complete chapter focus activity prior to class. Supplemental readings TBD depending on student interest or discipline	Determine how you will go about setting expectations and roles; welcoming conflict or disagreement; making power issues transparent.	Journal: Choose one of the reflexivity questions or suggested activities from the chapters to answer or complete.
5	**Gathering Data and Making Meaning:** Making traditional data collection and analysis approaches participatory	CPI Ch. 6 Complete chapter focus activity prior to class. Supplemental readings TBD depending on student interest or discipline	Discuss evidence and data collection with research collective—what does each person find compelling? Begin making data collection and analysis decisions with the collective.	Journal: Choose one of the reflexivity questions or suggested activities from the chapters to answer or complete.
6	**Gathering Data and Making Meaning:** Trying out participatory data collection and analysis processes	Additional readings (decided by class members, dependent on research interest and focus)	Engage in data collection and analysis with the collective.	Process documentation: Instructor will check online drop boxes for documentation of your CPI process to date.
	Gathering Data and Making Meaning: Arts-based data collection and analysis; practical and ethical concerns	CPI Ch. 7 Complete chapter focus activity prior to class. Supplemental readings TBD depending on student interest or discipline	Engage in data collection and analysis with the collective.	Journal: Choose one of the reflexivity questions or suggested activities from the chapters to answer or complete.

Week	Topic	Readings and Activities to be Completed Before Class	The Research Project	Post-Class Session Assignments
7	**Gathering Data and Making Meaning:** Trying out arts-based data collection and analysis	Additional readings (decided by class members, dependent on research interest and focus)	Engage in data collection and analysis with the collective.	Process documentation: Instructor will check online drop boxes for documentation of your CPI process to date.
8	**Gathering Data and Making Meaning:** Digital and multimedia data collection and analysis	CPI Ch. 8 Complete chapter focus activity prior to class. Supplemental readings TBD depending on student interest or discipline	Engage in data collection and analysis with the collective.	Journal: Choose one of the reflexivity questions or suggested activities from the chapters to answer or complete.
9	**Gathering Data and Making Meaning:** Trying out digital and multimedia data collection and analysis	Additional readings (decided by class members, dependent on research interest and focus)	Engage in data collection and analysis with the collective.	
10	*No class—work week (data collection and analysis)*			
11	**Taking Action and Sharing Findings:** Considering authorship/ ownership, **working** for change, and disseminating findings	CPI Ch. 9 Complete chapter focus activity prior to class. Supplemental readings TBD depending on student interest / discipline	Reflection. Share findings with broader community.	Journal: Choose one of the reflexivity questions or suggested activities from the chapters to answer or complete.
12	**Experiential opportunity (locate an organization or group in your area doing CPI work and meet with them offsite)**	Review organization's work online, e.g. website, publications, reports, or media coverage.	Reflection	Process documentation: Instructor will check online drop boxes for documentation of your CPI process to date.

(Continued)

(Continued)

Week	Topic	Readings and Activities to be Completed Before Class	The Research Project	Post-Class Session Assignments
13	**Staying Committed and in Solidarity:** Identifying opportunities for and implications of staying involved with co-researchers	CPI Ch. 10 Complete chapter focus activity prior to class. Supplemental readings TBD depending on student interest or discipline	Reflection	Journal: Choose one of the reflexivity questions or suggested activities from the chapters to answer or complete.
14	**Bringing Our CPI Experiences Back to the Group:** Sharing and reflecting on your learning and future directions		Plan and dialogue	Submit: participation self-evaluation (less than one page—assign points). Process documentation: Instructor will check online drop boxes for final documentation of your CPI process.

GLOSSARY

access: the opportunities we may or may not have to the knowledge, culture and language needed to understand a concept or truth claim

action research: an approach to research typically traced to social psychologist Kurt Lewin, which seeks to transform reality through a cyclical problem-solving process that includes planning, acting, observing, and reflecting

animators: those internal to a particular struggle who bring their own knowledge and methods as well as expertise gained from living through experiences, practices, and policies relevant to the struggle

bias: ideological commitments and sociopolitical values that may affect how one sees the world and conducts research

body mapping: tracing an individual's body and filling the outline in with representations of their identities and lived experiences

born-digital dissertation: a dissertation created and to be displayed online with multimedia and interactive components

brainwriting: an alternative to brainstorming or focus groups; composing thoughts in writing and then discussing them as a group

card (priority) sorting: a structured activity for organizing or ranking pieces of data written on individual cards

catalytic validity: an approach to validity that examines research quality as well as impact, that does not separate empirical and theoretical thought from the action sought through research, and that privileges the emancipatory aims of research and scholarship that seek social change

community-based participatory research: an approach to research that is distinguished by partnerships between university researchers, organizations, and community members formed to tackle community-identified problems; well established in the field of public health

community gatekeepers: people who are part of the community in which you are interested and who are recognized and trusted as leaders by that community

***conscientizaçao*:** a process of critical consciousness borne out of mutual respect

contact zones: interactions between people with different positionalities, life experiences, and cultures; often with unequal power dynamics

dialogical: characterized by dialogue, an open exchange of ideas

dialogue: the foundation of *conscientizaçao*, self-actualization, relationship building, mutual understanding, and action

digital storytelling: a participatory method of communicating lived experience through a combination of short audio-recorded narratives and photographs or other visuals

epistemicide: the erasure or destruction of knowledge systems

epistemological consistency: maintaining a consistent paradigm of knowledge throughout inquiry

epistemology: the theory or science of knowledge; how we know or come to know

evidence: any knowledge documented, gathered, or shared used to make truth claims

failure: structural, institutional, and/or contextual constraints on CPI and how we handle them

inquiry collective: a group of co-researchers who collaborate in CPI; forming trusting relationships, negotiating roles and power relationships, and sharing decision making are crucial to creating a strong collective

insider–outsider: positionality where a researcher belongs to the community in which they conduct inquiry in some ways and not others, which can facilitate access and mutual understanding while presenting unique dilemmas and critiques

intersectionality: how an individual's various identities produce a competing and interconnected web of oppression and discrimination

intersubjectivity/intersubjective understanding: reaching toward greater or better understanding of another's knowledge or experience through dialogue

knowledge creation: a social and educational process of establishing knowledge grounded in community realities, identities, and ways of knowing

knowledge democratization: a guiding concept in CPI and other participatory approaches that knowledge should be created in an equitable, accessible way that counters dominant positivist paradigms of research as an exclusive and sophisticated endeavor

known methods: data collection and analysis procedures that community members already use in their daily lives

method: the tools or techniques employed for data collection and analysis in a research study (e.g., survey, observation, interview)

methodology: an approach or philosophy about research that guides the selection of a method and design of procedures; guided by the researcher's paradigm about knowledge, the research question, the target population, and other considerations

mutual recognition: from the discipline of psychology and connected to the idea of intersubjectivity, this concept relates to an authentic, appreciative connectedness between two or more people, a "re-cognition" of an Other

objectivity: according to Habermas' Theory of Communicative Action, objectivity operates under the principle of multiple access, which means that many individuals have access to the knowledge, culture, and language needed to understand a concept

ontology: the study of existence or being; what can be known

ownership: power or control over decision making, the research process, and action in CPI

participatory action research: a form of action research that emphasizes the equitable and meaningful participation of community-based co-researchers throughout the research process

photovoice: a method developed by Caroline Wang to document community knowledge, assets, and/or needs and advocate for change through participant photography and short accompanying narratives

positionality: our position in this world, comprising intersecting, multiple, and evolving identities that involve both the totality and individuality of our experiences, our socialization, our physical markers, our privileges, and the ways in which we are socially, politically, and economically targeted

postpositivism: an ontological and epistemological stance toward knowledge that pursues an objective truth (which can only be understood probabilistically/imperfectly); amends the positivist paradigm by noting that a researcher's values can affect observations, although in practice narrowly defines what counts as valid knowledge and accepts only observable evidence as scientific

reciprocity: a mutual exchange; in traditional research often a small payment or gift in exchange for information

reflexivity: a process of critical self-reflection; for example, on relationships to other individuals and groups as well as social, political, and economic structures and systems

rigor: a measure of the quality or goodness of research in positivist and postpositivist research paradigms based on validity, reliability, and objectivity

ripples of change: a structured activity for defining and differentiating concepts using a set of concentric circles representing levels of change (e.g. personal, community, and policy)

storyworlding: a digital ethnographic method designed by a critical feminist research collective in Indiana, USA to collect life stories through in-depth interviews and meaningful artifacts

subjective claims: according to Habermas' Theory of Communicative Action, subjectivity operates under the principle of unique access, which means that there is limited access to the knowledge, culture, and language needed to understand a concept

sustainability: "development that meets the needs of the present without compromising the ability of future generations to meet their own needs" (WCED, 1987, p. 41)

***testimonios*:** first-person narratives of lived experience, often written as resistance or activism; originated by Latin American human rights activists

Theatre of the Oppressed: a group of performance-oriented practices developed by Augusto Boal to address the relationship between oppressor and oppressed through acting out and then re-enacting moments of oppression

thick reciprocity: reciprocity that supports collective and individual growth

thin reciprocity: reciprocity based on goals of mutual benefit through the exchange of resources

transactional relationships: relationships based on an exchange of information, goods, or services; common in traditional research

transformation: change that can occur through CPI at various levels (e.g., intrapersonal, community, institutional, and macrosystem) and in various forms, including cognitive, behavioral, and emotional

validity claims: assertions of truth, opinion, values, and norms communicated overtly or implicitly in human interaction (see also communicative action)

virtual and online ethnography: ethnographic methods adapted for online documentation of a culture or group through (participant) observation, interviews, and other documentation processes

***vivencia*:** lived experience

witnessing: a responsibility of the critical inquirer to document knowledge(s) and experiences through embracing methodological fluidity, actively negotiating power and positionality, and taking action in ways that honor community values and account for possible consequences

REFERENCES

CHAPTER 1

Antoine, A., Mason, R., Mason, R., Palahicky, S., & Rodriguez de France, C. (2018). *Pulling together: A guide for curriculum developers*. BCcampus. https://opentextbc.ca/indigenizationcurriculumdevelopers/

Arstein-Kerslake, A., Gooding, P., Mercer, S., Raymond, M., & McSherry, B. (2019). Implementing a participatory human rights-based research methodology: The unfitness to plead project. *Journal of Human Rights Practice*, *11*(3), 589–606. https://doi.org/10.1093/jhuman/huz034

Asirifi, M. A. (2019). Reflecting on leadership development through community based participatory action research. *International Journal of Nursing Education Scholarship*, *16*(1). https://doi.org/10.1515/ijnes-2018-0086

Bain, A. L., & Payne, W. J. (2016). Queer de-participation: Reframing the co-production of scholarly knowledge. *Qualitative Research*, *16*(3), 330–340. https://doi.org/10.1177/1468794115619002

Baird, M. B., Domian, E. W., Mulcahy, E. R., Mabior, R., Jemutai-Tanui, G., & Filippi, M. K. (2015). Creating a bridge of understanding between two worlds: Community-based collaborative-action research with Sudanese refugee women. *Public Health Nursing*, *32*(5), 388–396. https://doi.org/10.1111/phn.12172

Beatriz, E. D., Lincoln, A. K., Alder, J., Daley, N., Simmons, F., Ibeh, K., Figueroa, C., & Molnar, B. E. (2018). Evaluation of a teen dating violence prevention intervention among urban middle-school youth using youth participatory action research: Lessons learned from Start Strong Boston. *Journal of Family Violence*, *33*(8), 563–578. https://doi.org/10.1007/s10896-018-9981-4

Beh, A., Bruyere, B. L., & Lolosoli, S. (2013). Legitimizing local perspectives in conservation through community-based research: A photovoice study in Samburu, Kenya. *Society & Natural Resources*, *26*(12), 1390–1406. https://doi.org/10.1080/08941920.2013.805858

Bertrand, M. (2018). Youth participatory action research and possibilities for students of color in educational leadership. *Educational Administration Quarterly*, *54*(3), 366–395. https://doi.org/10.1177/0013161X18761344

Bhabha, J., Fuller, A., Matache, M., Vranješević, J., Chernoff, M. C., Spasić, B., & Ivanis, J. (2017). Reclaiming adolescence: A Roma youth perspective. *Harvard Educational Review*, *87*(2), 186–224, 301–305.

Binet, A., Gavin, V., Carroll, L., & Arcaya, M. (2019). Designing and facilitating collaborative research design and data analysis workshops: Lessons learned in the Healthy Neighborhoods Study. *International Journal of Environmental Research and Public Health*, *16*(3). https://doi.org/10.3390/ijerph16030324

Bishop, R., & Glynn, T. (2003). *Culture counts: Changing power relations in education*. Zed Books.

Boedecker, J., Odhiambo Odour, F., Lachat, C., Van Damme, P., Kennedy, G., & Termote, C. (2019). Participatory farm diversification and nutrition education increase dietary diversity in Western Kenya. *Maternal & Child Nutrition*, *15*(3). https://doi.org/10.1111/mcn.12803

Botha, C. S., & Hay, J. (2016). Narratives of adolescent girls journeying via feminist participatory action research through the aftermath of divorce. *Africa Education Review*, *13*(2), 165–180. https://doi.org/10.1080/18146627.2016.1224105

Boutwell, L. (2015). "I don't want to claim America": African refugee girls and discourses of othering. *Girlhood Studies*, *8*(2), 103–118. https://doi.org/10.3167/ghs.2015.080208

Bradford, L. (1967). Biography of an institution. *Journal of Applied Behavioral Science*, *3*, 127–143.

Brion-Meisels, G., & Alter, Z. (2018). The quandary of youth participatory action research in school settings: A framework for reflecting on the factors that influence purpose and process. *Harvard Educational Review*, *88*(4), 429–454. https://doi.org/10.17763/1943-5045-88.4.429

Brown, T. M., & Rodríguez, L. F. (2017). Collaborating with urban youth to address gaps in teacher education. *Teacher Education Quarterly*, *44*(3), 75–92. www.jstor.org/stable/90010904

Burke, K., & Greene, S. (2015). Participatory action research, youth voices, and civic engagement. *Language Arts*, *92*(6), 387–400.

Call-Cummings, M., & Martinez, S. (2016). Consciousness-raising or unintentionally oppressive? *The Qualitative Report*, *21*(5), 798–810. https://nsuworks.nova.edu/tqr/vol21/iss5/1

Call-Cummings, M., & Martinez, S. (2017). 'It wasn't racism; it was more misunderstanding.' White teachers, Latino/a students, and racial battle fatigue. *Race Ethnicity and Education*, *20*(4), 561–574. https://doi.org/10.1080/13613324.2016.1150830

Call-Cummings, M., Hauber-Özer, M., Byers, C., & Mancuso, G. P. (2019). The power of/in Photovoice. *International Journal of Research & Method in Education*, *42*(4), 399–413. https://doi.org/10.1080/1743727X.2018.1492536

Cammarota, J. (2011). From hopelessness to hope. *Urban Education*, *46*(4), 828–844. https://doi.org/10.1177/0042085911399931

Cammarota, J., & Fine, M. (2008). Youth participatory action research: A pedagogy for transformational resistance. In J. Cammarota & M. Fine (Eds.), *Revolutionizing education: Youth participatory action research in motion*. Routledge.

Campos, I. S., Alves, F. M., Dinis, J., Truninger, M., Vizinho, A., & Penha-Lopes, G. (2016). Climate adaptation, transitions, and socially innovative action-research approaches. *Ecology and Society*, *21*(1), Art. 13. https://doi.org/10.5751/ES-08059-210113

Carr, W., & Kemmis, S. (1986). *Becoming critical: Education, knowledge and action research*. Deakin University Press.

Chilisa, B. (2020). *Indigenous research methodologies* (2nd ed.). SAGE.

Collins, P. H. (2002). *Black feminist thought: Knowledge, consciousness, and the politics of empowerment*. Routledge.

Cook-Lynn, E. (1997). Who stole native American studies? *Wicazo Sa Review*, *12*(1), 9–28.

Crenshaw, K., Gotanda, N., Peller, G., & Thomas, K. (1995). *Critical race theory: The key writings that formed the movement*. The New Press.

Cueva, K., Revels, L., Cueva, M., Lanier, A. P., Dignan, M., Viswanath, K., Fung, T. T., & Geller, A. C. (2018). Culturally-relevant online cancer education modules empower Alaska's community health aides/practitioners to disseminate cancer information and reduce cancer risk. *Journal of Cancer Education*, *33*(5), 1102–1109. https://doi.org/10.1007/s13187-017-1217-4

Dazzo, G. P. (2016, September 1). *Reciprocity in research: Integrating evaluation and human rights methods to balance evaluator and community needs* [Webinar]. Search for Common Ground: DM&E for Peace. https://vimeo.com/181067904

de Sousa Santos, B. (2008). *Another knowledge is possible: Beyond northern epistemologies*. Verso.

Devine, A., Ignacio, R., Prenter, K., Temminghoff, L., Gill-Atkinson, L., Zayas, J., Marco, M. J., & Vaughan, C. (2017). "Freedom to go where I want": Improving access to sexual and reproductive health for women with disabilities in the Philippines. *Reproductive Health Matters*, *25*(50), 55–65. https://www.jstor.org/stable/26495932

Dewey, J. (1933). *How we think*. Heath and Company.

Dick, B. (2009). Action research literature 2006-2008: Themes and trends. *Action Research*, *7*(4), 423–441.

Evans-Agnew, R. A., & Rosemberg, M.-A. S. (2016). Questioning photovoice research: Whose voice? *Qualitative Health Research*, *26*(8), 1019–1030. https://doi.org/10.1177/1049732315624223

Fals-Borda, O., & Mora-Osejo, L. E. (2003). Context and diffusion of knowledge: A critique of Eurocentrism. *Action Research*, *1*(1), 29–37.

Fals-Borda, O. (1987). The application of participatory action-research in Latin America. *International Sociology, 2*(4), 329–347.

Fals-Borda, O. (2001). Participatory (action) research in social theory: Origins and challenges. In P. Reason & H. Bradbury, *Handbook of action research: Participative inquiry and practice* (pp. 27–37). SAGE.

Fals-Borda, O. (2006). The North-South convergence: 30-year first person assessment of PAR. *Action Research, 4*(3), 351–358.

Fast, E., Lefebvre, M., Reid, Christopher, Deer, B. W., Swiftwolfe, D., Clark, M., Boldo, V., Mackie, J., Mackie, R., & Tutanuak, K. (2021). Restoring our roots: Land-based community by and for indigenous youth. *International Journal of Indigenous Health, 16*(2), 120–138. https://doi.org/10.32799/ijih.v16i2.33932

Feldman, A. (2017). An emergent history of educational action research in the English-speaking world. In L. Rowell, C. D. Bruce, J. M. Shosh, & M. M. Riel, *The Palgrave international handbook of action research* (pp. 125–145). Palgrave Macmillan.

Fox, M., & Fine, M. (2015). Leadership in solidarity: Notions of leadership through critical participatory action research with young people and adults. *New Directions for Student Leadership, 2015*(148)., 45–58. https://doi.org/10.1002/yd.20152

Freire, P. (1970). *Pedagogy of the oppressed*. Herder & Herder.

Gardner, B. B. (1946). *Human relations in industry*. Richard Irwin.

Glassman, M., & Erdem, G. (2014). Participatory action research and its meanings: Vivencia, praxis, conscientization. *Adult Education Quarterly, 64*(3), 206–221. https://doi.org/10.1177/0741713614523667

Glassman, M., Erdem, G., & Bartholomew, M. (2013). Action research and its history as an adult education movement for social change. *Adult Education Quarterly, 63*(3), 272–288. https://doi.org/10.1177/0741713612471418

Greenwood, D., & Levin, M. (2007). *Introduction to action research: Social research for social change*. SAGE.

Guerrero, A. L., & Tinkler, T. (2010). Refugee and displaced youth negotiating imagined and lived identities in a photography-based educational project in the United States and Colombia. *Anthropology & Education Quarterly, 41*(1), 55–74. https://doi.org/10.1111/j.1548-1492.2010.01067.x

Hacker, K. (2013). *Community-based participatory research*. SAGE.

Hall, B. L., & Tandon, R. (2017). Decolonization of knowledge, epistemicide, participatory research and higher education. *Research for All, 1*(1), 6–19. https://doi.org/10.18546/RFA.01.1.02

Haraway, D. J. (1988). Situated knowledges: The science question in feminism and the privilege of partial perspective. *Feminist Studies, 14*(3), 575–599.

Hauber-Özer, M., & Call-Cummings, M. (2020). Empowerment or exposure? Ethical dilemmas of visual methods with vulnerable migrants. *Qualitative Research Journal, 20*(3), 329–340. https://doi.org/10.1108/QRJ-10-2019-0075

Houh, E. M. S., & Kalsem, K. (2015). Theorizing legal participatory action research: Critical race/feminism and participatory action research. *Qualitative Inquiry, 21*(3), 262–276. https://doi.org/10.1177/1077800414562897

Israel, B. A., Eng, E., Schulz, A. J., & Parker, E. A. (2005). *Methods in community-based participatory research for health*. Jossey-Bass.

Jackson, T. (1993). A way of working: Participatory research and the aboriginal movement in Canada. In P. Park, M. Brydon-Miller, B. Hall, & T. Jackson (Eds.), *Voices of change: Participatory research in the United States and Canada* (pp. 47–74). Bergin and Garvey.

Johnston-Goodstar, K. (2013). Indigenous youth participatory action research: Re-visioning social justice for social work with Indigenous youths. *Social Work, 58*(4), 314–320. https://doi.org/10.1093/sw/swt036

Kemmis, S., & McTaggart, R. (2005). Participatory action research: Communicative action and the public sphere. In N. Denzin & Y. Lincoln (Eds.), *Handbook of qualitative research* (3rd ed., pp. 559–604). SAGE.

Kemmis, S., McTaggart, R., & Nixon, R. (2014). *The action research planner: Doing critical participatory action research*. Springer.

Kim, M. A., Hong, J. S., Ra, M., & Kim, K. (2015). Understanding social exclusion and psychosocial adjustment of North Korean adolescents and young adult refugees in South Korea through Photovoice. *Qualitative Social Work*, *14*(6), 820–841. https://doi.org/10.1177/1473325015572940

Lather, P. (1986). Issues of validity in openly ideological research: Between a rock and a soft place. *Interchange*, *17*(4), 63–84. https://doi.org/10.1007/BF01807017

Lems, E., Hilverda, F., Sarti, A., van der Voort, L., Kegel, A., Pittens, C., Broerse, J., & Dedding, C. (2020). 'McDonald's is good for my social life': Developing health promotion together with adolescent girls from disadvantaged neighbourhoods in Amsterdam. *Children & Society*, *34*(3), 204–219. https://doi.org/10.1111/chso.12368

Letiecq, B. L., Grzywacz, J. G., Gray, K. M., & Eudave, Y. M. (2014). Depression among Mexican men on the migration frontier: The role of family separation and other structural and situational stressors. *Journal of Immigrant and Minority Health*, *16*(6), 1193–1200. https://doi.org/10.1007/s10903-013-9918-1

Letiecq, B., & Schmalzbauer, L. (2012). Community-based participatory research with Mexican migrants in a new rural destination: A good fit? *Action Research*, *10*(3), 244–259. https://doi.org/10.1177/1476750312443571

Lewin, K. (1943). Defining the "field at a given time." *Psychological Review*, *50*, 292–310.

Lewin, K. (1951). *Field theory in social science: Selected theoretical papers*. Harper & Row.

Lincoln, Y. S., Lynham, S. A., & Guba, E. G. (2011). Paradigmatic controversies, contradictions, and emerging confluences. In N. K. Denzin & Y. S. Lincoln (Eds.), *The SAGE handbook of qualitative research* (pp. 97–128). SAGE.

Lippitt, R., & Radke, M. (1946). New trends in the investigation of prejudice. *Annals of the (American) Academy of Political and Social Science*, *244*, 167–176.

Maguire, P. (1987). *Doing participatory research: A feminist approach*. University of Massachusetts, Center for International Education.

Maguire, P. (1996). Considering more feminist participatory research: What's congruency got to do with it?. *Qualitative Inquiry*, *2*(1), 106–118.

McTaggart, R. (1991). Principles for participatory action research. *Adult Education Quarterly*, *41*(3), 168–187. https://doi.org/10.1177/0001848191041003003

McTaggart, R. (1997). Guiding principles for participatory action research. In R. McTaggart (Ed.), *Participatory action research: International contexts and consequences* (pp. 25–44). State University of New York Press.

McTaggart, R., Nixon, R., & Kemmis, S. (2017). Critical participatory action research. In L. Rowell, C. D. Bruce, J. M. Shosh, & M. M. Riel (Eds.), *The Palgrave international handbook of action research* (pp. 21–35). Palgrave Macmillan.

Miled, N. (2020). Can the displaced speak? Muslim refugee girls negotiating identity, home and belonging through Photovoice. *Women's Studies International Forum*, *81*, 102381. https://doi.org/10.1016/j.wsif.2020.102381

Minkler, M., & Wallerstein, N. (2008). *Community-based participatory research for health: From process to outcomes* (2nd ed.). Jossey-Bass.

Ní Sheanáin, Ú. (2016). *Opening doors: A Gaelscoil approach to developing critical interculturalism* [Doctoral dissertation, National University of Ireland–Galway]. NUI Galway Theses (PhD Theses). https://hdl.handle.net/10379/5756

Nix, E., Paulose, J., Shrubsole, C., Altamirano-Medina, H., Belesova, K., Davies, M., Khosla, R., & Wilkinson, P. (2019). Participatory action research as a framework for transdisciplinary collaboration: Pilot study on healthy, sustainable, low-income housing in Delhi, India. *Global Challenges*, *3*(4), 1800054.

Olumide, A. O., Adebayo, E. S., & Ojengbede, O. A. (2018). Using photovoice in adolescent health research: A case-study of the Well-being of Adolescents in Vulnerable Environments (WAVE) Study in Ibadan, Nigeria. *International Journal of Adolescent Medicine and Health*, *30*(2), 1667–1676. https://doi.org/10.1515/ijamh-2016-0040

Payne, Y. A., & Bryant, A. (2018). Street participatory action research in prison: A methodology to challenge privilege and power in correctional facilities. *The Prison Journal*, *98*(4), 449–469. https://doi.org/10.1177/0032885518776378

Piaget, J. (1932). *The moral judgment of the child*. Kegan Paul, Trench, & Trubner.

Pillow, W. (2003). Confession, catharsis, or cure? Rethinking the uses of reflexivity as methodological power in qualitative research. *International Journal of Qualitative Studies in Education*, *16*(2), 175–196. https://doi.org/10.1080/0951839032000060635

Pyles, L. (2015). Participation and other ethical considerations in participatory action research in post-earthquake rural Haiti. *International Social Work*, *58*(5), 628–645. https://doi.org/10.1177/0020872815581912

Rahman, A. (2008). Some trends in the praxis of participatory action research. In P. Reason & H. Bradbury (Eds.), *Handbook of action research: Participative inquiry and practice* (pp. 49–62). SAGE.

Reid, C., & Frisby, W. (2008). Continuing the journey: Articulating dimensions of feminist participatory action research (FPAR). In P. Reason & H. Bradbury (Eds.), *The SAGE handbook of action research* (pp. 93–106). SAGE.

Reid, C., & Gillberg, C. (2014). Feminist participatory action research. In D. Coghlan & M. Brydon-Miller (Eds.), *The SAGE encyclopedia of action research* (pp. 344–347). SAGE. https://doi.org/10.4135/9781446294406

Sandwick, T., Fine, M., Greene, A. C., Stoudt, B. G., Torre, M. E., & Patel, L. (2018). Promise and provocation: Humble reflections on critical participatory action research for social policy. *Urban Education*, *53*(4), 473–502. https://doi.org/10.1177/0042085918763513

Santos, D. (2015). (Participatory) action research and the political realm. In B. Dennis, L. Carspecken, & P. F. Carspecken (Eds.), *Qualitative research: A reader in philosophy, core concepts, and practice* (pp. 492–513). Peter Lang.

Schensul, J. J. (2014). Youth participatory action research. In D. Coghlan & M. Brydon-Miller (Eds.), *The SAGE encyclopedia of action research* (pp. 831–834). SAGE.

Silver-Pacuilla, H. V. (2004). The meanings of literacy: A participatory action research project involving women with disabilities. *Women's Studies Quarterly*, *32*(1/2), 43–58.

Singh, A. A., Richmond, K., & Burnes, T. R. (2013). Feminist participatory action research with transgender communities: Fostering the practice of ethical and empowering research designs. *International Journal of Transgenderism*, *14*(3), 93–104. https://doi.org/10.1080/15532739.2013.818516

Sloane, J. A., & Wallin, D. (2013). Theatre of the Commons: A theatrical inquiry into the democratic engagement of former refugee families in Canadian public high school communities. *Educational Research*, *55*(4), 454–472. https://doi.org/10.1080/00131881.2013.844948

Smith, L. T. (1999). *Decolonizing methodologies: Research and indigenous peoples* (1st ed.). Zed Books.

Smith, L. T., Tuck, E., & Yang, K. W (Eds.). (2018). *Indigenous and decolonizing studies in education: Mapping the long view.* Routledge.

Solórzano, D. G., & Yosso, T. J. (2002). A critical race counterstory of race, racism, and affirmative action. *Equity & Excellence in Education*, *35*(2), 155–168. https://doi.org/10.1080/713845284

Spivak, G. C. (1981). French feminism in an international frame. *Yale French Studies*, *1981*(62)., 154–184. https://doi.org/10.2307/2929898

Stoudt, B. G., Fox, M., & Fine, M. (2012). Contesting privilege with critical participatory action research. *Journal of Social Issues*, *68*(1), 178–193. https://doi.org/10.1111/j.1540-4560.2011.01743.x

Swantz, M. (1982). Research as education for development: A Tanzanian case. In B. Hall, A. Gillette, & R. Tandon (Eds.), *Creating knowledge: A monopoly*? (pp. 113–126). Society for Participatory Research in Asia.

Swantz, M. L. (2008). Participatory action research as practice In P. Reason & H. Bradbury (Eds.), *The SAGE handbook of action research: Participative inquiry and practice* (pp. 31–48). SAGE.

Torre, M. E. (2009). Participatory action research and critical race theory: Fueling spaces for *nos-otras* to research. *The Urban Review*,

41(1), 106–120. https://doi.org/10.1007/s11256-008-0097-7

Torre, M. E., & Fine, M. (2006). Participatory action research (PAR) by youth. *Youth Activism: An International Encyclopedia*, *2*, 456–462.

Van Katwyk, T., & Seko, Y. (2019). Resilience beyond risk: Youth re-defining resilience through collective art-making. *Child and Adolescent Social Work Journal*, *36*(6), 609–619. https://doi.org/10.1007/s10560-018-0590-0

Vesely, C. K., Letiecq, B. L., Goodman, R. D., Marquez, M., Alves, L., Lazo, W., & Martinez, R. (2019). What does this mean to you? Partnering with Amigas de la Comunidad to analyze the housing conditions of undocumented Latina immigrants. In Á. Humble & E. Radina (Eds.), *How qualitative data analysis happens: Moving beyond "themes emerged"* (pp. 112–127). Taylor & Francis.

Wang, C. C., & Burris, M. A. (1997). Photovoice: Concept, methodology, and use for participatory needs assessment. *Health Education & Behavior*, *24*(3), 369–387. https://doi.org/10.1177/109019819702400309

Whyte, W. (1994). *Participant observer: An autobiography*. ILR Press.

Zubrzycki, J., Shipp, R., & Jones, V. (2017). Knowing, being, and doing: Aboriginal and Non-Aboriginal collaboration in cancer services. *Qualitative Health Research*, *27*(9), 1316–1329. https://doi.org/10.1177/1049732316686750

CHAPTER 2

Anderson, M. B., Brown, D., & Jean, I. (2012). *Time to listen: Hearing people on the receiving end of international aid*. CDA Collaborative Learning Projects.

Appadurai, A. (2006). The right to research. *Globalisation, Societies and Education*, *4*(2), 167–177.

Arnstein, S. R. (1969). A ladder of citizen participation. *Journal of The American Institute of Planners*, *35*(4), 216–224.

Arnstein, S. R. (2019). A ladder of citizen participation. *Journal of the American Planning Association*, *85*(1), 24–34. https://doi.org/10.1080/01944363.2018.1559388

Arstein-Kerslake, A., Gooding, P., Mercer, S., Raymond, M., & McSherry, B. (2019). Implementing a participatory human rights-based research methodology: The unfitness to plead project. *Journal of Human Rights Practice*, *11*(3), 589–606. https://doi.org/10.1093/jhuman/huz034

Burles, M., & Thomas, R. (2014). "I just don't think there's any other image that tells the story like [this] picture does": Researcher and participant reflections on the use of participant-employed photography in social research. *International Journal of Qualitative Methods*, *13*(1), 185–205. https://doi.org/10.1177/160940691401300107

Cahill, C. (2007). The personal is political: Developing new subjectivities through participatory action research. *Gender, Place & Culture*, *14*(3), 267–292. https://doi.org/10.1080/09663690701324904

Cahill, C., Cerecer, D. A. Q., Rivarola, A. R. R., Zamudio, J. H., & Gutiérrez, L. A. (2019). "Caution, we have power": Resisting the "school-to-sweatshop pipeline" through participatory artistic praxes and critical care. *Gender and Education*, *31*(5), 576–589. https://doi.org/10.1080/09540253.2019.1582207

Call-Cummings, M. (2017). Establishing communicative validity: Discovering theory through practice. *Qualitative Inquiry*, *23*(3), 192–200.

Call-Cummings, M. (2018). Claiming power by producing knowledge: The empowering potential of PAR in the classroom. *Educational Action Research*, *26*(3), 385–402. https://doi.org/10.1080/09650792.2017.1354772

Call-Cummings, M., & Dennis, B. (2019). Participation as entangled self-assertion. *Forum Qualitative Sozialforschung/Forum: Qualitative Social Research*, *20*(2). https://doi.org/10.17169/fqs-20.2.3203

Call-Cummings, M., Dennis, B., & Martinez, S. (2019). The role of researcher in participatory inquiry: Modeling intra-active reflexivity in conversational reflections. *Cultural Studies↔Critical Methodologies*, *19*(1), 68–76.

Call-Cummings, M., Hauber-Özer, M., & Dazzo, G. (2019). Examining researcher identity development within the context of a course on PAR: A layered narrative approach. *The Qualitative Report*, *24*(9), 2178–2196.

Call-Cummings, M., Hauber-Özer, M., & Ross, K. (2020). Struggling with/against the unintentional reproduction of power structures in participatory research: Using reconstructive horizon analysis. *Action Research*, *18*(2), 171–193. https://doi.org/10.1177/1476750319837324

Call-Cummings, M., & James, C. (2015). Empowerment for whom? Empowerment for what? Lessons from a participatory action research project. *Networks: An Online Journal for Teacher Research*, *17*(2), 615. https://doi.org/10.4148/2470-6353.1029

Cameron, J., & Gibson, K. (2005). Participatory action research in a poststructualist vein. *Geoforum*, *36*(3), 315–331.

Caxaj, C. S. (2015). Indigenous storytelling and participatory action research: Allies toward decolonization? Reflections from the peoples' international health tribunal. *Global Qualitative Nursing Research*, *2015*, 1–12. https://doi:10.1177/2333393615580764

Cornwall, A. (2003). Whose voices? Whose choices? Reflections on gender and participatory development. *World Development*, *31*(8), 1325–1342. https://doi.org/10.1016/S0305-750X(03)00086-X

Dazzo, G. P. (2020, May) Exploring the role of collective memory for reconciliation: A comparative case of Guatemala and Cambodia. *Beyond Intractability*.

Deeb-Sossa, N. (2019). Consejos y advertencias (Advice and warnings): Sustainability and community-based participatory research in Chicanx Studies. In N. Deeb-Sossa (Ed.), *Community-based participatory research: Testimonios from Chicana/o Studies* (pp. 225–238). University of Arizona Press.

Dennis, B., & Huf, C. (2016). *Children as researchers? Methodological considerations on participation in the context of childhood studies*. Paper presented at the Oxford Ethnography in Education Conference, September 17–19, Oxford, England.

Dodson, L., & Schmalzbauer, L. (2005). Poor mothers and habits of hiding: Participatory methods in poverty research. *Journal of Marriage and Family*, *67*(4), 949–959. https://www.jstor.org/stable/3600249

Erel, U., Reynolds, T., & Kaptani, E. (2017). Participatory theatre for transformative social research. *Qualitative Research*, *17*(3), 302–312. https://doi.org/10.1177/1468794117696029

Fals-Borda, O. (1979). Investigating reality in order to transform it: The Colombian experience. *Dialectical Anthropology*, *4*(1), 33–55.

Fals-Borda, O. (1987). The application of participatory action-research in Latin America. *International Sociology*, *2*(4), 329–347.

Fals-Borda, O. (1991). Some basic ingredients. In O. Fals-Borda & M. A. Rahman, *Action and knowledge: Breaking the monopoly with participatory action research* (pp. 3–12). The Apex Press.

Fals-Borda, O. (2001). Participatory (action) research in social theory: Origins and challenges. In P. Reason & H. Bradbury (Eds.), *Handbook of action research: Participative inquiry and practice* (pp. 27–37). SAGE.

Fals-Borda, O., & Rahman, M. A. (1991). *Action and knowledge: Breaking the monopoly with participatory action-research*. Apex.

Fine, M., & Torre, M. E. (2004). Re-membering exclusions: Participatory action research in public institutions. *Qualitative Research in Psychology*, *1*(1), 15–37.

Fine, M., Torre, M. E., Boudin, K., Bowen, I., Clark, J., Hylton, D., Martinez, M., Rivera, M., Roberts, R. A., Smart, P., & Upegui, D. (2001). Participatory action research: From within and beyond prison bars. In P. M. Camic, J. E. Rhodes, & L. Yardley (Eds.), *Qualitative research in psychology: Expanding perspective in methodology and design* (pp. 95–119). American Psychology Association.

Freire, P. (1970). *Pedagogy of the oppressed* (M. B. Ramos, Trans.). New York: Continuum, 2007.

Freire, P. (1972). *Pedagogy of the oppressed*. Herder & Herder.

Garcia, A., Mirra, N., Morrell, E., Martinez, A., & Scorza, D. (2015). The Council of Youth Research: Critical literacy and civic agency in the digital age. *Reading & Writing Quarterly*, *31*(2), 151–167. https://doi.org/10.1080/10573569.2014.962203

Gibbs, L., Block, K., MacDougall, C., Harms, L., Baker, E., Richardson, J., Ireton, G., Gallagher, H. C., Bryant, R.,

Lusher, D., Pattison, P., Watson, J., Gillett, J., Pirrone, A., Molyneaux, R., Sexton-Bruce, S., & Forbes, D. (2018). Ethical use and impact of participatory approaches to research in post-disaster environments: An Australian bushfire case study. *BioMed Research International*, *2018*, 1–11. https://doi.org/10.1155/2018/5621609

Giroux, H. A. (2002). Neoliberalism, corporate culture, and the promise of higher education: The university as a democratic public sphere. *Harvard Educational Review*, *72*(4), 425–463.

Greene, S., Burke, K. J., & McKenna, M. K. (2018). A review of research connecting digital storytelling, photovoice, and civic engagement. *Review of Educational Research*, *88*(6), 844–878. https://doi.org/10.3102/0034654318794134

Gubrium, A. C., Hill, A. L., & Flicker, S. (2014). A situated practice of ethics for participatory visual and digital methods in public health research and practice: A focus on digital storytelling. *American Journal of Public Health*, *104*(9), 1606–1614. https://doi.org/10.2105/AJPH.2013.301310

Guerrero, A. L., & Tinkler, T. (2010). Refugee and displaced youth negotiating imagined and lived identities in a photography-based educational project in the United States and Colombia. *Anthropology & Education Quarterly*, *41*(1), 55–74. https://doi.org/10.1111/j.1548-1492.2010.01067.x

Hannes, K., & Parylo, O. (2014). Let's play it safe: Ethical considerations from participants in a photovoice research project. *International Journal of Qualitative Methods*, *13*(1), 255–274.

Harper, S. G. (2016). Keystone characteristics that support cultural resilience in Karen refugee Parents. *Cultural Studies of Science Education*, *11*(4), 1029–1060.

Harper, S. G. (2017). Engaging Karen refugee students in science learning through a cross-cultural learning community. *International Journal of Science Education*, *39*(3), 358–376.

Hart, R. A. (1992). *Children's participation: From tokenism to citizenship*. UNICEF International Child Development Centre.

Hauber-Özer, M., & Call-Cummings, M. (2020). Empowerment or exposure? Ethical dilemmas of visual methods with vulnerable migrants. *Qualitative Research Journal*, *20*(3), 329–340. https://doi.org/10.1108/QRJ-10-2019-0075

hooks, b. (1995). *Killing rage: Ending racism*. Henry Holt and Company.

Kaba, M. (2021). *We do this 'til we free us: Abolitionist organizing and transforming social justice*. Haymarket Books.

Kemmis, S., & McTaggart, R. (2005). Participatory action research: Communicative action and the public sphere. In N. Denzin & Y. Lincoln (Eds.), *Handbook of qualitative research* (3rd ed., pp. 559–604). SAGE.

Kennedy, H. (2018). How adults change from facilitating youth participatory action research: Process and outcomes. *Children and Youth Services Review*, *94*, 298–305. https://doi.org/10.1016/j.childyouth.2018.10.010

Kilroy, W. (2011). From conflict to ownership: Participatory approaches to the re-integration of ex-combatants in Sierra Leone. *Irish Studies in International Affairs*, *22*, 127–144. https://www.jstor.org/stable/41413197

Lind, C. (2008). Knowledge development with adolescents in a PAR process. *Educational Action Research*, *16*(2), 221–233. https://doi.org/10.1080/09650790802011874

Marquez-Zenkov, K., Harmon, J., van Lier, P., & Marquez-Zenkov, M. (2007). If they'll listen to us about life, we'll listen to them about school: Seeing city students' ideas about "quality" teachers. *Educational Action Research*, *15*(3), 403–415. https://doi.org/10.1080/09650790701514457

Mayall, B. (2000). The sociology of childhood in relation to children's rights. *International Journal of Children's Rights*, *8*(3), 243–259. https://doi.org/10.1163/15718180020494640

McTaggart, R., Nixon, R., & Kemmis, S. (2017). Critical participatory action research. In L. Rowell, C. D. Bruce, J. M. Shosh, & M. M. Riel, *The Palgrave international handbook of action research* (pp. 21–35). Palgrave Macmillan.

Mirra, N., & Rogers, J. (2016). Institutional participation and social transformation: Considering the goals and tensions of university-initiated YPAR projects with K--12 youth. *International Journal of Qualitative Studies in Education*, *29*(10), 1255–1268. https://doi.org/10.1080/09518398.2016.1192697

Ochocka, J., Moorlag, E., & Janzen, R. (2010). A framework for entry: PAR values and engagement strategies in community research. *Gateways: International Journal of Community Research and Engagement*, *3*, 1–19. https://doi.org/10.5130/ijcre.v3i0.1328

Pittaway, E., Bartolomei, L., & Hugman, R. (2010). "Stop stealing our stories": The ethics of research with vulnerable groups. *Journal of Human Rights Practice*, *2*(2), 229–251. https://doi.org/10.1093/jhuman/huq004

Ponic, P., Reid, C., & Frisby, W. (2010). Cultivating the power of partnerships in feminist participatory action research in women's health: Cultivating partnerships. *Nursing Inquiry*, *17*(4), 324–335. https://doi.org/10.1111/j.1440-1800.2010.00506.x

Pratt, M. L. (1991). Arts of the contact zone. *Profession*, 33–40. https://www.jstor.org/stable/25595469

Quijada Cerecer, D. A., Cahill, C., & Bradley, M. (2013). Toward a critical youth policy praxis: Critical youth studies and participatory action research. *Theory Into Practice*, *52*(3), 216–223. https://doi.org/10.1080/00405841.2013.804316

Rahman, M. A. (1991). Glimpses of the "other Africa". In O. Fals-Borda & M. A. Rahman, *Action and knowledge: Breaking the monopoly with participatory action research* (pp. 84-108). The Apex Press.

Sahay, K. M., Thatcher, K., Núñez, C., & Lightfoot, A. (2016). "It's like we are legally, illegal": Latino/a youth emphasize barriers to higher education using photovoice. *The High School Journal*, *100*(1), 45–65. https://doi.org/10.1353/hsj.2016.0020

Salsberg, J., Macridis, S., Garcia Bengoechea, E., Macaulay, A. C., & Moore, S. (2017). Engagement strategies that foster community self-determination in participatory research: Insider ownership through outsider championship. *Family Practice*, *34*(3), 336–340. https://doi.org/10.1093/fampra/cmx001

Smyth, J., & McInerney, P. (2013). Whose side are you on? Advocacy ethnography: Some methodological aspects of narrative portraits of disadvantaged young people, in socially critical research. *International Journal of Qualitative Studies in Education*, *26*(1), 1–20. https://doi.org/10.1080/09518398.2011.604649" https://doi.org/10.1080/09518398.2011.604649

Sprague, L., Afifi, R., Ayala, G., & El-nasoor, M. L. (2019). Participatory praxis as an imperative for health-related stigma research. *BMC Medicine*, *17*(1), 32. https://doi.org/10.1186/s12916-019-1263-3

Teti, M. (2019). The murky ethics of visual qualitative methods: Picturing a clear path forward. *International Journal of Qualitative Methods*, *18*, 1–4. https://doi.org/10.1177/1609406919884810

Tilakaratna, S. (1991). Stimulation of self-reliant initiatives by sensitized agents: Some lessons from practice. In O. Fals-Borda & M.A. Rahman (Eds.), *Action and knowledge: Breaking the monopoly with participatory action research* (pp. 135–145). The Apex Press.

Tuck, E., & Del Vecchio, D. (2018). Representing refusals: Dilemmas in making photo-based research with migrant youth. In K. Gallagher (Ed.), *The methodological dilemma revisited: Creative, critical and collaborative approaches to qualitative research for a new era* (pp. 76–90). Routledge.

Wagaman, M. A., & Sanchez, I. (2017). Looking through the magnifying glass: A duoethnographic approach to understanding the value and process of participatory action research with LGBTQ youth. *Qualitative Social Work*, *16*(1), 78–95. https://doi.org/10.1177/1473325015595855

Wang, C. C., & Burris, M. A. (1994). Empowerment through photo novella: Portraits of participation. *Health Education Quarterly*, *21*(2), 171–186.

Wang, C. C., & Burris, M. A. (1997). Photovoice: Concept, methodology, and use for participatory needs assessment. *Health Education & Behavior*, *24*(3), 369–387. https://doi.org/10.1177/109019819702400309

Wang, C. C., & Redwood-Jones, Y. A. (2001). Photovoice ethics: Perspectives from Flint photovoice. *Health Education & Behavior*, *28*(5), 560–572. https://doi.org/10.1177/109019810102800504

CHAPTER 3

Aristotle. (1999). *Nicomachean ethics* (T. Irwin, Trans.). Hackett.

Atkinson, P., Coffey, A., & Delamont, A. (2003). *Key themes in qualitative research: Continuities and changes*. Altamira Press.

Bell Jr., D. A. (1987). *And we are not saved: The elusive quest for racial justice*. Basic Books.

Call-Cummings, M. (2017). Establishing communicative validity: Discovering theory through practice. *Qualitative Inquiry, 23*(3), 192–200.

Campbell, D. T., & Stanley, J. C. (1963). *Experimental and quasi-experimental designs for research*. Rand McNally & Company.

Carspecken, P. (1996). *Critical ethnography in educational research: A theoretical and practical guide*. Routledge.

Chilisa, B. (2012). *Indigenous research methodologies*. SAGE.

Cho, J., & Trent, A. (2006). Validity in qualitative research revisited. *Qualitative Research, 6*(3), 319–340. https://doi.org/10.1177/1468794106065006

Cochran-Smith, M., & Lytle, S. L. (1990). Research on teaching and teacher research: The issues that divide. *Educational Researcher, 19*(2), 2–11. https://doi.org/10.2307/1176596

Collins, P. H. (2010). *Black feminist thought: Knowledge, consciousness, and the politics of empowerment*. Routledge.

Cook, T. D., & Campbell, D. T. (1979). *Quasi-experimentation: Design and analysis issues for field settings*. Houghton Mifflin.

Crenshaw, K., Gotanda, N., Peller, G., & Thomas, K. (Eds.). (1995). *Critical race theory: The key writings that formed the movement*. New Press.

Creswell, J. W. (2007). *Qualitative inquiry and research design: Choosing among five approaches*. SAGE.

Cronbach, L. J., & Meehl, P. E. (1955). Construct validity in psychological tests. *Psychological Bulletin, 52*(4), 281–302. https://doi.org/10.1037/h0040957

De Sousa Santos, B. (2008). The World Social Forum and the Global Left. *Politics & Society, 36*(2), 247–270. https://doi.org/10.1177/0032329208316571

Delgado Bernal, D. (2002). Critical race theory, Latino critical theory, and critical raced-gendered epistemologies: Recognizing students of color as holders and creators of knowledge. *Qualitative Inquiry, 8*(1), 105–126.

Dennis, B. (2013). "Validity crisis" in qualitative research: Still? Movement toward a unified approach. In B. Dennis, L. Carspecken, & P. Carspecken (Eds.), *Qualitative research: A reader in philosophy, core concepts, and practice* (pp. 3–37). Peter Lang.

Dennis, B. (2018). Validity as research praxis: A study of self-reflection and engagement in qualitative inquiry. *Qualitative Inquiry, 24*(2), 109–118. https://doi.org/10.1177/1077800416686371

Erickson, F. (2011). A history of qualitative inquiry in social and educational research. In N. K. Denzin & Y. S. Lincoln (Eds.), *The SAGE handbook of qualitative research* (pp. 43–60). SAGE.

Fals-Borda, O., & Rahman, M. A. (1991). *Action and knowledge: Breaking the monopoly with participatory action-research*. Apex Press.

Fine, M. (2018). *Just research in contentious times: Widening the methodological imagination*. Teachers College Press.

Freire, P. (1972). *Pedagogy of the oppressed*. Herder and Herder.

Freire, P. (1982). Creating alternative research methods: Learning to do it by doing it. In B. Hall, A. Gillette, & R. Tandon (Eds.), *Creating knowledge: A monopoly?* (pp. 29–37). Society for Participatory Research in Asia. Reprinted in Kemmis, S., & McTaggart, R. (Eds.). (1988). *The action research reader* (pp. 291–313). Deakin University Press.

Fricker, M. (2007). *Epistemic injustice: Power and the ethics of knowing*. Oxford University Press.

Gaztambide-Fernández, R. A. (2012). Decolonization and the pedagogy of solidarity. *Decolonization: Indigeneity, Education & Society, 1*(1), 41–67.

Giroux, H. A. (1982). Power and resistance in the new sociology of education: Beyond theories of social and cultural reproduction. *Curriculum Perspectives, 2*(2), 1–12.

Giroux, H. (1983). Theories of reproduction and resistance in the new sociology of education: A critical analysis. *Harvard Education Review, 53*(3), 257–293.

Giroux, H. A. (2011). *On critical pedagogy*. Continuum International Publishing Group.

Gramsci, A. (1978). *Selections from the prison notebooks*. International Publishers.

Guba, E. (1981). Criteria for assessing the trustworthiness of naturalistic inquiries. *Educational Technology Research and Development*, *29*(2), 75–91. https://doi.org/10.1007/BF02766777

Guba, E. G., & Lincoln, Y. S. (1989). *Fourth generation evaluation*. SAGE.

Guillemin, M., & Gillam, L. (2004). Ethics, reflexivity and ethically important moments in research. *Qualitative Inquiry*, *10*(2), 261–280.

Habermas, J. (1984). *Theory of communicative action* (T. McCarthy, Trans.). Beacon Press.

Habermas, J. (1996). *Between facts and norms* (W. Rehg, Trans.). MIT Press.

Hall, B. L., & Tandon, R. (2017). Decolonization of knowledge, epistemicide, participatory research and higher education. *Research for All*, *1*(1), 6–19.

Harding, S. (1992). Rethinking standpoint epistemology: What is "strong objectivity"? *The Centennial Review*, *36*(3), 437–470. https://www.jstor.org/stable/23739232

Heron, J., & Reason, P. (1997). A participatory inquiry paradigm. *Qualitative Inquiry*, *3*(3), 274–294. https://doi.org/10.1177/107780049700300302

hooks, b. (1999). *Talking back: Thinking feminist, thinking black*. South End Press.

Horkheimer, M., & Adorno, T. W. (2002). *Dialectic of enlightenment: Philosophical fragments*. (G. S. Noerr, Ed., E. Jephcott, Trans.). Stanford University Press. (original work published 2006).

Jay, M. (1973). *The dialectical imagination. A history of the Frankfurt School and the Institute of Social Research 1923–1950*. Little Brown and Company.

Jay, M. (1996). *The dialectical imagination: A history of the Frankfurt School and the Institute of Social Research, 1923–1950* (10th ed.). University of California Press.

Kassam, Y., & Mustafa, K. (Eds.). (1982). *Participatory research: An emerging alternative methodology*. ICAE.

Kemmis, S., & McTaggart, R. (2005). Participatory action research: Communicative action and the public sphere. In N. K. Denzin & Y. S. Lincoln (Eds.), *Strategies of qualitative inquiry* (pp. 559–604). SAGE.

Kilgore, D. W. (2001). Critical and postmodern perspectives on adult learning. *New Directions for Adult and Continuing Education*, *2001*(89)., 53–62. https://doi.org/10.1002/ace.8

Kincheloe, J. L., McLaren, P., Steinberg, S. R., & Monzó, L. (2017). Critical pedagogy and qualitative research: Advancing the bricolage. In N. K. Denzin & Y. S. Lincoln (Eds.), *The SAGE handbook of qualitative research* (5th ed., pp. 235–260). SAGE.

Kovach, M. (2009). *Indigenous methodologies: Characteristics, conversations, and contexts*. University of Toronto Press.

Kvale, S. (1994). Ten standard objections to qualitative research interviews. *Journal of Phenomenological Psychology*, *25*(2), 147–173. https://doi.org/10.1163/156916294X00016

LatCrit. (2002). *LatCrit Primer: Volume 1*. LatCrit: Latina & Latino Critical Legal Theory, Inc. https://latcrit.org/wp-content/uploads/2020/07/lcprimeri.pdf

Lather, P. (1986). Issues of validity in openly ideological research: Between a rock and a soft place. *Interchange*, *17*(4), 63–84. https://doi.org/10.1007/BF01807017

Lincoln, Y. S., & Guba, E. G. (1985). *Naturalistic inquiry*. SAGE.

Lincoln, Y. S., Lynham, S. A., & Guba, E. G. (2011). Paradigmatic controversies, contradictions, and emerging confluences. In N. K. Denzin & Y. S. Lincoln (Eds.), *The SAGE handbook of qualitative research* (pp. 97–128). SAGE.

Massey, S. G., & Barreras, R. E. (2013). Introducing "impact validity". *Journal of Social Issues*, *69*(4), 615–632. https://doi.org/10.1111/josi.12032

Mertens, D. M. (2009). *Transformative research and evaluation*. Guilford Press.

Messick, S. (1989). Validity. In R. Linn (Ed.), *Educational measurement* (3rd ed., pp. 13–103). Macmillan.

Messick, S. (1995). Validity of psychological assessment: Validation of inferences from persons' responses and performances as scientific inquiry into score meaning. *American Psychologist*, *50*(9), 741–749. https://doi.org/10.1037/0003-066X.50.9.741

Nyoni, S. (1991). People's power in Zimbabwe. In O.

Fals-Borda & M. A. Rahman (Eds), *Action and knowledge: Breaking the monopoly with participatory action-research* (pp. 24–34). Apex Press.

Pihama, L., Tiakiwai, S.-J., & Southey, K. (Eds.). (2015). *Kaupapa rangahau: A reader. A collection of readings from the Kaupapa Rangahau workshops series* (2nd ed.). Te Kotahi Research Institute.

Pittaway, E., Bartolomei, L., & Hugman, R. (2010). 'Stop stealing our stories': The ethics of research with vulnerable groups. *Journal of Human Rights Practice*, *2*(2), 229–251. https://doi.org/10.1093/jhuman/huq004

Prilleltensky, I. (2003). Understanding, resisting, and overcoming oppression: Toward psychological validity. *American Journal of Community Psychology*, *31*(1/2), 195–201.

Prilleltensky, I. (2008). The role of power in wellness, oppression, and liberation: The promise of psychopolitical validity. *Journal of Community Psychology*, *36*(2), 116–136.

Rahman, M. A., & Fals-Borda, O. (1991). A self-review of PAR. In O. Fals-Borda & M. A. Rahman (Eds.), *Action and knowledge: Breaking the monopoly with participatory action-research* (pp. 24–34). Apex Press.

Simon, L. H. (Ed.). (1994). *Karl Marx: Selected writings*. Hackett, 1994.

Smith, G. H. (1992). Research issues related to Māori education. In *The issue of research and Māori*. Research Unit for Māori Education, University of Auckland.

Solórzano, D. G., & Yosso, T. J. (2002). Critical race methodology: Counter-storytelling as an analytical framework for education research. *Qualitative Inquiry*, *8*(1), 23–44. https://doi.org/10.1177/107780040200800103

Sprague Martinez, L., Carolan, K., O'Donnell, A., Diaz, Y., & Freeman, E. R. (2018). Community engagement in patient-centered outcomes research: Benefits, barriers, and measurement. *Journal of Clinical and Translational Science*, *2*(6), 371–376. https://doi.org/10.1017/cts.2018.341

Tandon, R. (1989). *Movement towards democratization of knowledge*. Society for Participatory Research in Asia.

Tanner, D. (2019). Opening communicative space: What do co-researchers contribute? *Qualitative Research*, *19*(3), 292–310. https://doi.org/10.1177/1468794118770076

Tuck, E., & Yang, K. W. (2012). Decolonization is not a metaphor. *Decolonization: Indigeneity, Education & Society*, *1*(1), 1–40.

Tuhiwai Smith, L. (2012). *Decolonizing methodologies: Research and Indigenous peoples*. Zed Books.

Wicks, P. G., & Reason, P. (2009). Initiating action research: Challenges and paradoxes of opening communicative space. *Action Research*, *7*(3), 243–262. https://doi.org/10.1177/1476750309336715

CHAPTER 4

Bettencourt, G. M. (2020). Embracing problems, processes, and contact zones: Using youth participatory action research to challenge adultism. *Action Research*, *18*(2), 153–170. https://doi.org/10.1177/1476750318789475

Boudreau Morris, K. (2016). Decolonizing solidarity: Cultivating relationships of discomfort *Settler* Colonial Studies, *7*(4), 456–473. https://doi.org/10.1080/2201473X.2016.1241210

Boxall, K., & Ralph, S. (2009). Research ethics and the use of visual images in research with people with intellectual disability. *Journal of Intellectual & Developmental Disability*, *34*(1), 45–54. https://doi.org/10.1080/13668250802688306

Call-Cummings, M., Hauber-Özer, M., Byers, C., & Mancuso, G. P. (2019). The power of/in Photovoice. *International Journal of Research & Method in Education*, *42*(4), 399–413. https://doi.org/10.1080/1743727X.2018.1492536

Call-Cummings, M., Hauber-Özer, M., & Ross, K. (2020). Struggling with/against the unintentional reproduction of power structures in participatory research: Using reconstructive horizon analysis. *Action Research*, *18*(2), 171–193. https://doi.org/10.1177/1476750319837324

Collins, P. (1989). The social construction of black feminist thought. *Signs*, *14*(4), 745–773.

Collins, P. H. (2010). *Black feminist thought: Knowledge,*

consciousness, and the politics of empowerment. Routledge.

Cook-Sather, A. (2006). Sound, presence, and power: 'Student voice' in educational research and reform. *Curriculum Inquiry*, *36*(4), 359–390. https://doi.org/10.1111/j.1467-873x.2006.00363.x

Dennis, B., & Huf, C. (2017). *Counteracting the adult–child binary: New perspectives on children's learning through critical ethnography.* Paper presented at the European Conference on Education Research, Copenhagen, Denmark.

Fanon, F. (1963/2014). *The wretched of the earth*. Grove Press.

Gallacher, L.-A., & Gallagher, M. (2008). Methodological immaturity in childhood research?: Thinking through 'participatory methods.' *Childhood*, *15*(4), 499–516. https://doi.org/10.1177/0907568208091672

Ghaffar-Kucher, A. (2015). Writing culture; inscribing lives: A reflective treatise on the burden of representation in native research. *International Journal of Qualitative Studies in Education*, *28*(10), 1186–1202. https://doi.org/10.1080/09518398.2014.974720

Guillemin, M., & Gillam, L. (2004). Ethics, reflexivity and ethically important moments in research. *Qualitative Inquiry*, *10*(2), 261–280. https://doi.org/10.1177/1077800403262360

Hannes, K., & Parylo, O. (2014). Let's play it safe: Ethical considerations from participants in a photovoice research project. *International Journal of Qualitative Methods*, *13*(1), 255–274. https://doi.org/10.1177/160940691401300112

Hart, R. A. (1992). *Children's participation: From tokenism to citizenship*. UNICEF International Child Development Centre.

Hauber-Özer, M. (2019). Yabancı: An autoethnography of migration. *Forum Qualitative Sozialforschung / Forum: Qualitative Social Research*, *20*(3). Art. 20. https://doi.org/10.17169/fqs-20.3.3328

Hauber-Özer, M., & Call-Cummings, M. (2020). Empowerment or exposure? Ethical dilemmas of visual methods with vulnerable migrants. *Qualitative Research Journal*, *20*(3), 329–240. https://doi.org/10.1108/QRJ-10-2019-0075

Herr, K., & Anderson, G. L. (2005). *The action research dissertation: A guide for students and faculty*. SAGE. https://doi.org/10.4135/9781452226644

Hugman, R., Bartolomei, L., & Pittaway, E. (2011). Human agency and the meaning of informed consent: Reflections on research with refugees. *Journal of Refugee Studies*, *24*(4), 655–671. https://doi.org/10.1093/jrs/fer024

Kohfeldt, D., Chhun, L., Grace, S., & Langhout, R. D. (2011). Youth empowerment in context: Exploring tensions in school-based YPAR. *American Journal of Community Psychology*, *47*(1–2), 28–45. https://doi.org/10.1007/s10464-010-9376-z

Limes-Taylor Henderson, K., & Esposito, J. (2019). Using others in the nicest way possible: On colonial and academic practice(s), and an ethic of humility. *Qualitative Inquiry*, *1*(14), 876-889. https://doi.org/10.1177/1077800417743528

Lincoln, Y. S., Lynham, S. A., & Guba, E. G. (2011). Paradigmatic controversies, contradictions, and emerging confluences. In N. K. Denzin & Y. S. Lincoln (Eds.), *The SAGE handbook of qualitative research* (pp. 97–128). SAGE.

Luttrell, W. (2010). *Qualitative educational research: Readings in reflexive methodology and transformative practice*. Routledge.

Luttrell, W., & Chalfen, R. (2010). Lifting up voices of participatory visual research. *Visual Studies*, *25*(3), 197–200. https://doi.org/10.1080/1472586X.2010.523270

Mackenzie, C., McDowell, C., & Pittaway, E. (2007). Beyond 'do no harm': The challenge of constructing ethical relationships in refugee research. *Journal of Refugee Studies*, *20*(2), 299–319. https://doi.org/10.1093/jrs/fem008

Miled, N. (2019). Muslim researcher researching Muslim youth: Reflexive notes on critical ethnography, positionality and representation. *Ethnography and Education*, *14*(1), 1–15. https://doi.org/10.1080/17457823.2017.1387063

Milner IV, H. R. (2007). Race, culture, and researcher positionality: Working through dangers seen, unseen, and unforeseen. *Educational Researcher*, *36*(7), 388–400.

Mosselson, J. (2010). Subjectivity and reflexivity: Locating the self in research on dislocation. *International Journal of*

Qualitative Studies in Education, 23(4), 479–494. https://doi.org/10.1080/09518398.2010.492771

Patel, L. (2012). Contact zones, problem posing and critical consciousness. *Pedagogies: An International Journal, 7*(4), 333–346. https://doi.org/10.1080/1554480x.2012.715738

Phillips, E. N., Berg, M. J., Rodriguez, C., & Morgan, D. (2010). A case study of participatory action research in a public New England middle school: Empowerment, constraints and challenges. *American Journal of Community Psychology, 46*(1–2), 179–194. https://doi.org/10.1007/s10464-010-9336-7

Pittaway, E., Bartolomei, L., & Hugman, R. (2010). 'Stop stealing our stories': The ethics of research with vulnerable groups. *Journal of Human Rights Practice, 2*(2), 229–251. https://doi.org/10.1093/jhuman/huq004

Popova, D. (2016). Decolonization of the self. In G. A. Tilley-Lubbs & S. B. Calva (Eds.), *Re-telling our stories. Imagination and praxis* (pp. 173–185). Sense. https://doi-org./10.1007/978-94-6300-567-8_13

Pratt, M. L. (1991). Arts of the contact zone. *Profession*, 33–40. https://www.jstor.org/stable/25595469

Sahay, K. M., Thatcher, K., Núñez, C., & Lightfoot, A. (2016). "It's like we are legally, illegal": Latino/a youth emphasize barriers to higher education using photovoice. *The High School Journal, 100*(1), 45–65. https://doi.org/10.1353/hsj.2016.0020

Surmiak, A. (2020). Ethical concerns of paying cash to vulnerable participants: The qualitative researchers' views. *The Qualitative Report, 25*(12), 4461–4481. https://doi.org/

Torre, M. E., Fine, M., Alexander, N., Billups, A. B., Blanding, Y., Genao, E., Marboe, E., Salah, T., & Urdang, K. (2008). Participatory action research in the contact zone. In J. Cammarota & M. Fine (Eds.), *Revolutionizing education: Youth participatory action research in motion* (pp. 23–44). Routledge.

Tuck, E., & Yang, K. W. (2012). Decolonization is not a metaphor. *Decolonization: Indigeneity, Education & Society, 1*(1), 1–40. https://doi.org/10.1080/09518398.2011.600274

CHAPTER 5

Altschuld, J. W., & Kumar, D. D. (2010). *Needs assessment: An overview (Book 1)*. SAGE.

Belenky, M. F., Clinchy, B. M., Goldberger, N. R., & Tarule, J. M. (1997). *Women's ways of knowing: The development of self, voice, and mind*. Basic Books.

Cahill, C., Cerecer, D. A. Q., Rivarola, A. R. R., Zamudio, J. H., & Gutiérrez, L. A. (2019). 'Caution, we have power': Resisting the 'school-to-sweatshop pipeline' through participatory artistic praxes and critical care. *Gender and Education, 31*(5), 576–589. https://doi.org/10.1080/09540253.2019.1582207

Call-Cummings, M. (2017). Establishing communicative validity: Discovering theory through practice. *Qualitative Inquiry, 23*(3), 192–200.

Call-Cummings, M., Hauber-Özer, M., Byers, C., & Mancuso, G. P. (2019). The power of/in Photovoice. *International Journal of Research & Method in Education, 42*(4), 399–413. https://doi.org/10.1080/1743727X.2018.1492536

Call-Cummings, M., Hauber-Özer, M., & Dazzo, G. (2019). Examining researcher identity development within the context of a course on PAR: A layered narrative approach. *The Qualitative Report, 24*(9), 2178–2196.

Caraballo, L., & Soleimany, S. (2019). In the name of (pedagogical) love: A conceptual framework for transformative teaching grounded in critical youth research. *The Urban Review, 51*(1), 81–100. https://doi.org/10.1007/s11256-018-0486-5

Cook-Sather, A. (2011). Layered learning: Student consultants deepening classroom and life lessons. *Educational Action Research, 19*(1), 41–57. https://doi.org/10.1080/09650792.2011.547680

DeNicolo, C. P., Yu, M., Crowley, C. B., & Gabel, S. L. (2017). Reimagining critical care and problematizing sense of school belonging as a response to inequality for immigrants and children of immigrants. *Review of Research in Education, 41*(1), 500–530. https://doi.org/10.3102/0091732X17690498

Dennis, B., Uttamchandani, S., Biery, S., & Blauvelt, A. (2019). LGBTQIA+ youth as multicultural educators. *Ethnography* and Education, 14(3), 360–376. https://doi.org/10.1080/17457823.2019.1578983

Fals-Borda, O., & Rahman, M. A. (1991). *Action and knowledge: Breaking the monopoly with participatory action-research*. Apex Press.

Freire, P. (1970). *Pedagogy of the oppressed*. Herder and Herder.

Fine, M. (2012). Troubling calls for evidence: A critical race, class and gender analysis of whose evidence counts. *Feminism & Psychology, 22*(1), 3–19. https://doi.org/10.1177/0959353511435475

Fricker, M. (2007). *Epistemic injustice: Power and the ethics of knowing*. Oxford University Press.

Garnett, B. R., Smith, L. C., Kervick, C. T., Ballysingh, T. A., Moore, M., & Gonell, E. (2019). The emancipatory potential of transformative mixed methods designs: Informing youth participatory action research and restorative practices within a district-wide school transformation project. *International Journal of Research & Method in Education, 42*(3), 305–316. https://doi.org/10.1080/1743727X.2019.1598355

Grosfoguel, R. (2007). The EPISTEMIC decolonial turn. *Cultural Studies, 21*(2–3), 211–223. https://doi.org/10.1080/09502380601162514

Groundwater-Smith, S., & Mockler, N. (2016). From data source to co-researchers? Tracing the shift from 'student voice' to student–teacher partnerships. *Educational Action Research, 24*(2), 159–176. https://doi.org/10.1080/09650792.2015.1053507

Hall, B. L., & Tandon, R. (2017). Decolonization of knowledge, epistemicide, participatory research and higher education. *Research for All, 1*(1), 6–19.

Haraway, D. (1988). Situated knowledges: The science question in feminism and the privilege of partial perspective. *Feminist Studies, 14*(3), 575–599. https://doi.org/10.2307/3178066

Jarldorn, M., & 'Deer.' (2017). Participatory action research with ex-prisoners: Using Photovoice and one woman's story told through poetry. *Action Research, 18*(3). https://doi.org/10.1177/1476750317719140

Kemmis, S., & McTaggart, R. (2005). Communicative action and the public sphere. In N. K. Denzin & Y. S. Lincoln (Eds.), *The SAGE handbook of qualitative research* (pp. 271–330). SAGE.

Lodge, C. (2005). From hearing voices to engaging in dialogue: Problematising student participation in school Improvement. *Journal of Educational Change, 6*(2), 125–146. https://doi.org/10.1007/s10833-005-1299-3

Martín-Baró, I. (1994). *Writings for a liberation psychology* (A. Aron & S. Corne, Eds.). Harvard University Press.

Mertens, D. M. (2009). *Transformative research and evaluation* (pp. 9–21). Guilford Press.

Pratt, M. L. (1991). Arts of the contact zone. *Profession*, 33–40.

Rotary International. (n.d.). *Community assessment tools: A resource for Rotary projects*. Rotary International. https://my.rotary.org/en/document/community-assessment-tools

Shahjahan, R. A. (2011). Decolonizing the evidence-based education and policy movement: Revealing the colonial vestiges in educational policy, research, and neoliberal reform. *Journal of Education Policy, 26*(2), 181–206. https://doi.org/10.1080/02680939.2010.508176

Smyth, J., & McInerney, P. (2013). Whose side are you on? Advocacy ethnography: Some methodological aspects of narrative portraits of disadvantaged young people, in socially critical research. *International Journal of Qualitative Studies in Education, 26*(1), 1–20. https://doi.org/10.1080/09518398.2011.604649

Student, R., Kendall, K., & Day, L. (2017). Being a refugee university student: A collaborative auto-ethnography. *Journal of Refugee Studies, 30*(4), 580–604. https://doi.org/10.1093/jrs/few045

Torre, M. E. (2010). Participatory action research in the contact zone. In *Revolutionizing education* (pp. 31–52). Routledge.

CHAPTER 6

Action Aid. (n.d.). *Ripples of change*. Reflection Action. https://www.reflectionaction.org/tools_and_methods/47/?from=ov

Blodgett, A. T., Schinke, R. J., Peltier, D., Wabano, M. J., Fisher, L. A., Eys, M.

A., & Pickard, P. (2010). Naadmaadmi: Reflections of Aboriginal community members engaged in sport psychology co-researching activities with mainstream academics. *Qualitative Research in Sport and Exercise, 2*(1), 56–76. https://doi.org/10.1080/19398440903510160

Braun, V., & Clarke, V. (2006). Using thematic analysis in psychology. *Qualitative Research in Psychology, 3*(2), 77–101. https://doi.org/10.1191/1478088706qp063oa

Carspecken, P. F. (1996). *Critical ethnography in educational research: A theoretical and practical guide*. Routledge.

Chambers, R. (2002). *Participatory workshops: A sourcebook of 21 sets of ideas & activities*. Earthscan.

Fine, M., Torre, M. E., Oswald, A. G., & Avory, S. (2021). Critical participatory action research: Methods and praxis for intersectional knowledge production. *Journal of Counseling Psychology, 68*(3), 344–356. https://doi.org/10.1037/cou0000445

Kovach, M. (2009). *Indigenous methodologies*. University of Toronto Press.

Merriam, S. B., & Tisdell, E. J. (2015). *Qualitative research: A guide to design and implementation*. Jossey-Bass.

Mertens, D. M. (2009). *Transformative research and evaluation*. Guilford Press.

Patton, M. Q. (2014). *Qualitative evaluation and research methods*. SAGE.

Stake, R. E. (1995). *The art of case study research*. SAGE.

Stoudt, B. (2014). Critical statistics. In T. Teo (Ed.), *Encyclopedia of critical psychology*. Springer Press.

Stoudt, B. G. (2016). Conversations on the margins: Using data entry to explore the qualitative potential of survey marginalia. *Qualitative Psychology, 3*(2), 186–208. https://doi.org/10.1037/qup0000060

Weiss, C. (1995). Nothing as practical as good theory: Exploring theory-based evaluation for comprehensive community initiatives for children and families. In J. Connell, A. Kubisch, L. Schorr, & C. Weiss (Eds.), *New approaches to evaluating community initiatives*. Aspen Institute.

CHAPTER 7

Alim, H. S. (2011). Global ill-literacies: Hip hop cultures, youth identities, and the politics of literacy. *Review of Research in Education, 35*(1), 120–146. https://doi.org/10.3102/0091732X10 383208

Atkinson, P., & Silverman, D. (1997). Kundera's immortality: The interview society and the invention of the self. *Qualitative Inquiry, 3*, 304–325.

Ball, H. K. (2008). Quilts. In J. G. Knowles & A. L. Cole (Eds.), *Handbook of the arts in qualitative research: Perspectives, methodologies, examples, and issues* (pp. 364–369). SAGE.

Bishop, E., & Willis, K. (2014). "Hope is that fiery feeling": Using poetry as data to explore the meanings of hope for young people. *Forum Qualitative Sozialforschung/Forum: Qualitative Social Research, 15*(1), Article 1. https://doi.org/10.17169/fqs-15.1.2013

Blumenfeld-Jones, D. (2008). Dance, choreography, and social science research. In J. G. Knowles & A. L. Cole (Eds.), *Handbook of the arts in qualitative research: Perspectives, methodologies, examples, and issues* (pp. 176–185). SAGE.

Boal, A. (1979). *Theatre of the Oppressed* (C. A. & M. L. McBride, Trans.). Theatre Communications Group, Inc. (Original work published 1974).

Boal, A. (2002). *Games for actors and non-actors* (A. Jackson, Trans.). Routledge. (Original work published 1992).

Boydell, K. (2011a). Using performative art to communicate research: Dancing experiences of psychosis. *Canadian Theatre Review, 146*(146), 12–17. https://doi.org/10.1353/ctr.2011.0042

Boydell, K. (2011b). Making sense of collective events: The co-creation of a research-based dance. *Forum Qualitative Sozialforschung/Forum: Qualitative Social Research, 12*(1), Article 1. https://doi.org/10.17169/fqs-12.1.1525

Boydell, K. (2019). The journey to a wider understanding of ways of knowing: Knowledge translation and the arts. *LEARNing Landscapes, 12*(1), 19–27.

Boydell, K. M., Bennett, J., Dew, A., Lappin, J., Lenette, C., Ussher, J., Vaughan, P., & Wells, R. (2020). Women and stigma: A protocol for understanding intersections of experience through body mapping. *International Journal of Environmental Research and Public Health, 17*(15), 5432. https://doi.org/10.3390/ijerph17155432

Bruner, J. (2001). Self-making and world-making. In J. Brockmeier & D. Cargbaugh (Eds.), *Narrative and identity: Studies in autobiography, self, and culture* (pp. 25–37). John Benjamins.

Butler-Kisber, L. (2008). Collage as inquiry. In J. Knowles & A. Cole, *Handbook of the arts in qualitative research: Perspectives, methodologies, examples, and issues* (pp. 265–277). SAGE.

Call-Cummings, M. (2015). *Exploring the intersections and implications of pedagogies of empowerment and critical PAR through youth research on racism in schools* [Doctoral dissertation, Indiana University].

Call-Cummings, M., Dazzo, G., Beardsley, L., & Blibo, J. (2021). Performance as transformation/transformative: Problematizing performance in PAR. *Educational Action Research*. Advance online publication. https://doi.org/10.1080/09650792.2021.2000879

Call-Cummings, M., Hauber-Özer, M., LePelch, V., DeSenti, K. L., Colandene, M., Sultana, K., & Scicli, E. (2020). "Hopefully this motivates a bout of realization": Spoken word poetry as critical literacy. *Journal of Adolescent and Adult Literacy, 64*(2), 191–199. https://doi.org/doi: 10.1002/jaal.1082

Cammarota, J., & Fine, M. (Eds.). (2008). *Revolutionizing education: Youth participatory action research in motion*. Routledge.

Coemans, S., & Hannes, K. (2016, August) Applying a multi-sensory methods base in collaborative research practice: Solid "Dare it" (y) [Conference presentation abstract]. TISSA PhD & Plenum Conference, Ghent, Belgium. https://lirias.kuleuven.be/handle/123456789/543674

Crawford, A. (2010). If "the body keeps score": Mapping the dissociated body in trauma narrative, intervention and theory. *University of Toronto Quarterly, 79*(2), 702–719. http://documents.mx/documents/mapping-the-ed-body-in-trauma-narrative-and-intervention.html

Dazzo, G. P. (2016, September 1). Reciprocity in research: Integrating evaluation & human rights methods to balance evaluator & community needs. [Webinar]. *Search for Common Ground Thursday Talks*. https://vimeo.com/181067904

de Cosson, A. F. (2008). Textu(r)al walking/writing through sculpture. In J. Knowles & A. Cole (Eds.), *Handbook of the arts in qualitative research: Perspectives, methodologies, examples, and issues* (pp. 278–287). SAGE.

de Jager, A., Tewson, A., Ludlow, B., & Boydell, K. (2016). Embodied ways of storying the self: A systematic review of body-mapping. *Forum: Qualitative Social Research, 17*(2). https://doi.org/10.17169/fqs-17.2.2526

Dennis, B., Call-Cummings, M., Ross, K., & Shah, P. (2017, March 5–9). *Acting out: Challenging inequalities in the researcher-participant relationship: A workshop addressing methodological challenges in international contexts* [Co-facilitated workshop]. Comparative and International Education Society (CIES) Conference, Atlanta, GA, United States.

Ellis, C., & Berger, L. (2002). Their story/my story/our story: Including the researcher's experience in interview research. In J. F. Gubrium & J. A. Holstein (Eds.), *Handbook of interview research: Context and method* (pp. 849–875). SAGE.

Endsley, C. L. (2014). Performing Blackness: Spoken word poetry and performance. *Transformations: The Journal of Inclusive Scholarship and Pedagogy, 24*(1–2), 110–120. http://www.jstor.org/stable/10.5325/trajincschped.24.1-2.0110

Fernández, J. S. (2018). Toward an ethical reflective practice of a theory in the flesh: Embodied subjectivities in a youth participatory action research mural project. *American Journal of Community Psychology, 2018*(62)., 221–232. https://doi.org/10.1002/ajcp.12264

Fisher, M. T. (2003). Open mics and open minds: Spoken word poetry in African Diaspora Participatory Literacy Communities. *Harvard Educational Review, 73*(3), 362–389. https://doi.org/10.17763/haer.73.3.642q2 564m1k90670

Fisher, M. T. (2005). From the coffee house to the school house: The promise and potential of spoken word poetry in school contexts. *English Education, 37*(2), 115–131.

Fisher, M. T. (2007). *Writing in rhythm: Spoken word poetry in urban classrooms*. Teachers College Press.

Fobear, K. (2017). "This painting is nice, but I wish it were more political." Exploring the challenges and dilemmas of community art with LGBT refugees. *Women's Studies International Forum*, *62*(May–June 2017), 52–60. https://doi.org/10.1016/j.wsif.2017.02.002

Freire, P. (1970). *Pedagogy of the oppressed*. Herder & Herder.

Galvin, K. T., & Prendergast, M. (Eds.). (2016). *Poetic inquiry II—seeing, caring, understanding: Using poetry as and for inquiry*. Springer.

Gaventa, J. (1991). Toward a knowledge democracy: Viewpoints on participatory research in North America. In O. Fals-Borda & M. A. Rahman (Eds), *Action and knowledge: Breaking the monopoly with participatory action-research* (pp. 121–131). Apex Press.

Glesne, C. (1997). That rare feeling: Re-presenting research through poetic transcription. *Qualitative Inquiry*, *3*(2), 202–221.

Gorman, A. (2021). *The hill we climb: An inaugural poem for the country*. Penguin.

Guenette, F., & Marshall, A. (2009). Time line drawings: Enhancing participant voice in narrative interviews on sensitive topics. *International Journal of Qualitative Methods*, *8*(1), 85–92. https://doi.org/10.1177/160940690900800108

Haug, F. (1987). *Female sexualization: A collective work of memory* (E. Carter, Trans.). Verso.

Hurston, Z. N. (1927). Cudjoe's own story of the last African slaver. *Journal of Negro History*, *12*(4), 648–663. https://doi.org/10.2307/2714041

Impey, A. (2002). Culture, conservation and community reconstruction: Explorations in advocacy: Ethnomusicology and participatory action research in Northern Kwazulu Natal. *Yearbook for Traditional Music*, *34*(2002)., 9–24.

Jocson, K. M. (2005). "Taking it to the mic": Pedagogy of June Jordan's Poetry for the People and partnership with an urban high school. *English Education*, *37*(2), 132–148.

Jocson, K. M. (2006). "There's a better word": Urban youth rewriting their social worlds through poetry. *Journal of Adolescent & Adult Literacy*, *49*(8), 700–707. https://doi.org/10.1598/JAAL.49.8.6

Jocson, K. M. (2008). *Youth poets: Empowering literacies in and out of the classroom*. Peter Lang.

Johnson, J. (2017). *Killing poetry: Blackness and the making of slam and spoken word communities*. Rutgers University Press.

Kasat, P. (2014). Tools for social transformation: Making the personal creative and political. *Griffith Review*, *44*.

Lahman, M. K. E., Geist, M. R., Rodriguez, K. L., Graglia, P. E., Richard, V. M., & Schendel, R. K. (2010). Poking around poetically: Research, poetry, and trustworthiness. *Qualitative Inquiry*, *16*(1), 39–48. https://doi.org/10.1177/1077800409350061

Laimikis Urban Games & Research. (2021, August 25). *Street mosaic workshop*. http://laimikis.lt/street-mosaic-workshop/

Lapadat, J. C. (2009). Writing our way into shared understanding: Collaborative autobiographical writing in the qualitative methods class. *Qualitative Inquiry*, *15*(6), 955–979. https://doi.org/10.1177/1077800409334185

Lather, P. (2007). *Getting lost: Feminist efforts toward a double(d) science*. SUNY.

Lavrinec, J. (2014). Community art initiatives as a form of participatory research: the case of street mosaic workshop. *Creativity Studies*, *7*(1), 55–68. https://doi.org/10.3846/20297475.2014.933365

Lawton, P. H. (2010). Hand-in hand, building community on common ground. *Art Education*, *63*(6), 6–12. http://www.jstor.org/stable/20799848

Leavy, P. (2009). *Method meets art: Arts-based research practice*. Guilford Press.

Leggo, C. (2008). Astonishing silence: Knowing in poetry. In J. Knowles & A. Cole, *Handbook of the arts in qualitative research: Perspectives, methodologies, examples, and issues* (pp. 166–175). SAGE. https://doi.org/10.4135/9781452226545.n14

Leung, P. P. Y. (2010). Autobiographical timeline: A narrative and life story approach in understanding meaning-making in cancer patients. *Illness, Crisis & Loss*, *18*(2), 111–127. https://doi.org/10.2190/IL.18.2.c

Lincoln, Y. S., Lynham, S. A., & Guba, E. G. (2011).

Paradigmatic controversies, contradictions, and emerging confluences. In N. K. Denzin & Y. S. Lincoln (Eds.), *The SAGE handbook of qualitative research* (pp. 97–128). SAGE.

MacCormack, C. P., & Draper, A. (1987). Social and cognitive aspects of female sexuality in Jamaica. In P. Caplan (Ed.), *The cultural construction of sexuality* (pp. 143–165). Routledge.

MacGregor, H. N., & Mills, E. (2011). Framing rights and responsibilities: Accounts of women with a history of AIDS activism. *Bio Med Central International Health & Human Rights*, *11*(S7), 1–11. http://www.ncbi.nlm.nih.gov/pmc/articles/PMC3287463/

Macken, S., Nathan, S., Jersky, M., Boydell, K. M., & Gibson, A. (2021). Body mapping in a drug and alcohol treatment program: Eliciting new identity and experience. *International Journal of Environmental Research and Public Health*, *18*(9), 4942. https://doi.org/10.3390/ijerph18094942

Mitchell, C., & Allnutt, S. (2008). 21 photographs and/as social documentary. In J. G. Knowles & A. L. Cole (Eds.), *Handbook of the arts in qualitative research: Perspectives, methodologies, examples, and issues* (pp. 252–264). SAGE. https://www.doi.org/10.4135/9781452226545.n21

Morrell, E. (2002). Toward a critical pedagogy of popular culture: Literacy development among urban youth. *Journal of Adolescent & Adult Literacy*, *46*(1), 72–77. http://www.jstor.org/stable/40017507

Morrell, E., & Duncan-Andrade, J. (2004). What they do learn in school: Hip-hop as a bridge to canonical poetry. In J. Mahiri (Ed.), *What they don't learn in school: Literacy in the lives of urban youth* (pp. 247–268). Peter Lang.

Na, K.-A., Park, H.-J., & Han, S. J. (2016). Designing a community-based dance programme for North Korean female refugees in South Korea. *Research in Dance Education*, *17*(1), 3–13. https://doi.org/10.1080/14647893.2016.1139076

Pittaway, E., Bartolomei, L., & Hugman, R. (2010). 'Stop stealing our stories': The ethics of research with vulnerable groups. *Journal of Human Rights Practice*, *2*(2), 229–251. https://doi.org/10.1093/jhuman/huq004

Prendergast, M. (2009). Poem is what? Poetic inquiry in qualitative social science research. *International Review of Qualitative Research*, *1*(4), 541–568.

Prendergast, M. (2015). Poetic inquiry, 2007-2012: A surrender and catch found poem. *Qualitative Inquiry*, *21*(8), 678–685. https://doi.org/10.1177/1077800414563806

Santen, B. (2014). Into the fear-factory: Connecting with the traumatic core. *Person-Centred & Experiential Psychotherapies*, *13*(2), 75–93.

Santen, B. (2015). Treating dissociation in traumatized children with body maps. In C. Malchiodi (Ed.), *Creative interventions with traumatized children* (pp. 126–149). Guilford Press.

Skinner, E., & Masuda, J. R. (2013). Right to a healthy city? Examining the relationship between urban space and health inequity by Aboriginal youth artist-activists in Winnipeg. *Social Science & Medicine*, *91*, 210–218. https://doi.org/10.1016/j.socscimed.2013.02.020

Solomon, J. (2002). "Living with X": A body mapping journey in time of HIV and AIDS. *Facilitator's Guide. Psychosocial Wellbeing Series*. REPSSI.

Stapleton, S. R. (2021). Data analysis in participatory action research: Using poetic inquiry to describe urban teacher marginalization. *Action Research*, *19*(2), 449–471. https://doi.org/10.1177/1476750318811920

Tanner, S. J. (2014). *A youth participatory action research (YPAR), theatrical inquiry into whiteness* [Doctoral dissertation]. https://conservancy.umn.edu/handle/11299/165091

Tanner, S. J. (2016). Accounting for whiteness through collaborative fiction. *Research in Drama Education*: The Journal of Applied Theatre and Performance, *21*(2), 183–195. https://doi.org/10.1080/13569783.2016.1155404

Tanner, S. J. (2018). My teaching, my whiteness. *Journal of Curriculum Theorizing*, *32*(3), 79–92.

Thompson, T. (2013, August 21). NYPD's Infamous stop-and-frisk policy found unconstitutional. *The Leadership Conference Education Fund*. https://civilrights.org/edfund/resource/nypds-infamous-stop-and-frisk-policy-found-unconstitutional/

Travlou, P., Owens, P. E., Thompson, C. W., & Maxwell,

L. (2008). Place mapping with teenagers: Locating their territories and documenting their experience of the public realm. *Children's Geographies*, *6*(3), 309–326.

Tucker-Raymond, E., Rosario-Ramos, E. M., & Rosario, M. L. (2011). Cultural persistence, political resistance, and hope in the community and school-based art of a Puerto Rican diaspora neighborhood. *Equity & Excellence in Education*, *44*(2), 270–286. https://doi.org/10.1080/10665684.2011.563678

Wang, Q., Coemans, S., Siegesmund, R., & Hannes, K. (2017). Arts-based methods in socially engaged research practice: A classification framework. *Art/Research International: A Transdisciplinary Journal*, *2*(2), 5–39.

WBUR. (2021, January 18). *Poet Amanda Gorman on using her art as a tool for activism*. https://www.wbur.org/hereandnow/2021/01/18/poet-amanda-gorman-activism

CHAPTER 8

Akom, A., Shah, A., Nakai, A., & Cruz, T. (2016). Youth Participatory Action Research (YPAR) 2.0: How technological innovation and digital organizing sparked a food revolution in East Oakland. *International Journal of Qualitative Studies in Education*, *29*(10), 1287–1307. https://doi.org/10.1080/09518398.2016.1201609

Berman, H., Ford-Gilboe, M., Moutrey, B., & Cekic, S. (2016). Portraits of pain and promise: A photographic study of Bosnian youth. *Canadian Journal of Nursing Research Archive*, *32*(4), 21–41.

Bhaskar, R. (1987). *Scientific realism and human emancipation*. Verso.

Call-Cummings, M. (2017). "It's too political": The overt and covert silencing of critical Latino/a voices. *Latino Studies*, *15*(4), 532–540. https://doi.org/10.1057/s41276-017-0086-7

Call-Cummings, M., Hauber-Özer, M., Byers, C., & Mancuso, G. P. (2019). The power of/in Photovoice. *International Journal of Research & Method in Education*, *42*(4), 399–413. https://doi.org/10.1080/1743727X.2018.1492536

Call-Cummings, M., Hauber-Ozer, M., Rowell, L., & Ross, K. (2020). The roles and responsibilities of action research networks in times of crisis: Lessons from the Action Research Network of the Americas. *The Canadian Journal of Action Research*, *20*(3), 19–35. https://doi.org/10.33524/cjar.v20i3.486

Dennis, B., Carspecken, L., Zhao, P., Silberstein, S., Saxena, P., Bose, S., Palmer, D., Washington, S., & Elfreich, A. (2020). Digital migrating and storyworlding with women we love: A feminist ethnography. *Journal of Contemporary Ethnography*, *49*(6), 745–776.

Doyumğaç, İ., Tanhan, A., & Kiymaz, M. S. (2021). Understanding the most important facilitators and barriers for online education during COVID-19 through online photovoice methodology. *International Journal of Higher Education*, *10*(1), 166–199. https://doi.org/10.5430/ijhe.v10n1p166

Dumbrill, G. C. (2009). Your policies, our children: Messages from refugee parents to child welfare workers and policymakers. *Child Welfare*, *88*(3), 145–168.

Dutton, S., Davison, C. M., Malla, M., Bartels, S., Collier, K., Plamondon, K., & Purkey, E. (2019). Biographical collage as a tool in Inuit community-based participatory research and capacity development. *International Journal of Qualitative Methods*, *18*(2019)., 1–10. https://doi.org/10.1177/1609406919877307

Fairclough, N. (Ed.). (2001). *Critical discourse analysis as a method in social scientific research*. SAGE.

Freire, P. (1972). *Pedagogy of the oppressed*. Herder & Herder.

Gubrium, A., & Harper, K. (2009). Visualizing change: Participatory digital technologies in research and action. *Practicing Anthropology*, *31*(4), 2–4.

Hauber-Özer, M., & Call-Cummings, M. (2020). Empowerment or exposure? Ethical dilemmas of visual methods with vulnerable migrants. *Qualitative Research Journal*, *20*(3), 329–340. https://doi.org/10.1108/QRJ-10-2019-0075

Hidalgo, L. (2015). Augmented Fotonovelas: Creating new media as pedagogical and social justice tools. *Qualitative Inquiry*, *21*(3), 300–314. https://doi.org/10.1177/1077800414557831

Hugman, R., Bartolomei, L., & Pittaway, E. (2011). Human agency and the meaning of informed consent: Reflections on research with refugees. *Journal of Refugee Studies*, *24*(4), 655–671. https://doi.org/10.1093/jrs/fer024

Jarldorn, M., & 'Deer.' (2017). Participatory action research with ex-prisoners: Using Photovoice and one woman's story told through poetry. *Action Research*, *18*(3), 318–335. https://doi.org/10.1177/1476750317719140

Kay, L. (2013). Bead collage: An arts-based research method. *International Journal of Education & the Arts*, *14*, Art. 3.

Mayorga, E. (2014). Toward digital, critical, participatory action research: Lessons from the #BarrioEdProj. *Journal of Interactive Technology & Pedagogy*, *5*.

McKenzie, C. (2008). Radio in/for research: Creating knowledge waves. In J. G. Knowles & A. L. Cole (Eds.), *Handbook of the arts in qualitative research: Perspectives, methodologies, examples, and issues* (pp. 337–350). SAGE.

Monea, B., Andrade, J., Gonzalez, P., & Pozo, M. (2020). Beyond words: Reimagining education through arts and activism. *Perspectives in Urban Education*, *18*(1). https://urbanedjournal.gse.upenn.edu/archive/volume-18-issue-1-fall-2020/beyond-words-reimagining-education-through-art-and-activism

Oh, S.-A. (2012). Photofriend: Creating visual ethnography with refugee children. *Area*, *44*(3), 382–288. https://doi.org/10.1111/j.1475-4762.2012.01111.x

Robinson, C. J. (2000). *Black Marxism: The making of the Black radical tradition*. University of North Carolina Press.

Sahay, K. M., Thatcher, K., Núñez, C., & Lightfoot, A. (2016). "It's like we are legally, illegal": Latino/a youth emphasize barriers to higher education using photovoice. *The High School Journal*, *100*(1), 45–65. https://doi.org/10.1353/hsj.2016.0020

Scott-Jones, J. (2010). Origins and ancestors: A brief history of ethnography. In Scott-Jones, J., & Watt, S. (Eds.), *Ethnography in social science practice* (pp. 13–27). Taylor & Francis.

Sharpe, P. A., Greaney, M. L., Lee, P. R., & Royce, S. W. (2000). Assets-oriented community assessment. *Public Health Reports*, *115*(2–3), 205–211.

Smith, R., Danford, M., Darnell, S. C., Larrazabal, M. J. L., & Abdellatif, M. (2021). 'Like, what even is a podcast?' Approaching sport-for-development youth participatory action research through digital methodologies. *Qualitative Research in Sport, Exercise and Health*, *13*(1), 128–145.

Smyth, J., & McInerney, P. (2013). Whose side are you on? Advocacy ethnography: Some methodological aspects of narrative portraits of disadvantaged young people, in socially critical research. *International Journal of Qualitative Studies in Education*, *26*(1), 1–20. https://doi.org/10.1080/09518398.2011.604649

Solórzano, D. G., & Yosso, T. J. (2002). Critical race methodology: Counter-storytelling as an analytical framework for education research. *Qualitative Inquiry*, 8(1), 23–54.

Tanhan, A. (2020). Utilizing online photovoice (OPV) methodology to address biopsychosocial spiritual economic issues and wellbeing during COVID-19: Adapting OPV to Turkish. *Journal of Turkish Studies*, *15*(4), 1029–1086. https://doi.org/10.7827/TurkishStudies.44451

Tanhan, A., & Strack, R. W. (2020). Online photovoice to explore and advocate for Muslim biopsychosocial spiritual wellbeing and issues: Ecological systems theory and ally development. *Current Psychology*. Advance online publication. https://doi.org/10.1007/s12144-020-00692-6

Toroyan, T., & Reddy, P. S. (2005). Participation of South African youth in the design and development of AIDS photocomics. *International Quarterly of Community Health Education*, *25*(1–2), 149–163.

Trentham, B., Sokoloff, S., Tsang, A., & Neysmith, S. (2015). Social media and senior citizen advocacy: An inclusive tool to resist ageism? *Politics, Groups, and Identities*, *3*(3), 558–571. https://doi.org/10.1080/21565503.2015.1050411

Villanueva, G., Broad, G., Gonzalez, C., Ball-Rokeach, S., & Murphy, S. (2016). Communication asset mapping: An ecological field application toward building healthy communities. *International Journal of Communication*, *10*(21), 2704–2724. https://ijoc.org/index.php/ijoc/article/view/5335/1674

Wang, C. C., & Burris, M. A. (1994). Empowerment through photo novella: Portraits of participation. *Health Education Quarterly*, *21*(2), 171–186. https://doi.org/10.1177/109019819402100204

Wang, C. C., & Burris, M. A. (1997). Photovoice: Concept, methodology, and use for participatory needs assessment. *Health Education & Behavior*, *24*(3), 369–387.

Wang, C. C., & Redwood-Jones, Y. A. (2001). Photovoice ethics: Perspectives from Flint photovoice. *Health Education & Behavior*, *28*(5), 560–572.

Wodak, R. (Ed.). (2001). *What CDA is about: A summary of its history, important concepts and its developments*. SAGE.

Wodak, R., & Meyer, M. (Eds.). (2001). *Methods of critical discourse analysis*. SAGE.

Wright, A., Wahoush, O., Ballantyne, M., Gabel, C., & Jack, S. (2016). Qualitative health research involving indigenous peoples: Culturally appropriate data collection methods. *The Qualitative Report*, *21*(12), 2230–2245. https://doi.org/10.46743/2160-3715/2016.2384

Zenkov, K., Ewaida, M., Lynch, M. R., Bell, A., Harmon, J., Pellegrino, A., & Sell, C. (2014). Shooting back and 'looking for life' in the USA and Haiti: Seeing the ethics of visual research methods through a development lens. *International Journal of Research & Method in Education*, *37*(1), 63–86. https://doi.org/10.1080/1743727X.2013.795530

CHAPTER 9

Bertrand, M. (2019). "I was very impressed": Responses of surprise to students of color engaged in youth participatory action research. *Urban Education*, *54*(9), 1370–1397. https://doi.org/10.1177/0042085916648744

Boal, A. (1979). *Theatre of the oppressed*. Pluto Press.

Bronfenbrenner, U. (1979). *The ecology of human development: Experiments by nature and design*. Harvard University Press.

Brown, T. M., & Rodriguez, L. F. (2017). Collaborating with urban youth to address gaps in teacher education. *Teacher Education Quarterly*, *44*(3), 75–92.

Call-Cummings, M. (2021, June) A reflection from the action research podcast episode 19. *Social Publishers Foundation*. https://www.socialpublishersfoundation.org/knowledge_base/a-reflection-from-the-action-research-podcast-episode-19/

Call-Cummings, M., Dazzo, G. P., Beardsley, L., & Blibo, J. (2021). Performance as transformation/transformative: Problematizing performance in PAR. *Educational Action Research*. Advance online publication. https://doi.org/10.1080/09650792.2021.2000879

Call-Cummings, M., Hassell-Goodman, S., Dazzo, G., Scicli, E., Sultana, K., Elfaki, M., Clyde, A., Beardsley, L., & Hauber-Özer, M. (2022). The 'Impact' of YPAR: In their own words. *Educational Action Research*, 1-11.

Cameron, J. (2008). Linking participatory research to action: Institutional challenges. In S. Kindon, R. Pain, & M. Kesby (Eds.), *Participatory action research approaches and methods: Connecting people, participation and place* (pp. 206–215). Routledge.

Conquergood, D. (1985). Performing as a moral act: Ethical dimensions of the ethnography of performance. *Literature in Performance*, *5*(1), 1–13.

Conquergood, D. (1998). Beyond the text: Toward a performative cultural politics. In S. J. Dailey (Ed.), *The future of performance studies: Visions and revisions* (pp. 25–36). National Communication Association.

Dazzo, G. P. (2016, September 1). Reciprocity in research: Integrating evaluation & human rights methods to balance evaluator & community needs. [Webinar]. *Search for Common Ground Thursday Talks*. https://vimeo.com/181067904

Dazzo, G. P. (2017, March 27). Interactive strategies + deliberative democracy = meaningful measures. *AEA365*. https://aea365.org/blog/dg-tig-week-interactive-strategies-deliberative-democracy-meaningful-measures-by-giovanni-dazzo/

Dazzo, G. P. (2019, December) Courageous conversations: Ripples / theories of change. *Project Empowerment*. http://researchforempowerment.com/courageous-conversations-ripples-theories-of-change/

Dazzo, G. P. (2020, May) Exploring the role of collective memory for reconciliation: A comparative case of Guatemala and Cambodia. *Beyond Intractability*. https://www.beyondintractability.org/casestudy/dazzo-collective-memory

Dazzo, G. P. (2021, June 2). Restorative validity: Confronting barriers to participation and self-realization through participatory and collaborative moments in Guatemala. *AEA365*. https://aea365.org/blog/icce-tig-week-restorative-validity-confronting-barriers-to-participation-and-self-realization-through-participatory-and-collaborative-moments-in-guatemala-by-giovanni-dazzo/

Dworski-Riggs, D., & Langhout, R. D. (2010). Elucidating the power in empowerment and the participation in participatory action research: A story about research team and elementary school change. *American Journal of Community Psychology*, *45*(3–4), 215–230. https://doi.org/10.1007/s10464-010-9306-0

Endsley, C. L. (2014). Performing Blackness: Spoken word poetry and performance. *Transformations: The Journal of Inclusive Scholarship and Pedagogy*, *24*(1/2), 110–120.

Fisher, M. T. (2007). *Writing in rhythm: Spoken word poetry in urban classrooms*. Teachers College Press.

Freire, P. (1970). *Pedagogy of the oppressed*. Herder & Herder.

Habermas, J. (1996). *Between facts and norms* (W. Rehg, Trans.). MIT Press.

Hauber-Özer, M. (2020a, May 5). *Solidarity with migrants amidst the pandemic*. https://knowledgedemocracy.org/2020/05/05/solidarity-with-migrants-amidst-the-pandemic/

Hauber-Özer, M. (2020b, July 6). *Change of plans: Participatory migration research during a global crisis*. https://www.imiscoe.org/news-and-blog/phd-blog/1094-change-of-plans-participatory-migration-research-during-a-global-crisis

Hauber-Özer, M. (2020c, December 16). *Suriyeli üniversite öğrencilerinin Türkçe öğrenme stratejileri: Türkçe kursları ve gerçek hayat* [Syrian university students' Turkish learning strategies: Turkish courses and real life] [Webinar]. Yabancı Dil Olarak Türkçe Eğitim Derneği [Turkish as a Foreign Language Education Association] (YADOT). https://www.youtube.com/watch?v=lZ2VewRh1Q8

Hauber-Özer, M., & Call-Cummings, M. (2020, September) Looking ahead into a murky future, holding on to solidarity. *Knowledge Democracy Initiative, Action Research Network of the Americas*. https://knowledgedemocracy.org/2020/09/14/looking-ahead-into-a-murky-future-holding-on-to-solidarity/

The Illuminator. (2012, September 21). *Stop and frisk in the South Bronx* [Video]. YouTube. https://www.youtube.com/watch?v=mliulSC2hJk

Kilroy, W. (2011). From conflict to ownership: Participatory approaches to the re-integration of ex-combatants in Sierra Leone. *Irish Studies in International Affairs*, *22*, 127–144. https://doi.org/10.3318/isia.2011.22.127

Madison, D. S. (1998). Performances, personal narratives, and the politics of possibility. In S. J. Dailey (Ed.), *The future of performance studies: Visions and revisions* (pp. 276–286). National Communication Association.

McDougal, S. (2014). *Research methods in Africana studies*. Peter Lang.

Morris Justice Project. (n.d.). *Dear NYPD (AKA The Illuminator)*. Morris Justice: A Public Science Project. https://morrisjustice.org/dear-nypd/

Payne, Y. A., & Bryant, A. (2018). Street participatory action research in prison: A methodology to challenge privilege and power in correctional facilities. *The Prison Journal*, *98*(4), 449–469. https://doi.org/10.1177/0032885518776378

Reich, J., Liebenberg, L., Denny, M., Battiste, H., Bernard, A., Christmas, K., Dennis, R., Denny, D., Knockwood, I., Nicholas, R., & Paul, H. (2017). In this together: Relational accountability and meaningful research and dissemination with youth. *International Journal of Qualitative Methods*, *16*(1). https://doi.org/10.1177/1609406917717345

Ross, K., & Call-Cummings, M. (2019). Acknowledging and transcending 'failure': Lifeworld possibilities and system constraints. *International Journal of Social Research Methodology*, *22*(1), 97–109. https://doi.org/10.1080/13645579.2018.1501642

Stoudt, B. G., & Torre, M. E. (2014). The Morris Justice Project: Participatory action research. In P. Brindle (Ed.),

SAGE cases in methodology. SAGE. https://doi.org/10.4135/97814462730501453358

Stoudt, B. G., Torre, M. E., Bartley, P., Bracy, F., Caldwell, H., Downs, A., Greene, C., Haldipur, J., Hassan, P., Manoff, E., Sheppard, N., & Yates, J. (2015). Participatory action research and policy change. In C. Durose & L. Richardson (Eds.), *Designing public policy for co-production: Theory, practice and change* (pp. 125–137). Policy Press.

VanCleave, J. (Host). (2021, May 11). Episode 25: "Disruption, interruption, change . . . it's not enough. What we need is sabotage.": Critical participatory inquiry as sabotage in/of the academy [Audio podcast episode]. *Qualitative Conversations*. https://podtail.com/podcast/qualitative-conversations/episode-25-episode-25-critical-participatory-inqui/

CHAPTER 10

AIATSIS (Australian Institute of Aboriginal and Torres Strait Islander Studies). (2020). AIATSIS Code of Ethics for Aboriginal and Torres Strait Islander Research. https://aiatsis.gov.au/sites/default/files/2020-10/aiatsis-code-ethics.pdf

Behar, R. (1996). *The vulnerable observer: Anthropology that breaks your heart*. Beacon Press.

Cahill, C. (2007). Repositioning ethical commitments: Participatory action research as a relational praxis of social change. *ACME: An International E-Journal for Critical Geographies*, *6*(3), 360–373.

Caldwell, J. Y., Davis, J. D., Du Bois, B., Echo-Hawk, H., Erickson, J. S., Goins, R. T., Hill, C., Hillabrant, W., Johnson, S. R., Johnson, S. R., Kendall, E., Keemer, K., Manson, S. M., Marshall, C. A., Running Wolf, P., Santiago, R. L., Schacht, R., & Stone, J. B. (2005). Culturally competent research with American Indians and Alaska Natives: Findings and recommendations of the first symposium of the work group on American Indian Research and Program Evaluation Methodology. *American Indian and Alaska Native Mental Health Research*, *12*(1), 1–21. https://doi.org/10.5820/aian.1201.2005.1

Call-Cummings, M., & Hauber-Özer, M. (2022). Care as resistance and epistemological necessity in YPAR. In P. Nagarajan, N. Gross, V. Vasudevan, & K. Clonan-Roy (Eds.), *Care-based methodologies: Reimagining qualitative research with youth in US schools* (pp. 45–56). Bloomsbury.

Collins, P. H. (2010). *Black feminist thought: Knowledge, consciousness, and the politics of empowerment*. Routledge.

Craps, S. (2013). *Postcolonial witnessing: Trauma out of bounds*. Palgrave Macmillan.

Erickson, F. (2011). A history of qualitative inquiry in social and educational research. In N. K. Denzin, & Y. S. Lincoln (Eds.), *The SAGE handbook of qualitative research* (pp. 43–60). SAGE.

Fine, M., & Torre, M. E. (2004). Re-membering exclusions: Participatory action research in public institutions. *Qualitative Research in Psychology*, *1*(1), 15–37. https://doi.org/10.1191/1478088704qp003oa

Gaztambide-Fernández, R. A. (2012). Decolonization and the pedagogy of solidarity. *Decolonization: Indigeneity, Education & Society*, *1*(1), 41–67.

Grenberg, J. (2005). *Kant and the ethics of humility: A story of dependence, corruption and virtue*. Cambridge University Press.

Guillemin, M., & Gillam, L. (2004). Ethics, reflexivity, and "ethically important moments" in research. *Qualitative Inquiry*, *10*(2), 261–280. https://doi.org/10.1177/1077800403262360

Guishard, M. A., Halkovic, A., Galletta, A., & Li, P. (2018). Toward epistemological ethics: Centering communities and social justice in qualitative research. *Forum Qualitative Sozialforschung / Forum: Qualitative Social Research*, *19*(3). https://doi.org/10.17169/fqs-19.3.3145

Habermas, J. (1996). *Between facts and norms* (W. Rehg, Trans.). MIT Press.

Jamesson, J. K., Clayton, P. H., & Jaeger, A. J. (2011). Community-engaged scholarship through mutually transformative partnerships. In L. Harter, J. Hamel-Lambert, & J. Millesen (Eds.), *Participatory partnerships for social action and research* (pp. 259–277). Kendall Hunt.

Jones, C. H., & Whittle, R. (2021). Researcher self-care and caring in the research community. *Area*, *53*(2),

381–388. https://doi.org/10.1111/area.12703

Limes-Taylor Henderson, K., & Esposito, J. (2019). Using others in the nicest way possible: On colonial and academic practice(s), and an ethic of humility. *Qualitative Inquiry, 25*(9–10), 876–889. https://doi.org/10.1177/1077800417743528

Native Governance Center. (2021). *A guide to indigenous wealth building*. https://nativegov.org/resources/indigenous-wealth-guide/

Ropers-Huilman, B. (1999). Witnessing: Critical inquiry in a poststructural world. *International Journal of Qualitative Studies in Education, 12*(1), 21–35. https://doi.org/10.1080/095183999236312

Ross, K., Li, P., & Call-Cummings, M. (2022). Solidarity as methodological praxis. *Qualitative Research*. https://doi.org/10.1177/14687941221098919

Schensul, J. J., & Berg, M. (2004). Youth participatory action research: A transformative approach to service-learning. *Michigan Journal of Community Service Learning, Summer 2004*, 76–88.

Tilakaratna, S. (1991). Stimulation of self-reliant initiatives by sensitized agents: Some lessons from practice. In O. Fals-Borda & M. A. Rahman (Eds.), *Action and knowledge: Breaking the monopoly with participatory action research* (pp. 135–145). The Apex Press.

Tuhiwai Smith, L. (1999/2012). *Decolonizing methodologies: Research and indigenous peoples*. Zed Books.

WCED (World Commission on Environment and Development). (1987). *Report of the World Commission on Environment and Development: Our common future*. Oxford University Press. https://sustainabledevelopment.un.org/content/documents/5987our-common-future.pdf

Vincett, J. (2018). Researcher self-care in organizational ethnography. *Journal of Organizational Ethnography, 7*(1), 44–58. https://doi.org/10.1108/JOE-09-2017-0041

Zuchowski, I., Gopalkrishnan, N., King, J., & Francis, A. (2017). Reciprocity in international student exchange: Challenges posed by neo-colonialism and the dominance of the Western voice. *Aotearoa New Zealand Social Work, 29*(1), 77–87.

APPENDIX: CASE STUDIES

CASE STUDY 1

Abrego, L. (2014). *Sacrificing families: Navigating laws, labor, and love across borders*. Stanford University Press.

Asad, A., & Clair, M. (2018). Racialized legal status as a social determinant of health. *Social Science & Medicine (1982)., 199*, 19–28. https://doi.org/10.1016/j.socscimed.2017.03.010

Collins, P. H. (2019). *Intersectionality as critical social theory*. Duke University Press.

Cornwall, A., & Jewkes, R. (1995). What is participatory research? *Social Science and Medicine, 41*(12), 1667–1676. https://doi.org/10.1016/0277-9536(95)00127-S

De Genova, N., & Peutz, N. (Eds.). (2010). *The deportation regime: Sovereignty, space, and freedom of movement*. Duke University Press.

Del Real, D. (2019). Toxic ties: The reproduction of legal violence within mixed-status intimate partners, relatives, and friends. *International Migration Review, 53*(2), 548–570. https://doi.org/10.1177/0197918318769313

Enriquez, L. (2015). Multigenerational punishment: Shared experiences of undocumented immigration status within mixed-status families. *Journal of Marriage and Family, 77*(4), 939–953. https://doi.org/10.1111/jomf.12196

Fals-Borda, O. (2001). Participatory (action) research in social theory: Origins and challenges. In P. Reason & H. Bradbury (Eds.), *Handbook of action research* (pp. 27–27). SAGE.

Fals-Borda, O., & Rahman, M. A. (1991). *Action and knowledge: Breaking the monopoly with participatory action-research*. Apex Press.

Freire, P. (1982). Creating alternative research methods: Learning to do it by doing it. In B. Hall, A. Gillette, & R. Tandon (Eds.), *Creating knowledge: A monopoly? Participatory research in development* (pp. 29–37). Participatory Research Network Series 1.

Golash-Boza, T., & Hondagneu-Sotelo, P. (2013). Latino immigrant men and the deportation crisis: A gendered racial removal program. *Latino Studies, 11*(3), 271–292. https://doi.org/10.1057/lst.2013.14

Letiecq, B. L., Mehta, S., Vesely, C. K., Marquez, M., Goodman, R. D., & Moron, L. (2019). Central American immigrant mothers' mental health in the context of illegality: Structural stress, parental concern, and trauma. *Journal of Family and Community Health, 42*, 271–282.

Letiecq, B., & Schmalzbauer, L. (2012). Community-based participatory research with Mexican migrants in a new rural destination: A good fit? *Action Research Journal, 10*(3), 244–259. https://doi.org/10.1177/1476750312443571

Letiecq, B. L., Vesely, C. K., & Goodman, R. (2022). Participatory action research with, by, and for families. In K. Adamson, A. Few-Demo, C. Proulx, & K. Roy (Eds.), *Sourcebook of family theories and methodologies*. Springer.

Letiecq, B., Davis, E., Vesely, C., Goodman, R., Zeledon, D. & Marquez, M. (2022). Central American immigrant mothers' narratives of intersecting oppressions: A resistant knowledge project. *Journal of Marriage & Family*, 1-3. 3. *https://doi.org/10.1111/jomf.12854*

Logan, R., Melo, M. A., & Castañeda, H. (2021). Familial vulnerability: Legal status and mental health within mixed-status families. *Medical Anthropology, 40*(7), 639–652. https://doi.org/10.1080/01459740.2021.1879061

Menjívar, C., Abrego, L. J., & Schmalzbauer, L. (2016). *Immigrant families*. Polity Press.

Ortiz, F. A. (2020). Self-actualization in the Latino/Hispanic culture. *Journal of Humanistic Psychology, 60*, 418–435.

Parrado, E. A., Flippen, C. A., & McQuiston, C. (2005). Migration and relationship power among Mexican women. *Demography, 42*(2), 347–372. www.jstor.org/stable/4147350

Reason, P., & Bradbury, H. (Eds.). (2008). *Action research: Participative inquiry and practice*. SAGE.

Vaughn, L. M., Jacquez, F., Linquist-Gantz, R., Parsons, A., & Milink, K. (2016). Immigrants as research partners: A review of immigrants in community-based participatory research (CBPR). *Journal of Immigrant and Minority Health, 19*, 1457–1468. https://doi.org/10.1007/s10903-016-0474-3

Vesely, C. K., DeMulder, E., Sansbury, A., Davis, E., Letiecq, B. L., Willard, I., Goodman, R., & Amigas de la Comunidad. (2021a). 'A place where my children could learn to read, write, and play': The search for early care and education among undocumented Central American immigrant mothers. *Early Childhood Research Quarterly, 56*, 306–319.

Vesely, C. K., Letiecq, B. L., Davis, E., Goodman, R. D., & Amigas de la Comunidad. (2021b, March). *Central American immigrant families during COVID: Childcare, education, and work experiences*. In D. Crosby, Families' work-childcare coordination in the context of low-wage work, precarious schedules and the COVID-19 pandemic. Paper symposium at the Society for Research in Child Development biennial meeting. (virtual due to COVID).

Vesely, C. K., Letiecq, B. L., & Goodman, R. D. (2017). Immigrant family resilience in context: Using a community-based approach to build a new conceptual model. *Journal of Family Theory and Review, 9*, 93–110. https://doi.org/10.1111/jftr.12177

Vesely, C. K., Letiecq, B. L., Goodman, R. D., Marquez, M., Alves, L., Lazo, W., & Martinez, R. (2019). What does this mean to you? Partnering with Amigas de la Comunidad to analyze the housing conditions of undocumented Latina immigrants. In Á. Humble & E. Radina (Eds.), How qualitative data analysis happens: Moving beyond "themes emerged" (pp. 112–127). Taylor & Francis.

Yosso, T. J. (2005). Whose culture has capital? A critical race theory discussion of community cultural wealth. *Race, Ethnicity and Education, 8*, 69–91.

Wallerstein, N., Duran, B., Oetzel, J., & Minkler, M. (Eds.). (2018). *Community-based participatory research for health* (3rd ed). Jossey-Bass.

CASE STUDY 2

Mortari, L. (2015). Reflexivity in research practice: An overview of different perspectives. *International Journal of Qualitative Methods, 14*(5), 1–9. https://doi.org/10.1177/1609406915618045

Perkins, D. D., & Zimmerman, M. A. (1995). Empowerment theory, research and application. *American Journal of Community Psychology*, *23*(5), 569–579.

Rappaport, J. (1981). In praise of paradox: A social policy of empowerment over prevention. *American Journal of Community Psychology*, *9*, 1–25.

Rappaport, J. (1984). Studies in empowerment: Introduction to the issue. *Prevention in Human Services*, *3*, 1–7.

Substance Abuse and Mental Health Services Administration (SAMHSA). (2014). *SAMHSA's Concept of Trauma and Guidance for a Trauma-Informed Approach*. https://ncsacw.samhsa.gov/userfiles/files/SAMHSA_Trauma.pdf

CASE STUDY 3

Call-Cummings, M., Hauber-Òl^zer, M., Byers, C., & Mancuso, G. (2019). The power of/in photovoice. *International Journal of Research and Method in Education*, *42*(4), 399–413. https://doi.org/10.1080/1743727X.2018.1492536

Cheak-Zamora, N. C., Teti, M., & Maurer-Batjer, A. (2018). Capturing experiences of youth with ASD via photo exploration: Challenges and resources becoming an adult. *Journal of Adolescent Research*, *33*, 117–145. https://doi.org/10.1177%2F0743558416653218

Clandinin, D. J., & Connelly, F. M. (1990). *Narrative inquiry: Experience and story in qualitative research*. Jossey-Bass.

Fals-Borda, O., & Rahman, M. A. (1991). *Action and knowledge: Breaking the monopoly with participatory action-research*. Apex Press.

Fine, M., & Torre, M. E. (2004). Re-membering exclusions: Participatory action research in public institutions. *Qualitative Research in Psychology*, *1*(1), 15–37.

Francis, G. L., Reed, A. S., & Howard, M. E. (2020). Interactions with and between families and professionals in college: Perspectives of young adults with intellectual and developmental disabilities. *Inclusion*, *8*(2), 163–179. https://doi.org/10.1352/2326-6988-8.2.163

Freire, P. (1970). *Pedagogy of the oppressed*. Continuum International.

Jurkowski, J. (2008). Photovoice as action research tool for engaging people with intellectual disabilities in research and program development. *Intellectual and Developmental Disabilities*, *46*, 1–11. https://doi.org/10.1352/0047-6765(2008)46[1:PAPART]2.0.CO;2

Kemmis, S., & McTaggart, R. (2005). Participatory action research: Communicative action and the public sphere. In N. K. Denzin & Y. S. Lincoln (Eds.), *The SAGE handbook of qualitative research* (3rd ed., pp. 559–603). SAGE.

Limes-Taylor Henderson, K., & Esposito, J. (2019). Using others in the nicest way possible: On colonial and academic practice(s), and an ethic of humility. *Qualitative Inquiry*, *25*(9–10), 876–889. https://doi.org/10.1177/1077800417743528

McDonald, E. E., Kidney, C. A., & Patka, M. (2012). "You need to let your voice be heard": Research participants' views on research. *Journal of Intellectual Disability Research*, *57*(3), 216–225. https://doi.org/10.1111/j.1365-2788.2011.01527.x

McDonald, K. E., Conroy, N. E., & Olick, R. S. (2016). Is it worth it? Benefits in research with adults with intellectual disability. *Intellectual and Developmental Disability*, *54*, 440–453. https://doi.org/10.1352/1934-9556-54.6.440

Povee, K., Bishop, B. J., & Roberts, L. D. (2014). The use of photovoice with people with intellectual disabilities: Reflections, challenges, and opportunities. *Disability and Society*, *29*(6), 893–907. https://doi.org/10.1080/09687599.2013.874331

Prohn, S. (2014). A grounded theory of social inclusion for postsecondary education students with intellectual disability. (UMI Nol 3690350). [Doctoral dissertation]. ProQuest Dissertations and Theses.

Strnadová, I., & Walmsley, J. (2017). Peer-reviewed articles on inclusive research: Do co-researchers with intellectual disabilities have a voice? *Journal of Applied Research in Intellectual Disabilities*, *31*(1), 132–141. https://doi.org/10.1111/jar.12378

Strauss, A., & Corbin, J. (1998). *Basics of qualitative research: Techniques and procedures for developing grounded theory* (2nd ed.). SAGE.

Turnbull, H. R., & Turnbull, A. P. (2000). Newly in pursuit of an old philosophy: Rebalancing liberty, equality, and community. In M. L. Wehmeyer & J. Patton (Eds.), *Mental retardation in the 21st century* (pp. 413–430). PRO-ED.

Tuck, E. (2010). Breaking up with Deleuze: Desire and valuing the irreconcilable. *The International Journal of Qualitative Studies in Education*, *23*(5), 635–650. https://doi.org/10.1080/09518398.2010.500633

Tuck, E., & Yang, K. W. (2014). R-words: Refusing research. In D. Paris & M. T. Winn (Eds.), *Humanizing research* (pp. 223–247). SAGE.

Wang, C. C. (1999). Photovoice: A participatory action research strategy applied to women's health. *Journal of Women's Health*, *8*(2). https://doi.org/10.1089/jwh.1999.8.185

Wang, C. C. (2006). Youth participation in photovoice as a strategy for community change. *Journal of Community Practice*, *14*, 147–161. https://doi.org/10.1300/J125v14n01_09

Wang, C. C. & Burris, M. A. (1997). Photovoice: Concept, methodology, and use for participatory needs assessment. *Health Education & Behavior*, *24*(3), 369–387. https://doi.org.10.1177_109019819702400309

INDEX

J

K

L

M

N

O

P

Q

R

S

T

U

V

W

Y

Z